INFECTION CONTROL IN LONG-TERM CARE FACILITIES

INFECTION CONTROL IN LONG-TERM CARE FACILITIES

Edited by

Philip W. Smith, M.D.
Hospital Epidemiologist
Bishop Clarkson Memorial Hospital
Assistant Professor of Internal Medicine
University of Nebraska Medical Center
Consultant to the State of Nebraska Department of Health
for Infectious Diseases and Nosocomial Infections
Omaha, Nebraska

A WILEY MEDICAL PUBLICATION
JOHN WILEY & SONS
New York · Chichester · Brisbane · Toronto · Singapore

Cover design: Wanda Lubelska
Production Supervisor: Audrey Pavey

Library of Congress Cataloging in Publication Data:

Main entry under title:

Infection control in long-term care facilities.

(A Wiley medical publication)
Includes index.
1. Long-term care facilities—Sanitation. 2. Nursing
homes—Sanitation. 3. Nosocomial infections—Prevention.
4. Aged—Diseases—Prevention. I. Smith, Philip W.
II. Series. [DNLM: 1. Nursing homes. 2. Infection—
Prevention and control. WT 27.1 143]
RA999.S36I64   1984   614.4'4   83-21756
ISBN 0-471-89520-2

Printed in the United States of America

10 9 8 7 6

To the elderly we serve, who can show us both where we have been and where we will be.

CONTRIBUTORS

Nancy J. Haberstich, R.N.
Infection Control Nurse
Lincoln General Hospital
Lincoln, Nebraska

Brenda L. W. Hagan, R.N., C.R.N.P.
Nurse Epidemiologist
Lower Bucks Hospital
Bristol, Pennsylvania

Walter J. Hierholzer, Jr., M.D.
Hospital Epidemiologist and
Associate Professor of Internal Medicine
University of Iowa Hospitals and Clinics
Iowa City, Iowa

R. Michael Massanari, M.D.
Associate Professor of Internal Medicine
University of Iowa Hospitals and Clinics
Iowa City, Iowa

Susan G. Miller, R.N.
Assistant Nurse Epidemiologist
Bishop Clarkson Memorial Hospital
Omaha, Nebraska

Robert G. Penn, M.D.
Hospital Epidemiologist
Methodist and Childrens Hospitals
Clinical Assistant Professor
Department of Microbiology
Creighton University School of Medicine
Omaha, Nebraska

Jane F. Potter, M.D.
Assistant Professor
Chief, Section of Geriatrics and Gerontology
Department of Internal Medicine
University of Nebraska Medical Center
Omaha, Nebraska

Dorothy A. Rasley, R.N.
Nurse Epidemiologist
University of Iowa Hospitals and Clinics
Iowa City, Iowa

Patricia G. Rusnak, R.N.
Nurse Epidemiologist
Bishop Clarkson Memorial Hospital
Omaha, Nebraska

Ian M. Smith, M.D.
Professor, Departments of Internal Medicine
and Family Practice
University of Iowa Hospitals and Clinics
Iowa City, Iowa

Philip W. Smith, M.D.
Hospital Epidemiologist
Bishop Clarkson Memorial Hospital
Assistant Professor of Internal Medicine
University of Nebraska Medical Center
Consultant to the State of Nebraska
Department of Health for Infectious Diseases
and Nosocomial Infections
Omaha, Nebraska

V. Delight Wreed, R.N., B.S.N.
Health Services Consultant
Nebraska Health Care Association
Lincoln, Nebraska

PREFACE

There has been an exponential increase in the attention and literature devoted to the problems of the elderly, including those in long-term care facilities. In the course of giving seminars about infection control throughout Nebraska, I was impressed with the interest of nursing home staff in the infectious disease problems within their facilities. Although the field of hospital infection control is well established, there has been very little material available to help nursing home staff solve their unique infection control problems.

Infection Control in Long-Term Care Facilities is written to provide a thorough but practical background in nursing home infection control. Basic concepts in diagnosis, transmission, and prevention of infection are presented. Although ideas were drawn from the hospital infection control literature, every effort was made to focus specifically on the problems of long-term care facilities. This book is intended for nursing home nurses, ancillary nursing home staff, those in geriatric training programs, state surveyors, and physicians who practice in nursing homes.

The book is divided into sections for easy reference. Section I provides a background in aspects of infectious diseases relevant to the elderly person. Section II deals with infectious diseases that occur in the nursing home. The organization and major components of an infection control program for nursing homes are discussed in Section III, while Section IV covers specific measures to control and prevent infections in the long-term care facility.

I would like to acknowledge the valuable assistance of Patricia Rusnak, R.N., in the development of this book and the great editorial assistance of Andrea Stingelin, Janet Foltin, Megan Thomas, Audrey Pavey, and Bill Green of John Wiley & Sons. Many individuals assisted with the typing of this manuscript, and many reviewers provided thoughtful criticism of the contents. I am extremely grateful to them all. Finally, I wish to acknowledge the great support and assistance of my lovely wife, Sharon.

Philip W. Smith

CONTENTS

INFECTION CONTROL IN LONG-TERM CARE FACILITIES

SECTION I

GENERAL BACKGROUND

CHAPTER 1

A FEW BASICS ABOUT INFECTIONS

Philip W. Smith

FACTORS INVOLVED IN INFECTION

Infection involves the interaction between a microorganism, the environment, and the host.

Microorganisms

Organisms that cause infectious diseases in humans form a large spectrum in terms of size and complexity. Viruses have a mean size of 0.1 μm (0.0000001 meter) and cannot be seen under the average laboratory microscope. Bacteria average about 1 μm in size and can be visualized by high-power microscopy. The largest agents that cause infection in humans are the helminths, or worms. Organisms are most often named by genus (e.g., *Staphylococcus*) and species (e.g., *aureus*).

Although we tend to associate microorganisms with disease, they are beneficial to humans in many ways. Bacteria found on the surface of the skin and mucous membranes, the normal bacterial flora, are very important because they inhibit the growth of potential pathogens. Bacteria are also involved in the metabolism of vitamin K in the human intestine.

Immunity

Immunity is resistance of the host to infection. Local defenses form the first barrier against potential invaders and are an important aspect of immunity. Examples of local defenses include intact skin, gastric acidity, and the normal bacterial flora of skin, mouth, gut, and vagina.

The normal host has several lines of defense against pathogenic microorganisms, including white blood cells, antibodies, complement, and interferon. These are reviewed in Chapter 2.

3

Pathogenesis of Infection

The interaction of the organism and the host may have several outcomes. **Infection** may be defined as invasion of the host by microorganisms; infection requires the replication of organisms in the tissues of the host. Whether or not infection develops depends upon the **virulence** (ability of the organism to produce disease) of the pathogen as well as host defenses against the pathogen. Related organisms may vary greatly in virulence. *Staphylococcus aureus* is a virulent organism and an important cause of infections, for example, whereas S. *epidermidis* is a relatively benign organism that is part of normal skin flora.

Virulence operates by several mechanisms. First, the organism may produce disease by direct invasion of tissues. Invasiveness of bacteria may be enhanced by antiphagocytic capsules (pneumococci) or enzymes that promote the spread of organisms through connective tissue (staphylococci). A second mechanism involves the injury of the host by production of toxins by the invading organism. Botulism, tetanus, diphtheria, and cholera are examples of toxin-related diseases. Finally, tissue damage may be caused by the response of the host to the organism. This mechanism is typified by the delayed hypersensitivity response of the host to infection with *Mycobacterium tuberculosis.*

Disease production also depends upon the portal of entry of the organism. For instance, *Legionella pneumophila* produces severe pneumonia when inhaled, but has little effect on the skin. S. *aureus* produces severe cutaneous infections, but rarely causes pharyngitis.

Infection requires an imbalance among the host, the environment, and the organism. **Immunity,** the resistance of the host to infection, is most important in determining response to an organism. Specific immunity develops after exposure to a particular organism. A host that is not immune to a specific infectious disease is called **susceptible.**

Colonization is the coexistence of microorganisms and the host without injury to or reaction by the host. A person who is colonized with a particular organism may be referred to as a **carrier** of that organism.

Manifestations of Infection

The infected host may be asymptomatic or may develop clinical manifestations of infection. The most universal manifestation of infection is **fever,** which is defined as an oral temperature above 99°F or 37.2°C. Rectal temperatures are 0.5°C higher. There are causes of fever other than infection, including neoplasms, autoimmune diseases, endocrine disturbances, vascular accidents, drugs, and neurologic disorders.

The host generally manifests organ-specific symptoms of infection.

Urinary tract infections cause dysuria; cutaneous infections cause redness, warmth, and tenderness of the skin; infectious gastroenteritis results in diarrhea; and individuals with pneumonia manifest cough and shortness of breath. These symptoms provide a clue to the underlying cause of the infection.

Patients with severe or prolonged infection develop other generalized symptoms or signs, such as weakness, weight loss, fatigue, and anemia. The elderly may present with unusual symptoms, making the diagnosis of infection more difficult (1). For instance, the elderly may not develop the normal febrile response to bacterial sepsis but often first present with confusion or tachypnea.

Diagnosis of Infection

The diagnosis of an infection may be made on clinical grounds or by laboratory tests. Clinical observation of signs and symptoms will reliably diagnose a number of infections, such as chickenpox. However, laboratory assistance is usually required to determine the specific organism causing an infection. The organism may be identified either directly or indirectly (by measuring the host response to the organism).

There are several ways to directly identify a microorganism in the laboratory. The standard method is isolation and identification of an organism in an appropriate culture medium. Collection of specimens from normally sterile body fluids such as spinal fluid and blood should be preceded by cleansing of the skin with alcohol and iodine solution. Specimens that are contaminated by normal bacterial flora pose special problems. When culturing urine, for example, a clean-catch, quantitative midstream culture is necessary to distinguish contamination from infection. Other direct means of organism identification include direct visualization by staining techniques (e.g., acid-fast staining for diagnosis of tuberculosis) and detection of components or antigens of the organism (e.g., radioimmunoassay for hepatitis B surface antigen). Alternatively, the laboratory may diagnose an infection indirectly by measurement of host response to a specific organism. Examples include detection of measles antibody by complement fixation technique and measurement of skin test reaction to a protein extract of *M. tuberculosis* (purified protein derivative, PPD).

Serum antibody levels or titers against organisms can be measured by a variety of techniques. A single antibody titer is rarely diagnostic. Hence, every effort should be made to obtain two samples, preferably two to three weeks apart, to look for a diagnostic rise in antibody titer. A fourfold or greater rise in titer is generally considered to be of diagnostic significance.

Table 1.1.   Mode of Diagnosis of Viral Infections

Organism	Mode of Diagnosis
Respiratory viruses	
Influenza	Cl, Ab
Parainfluenza	Ab
Respiratory syncytial virus (RSV)	Ab
Rhinovirus	Cl
Gastrointestinal viruses	
Enterovirus	Ab
Rotavirus	Ag, Ab
Norwalk virus	Ab
Hepatitis A	Ab
Hepatitis B	Ag
Mucocutaneous viruses	
Herpes simplex	Cl
Herpes zoster	Cl
Rubella	Ab
Measles	Cl

KEY: *Cl, clinical; Ag, antigen; Ab, antibody.*

BASIC MICROBIOLOGY

Viruses

Viruses are the smallest infectious agents. The basic structure of the virus is a central core of nucleic acid (DNA or RNA) wrapped in a protective protein coat. Some viruses also have an outer envelope. Replication requires the use of the host cell.

Viral infections are difficult to confirm microbiologically. Viruses grow only in tissue culture, a procedure that is quite expensive and technically difficult and is available only at certain reference laboratories. Thus the diagnosis of viral infection frequently depends on measurement of host antibodies against the virus (see Table 1.1). Antibody testing for herpesvirus infections is often unsatisfactory, but fortunately these infections may usually be diagnosed clinically.

Bacteria

Bacteria, unlike viruses, may survive and reproduce independent of the host cell. They have a rigid cell wall that surrounds the cell membrane and protects it from mechanical damage. Bacteria multiply by binary fission. Some bacteria form endospores that are resistant to adverse en-

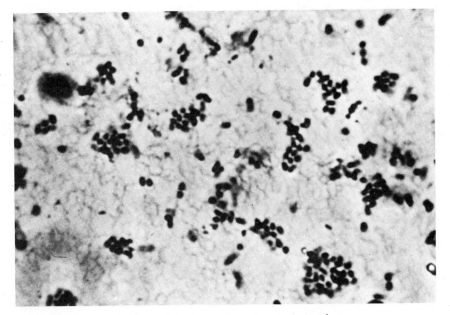

Figure 1.1. *Staphylococcus aureus* in Gram stain of a wound.

Table 1.2. **Bacterial Classification**

Aerobic	Anaerobic
Gram-positive	
Cocci	Cocci
Staphylococcus	*Peptococcus*
Streptococcus	*Peptostreptococcus*
Bacilli	Bacilli
Lactobacillus	*Clostridium*
Corynebacterium	*Propionibacterium*
Listeria	
Gram-negative	
Cocci	
Neisseria	
Bacilli	Bacilli
Escherichia	*Bacteroides*
Klebsiella	*Fusobacterium*
Proteus	
Pseudomonas	
Salmonella	
Shigella	
Serratia	
Hemophilus	
Acid-fast	
Bacilli	
Mycobacterium	

Source: Adapted from Smith PW: Infectious diseases, in Kochar MS (ed): *Textbook of General Medicine*, 1st ed., New York, Wiley, 1983.

vironmental conditions: *Clostridium* and *Bacillus* species are the most important spore formers.

Bacteria are classified on the basis of shape, staining characteristics, and oxygen tolerance. Most bacteria are either round (cocci) or rod-shaped (bacilli). Staphylococci, for instance, form clusters of gram-positive cocci (Fig. 1.1). Aerobic bacteria grow in the presence of oxygen, whereas anaerobic bacteria are inhibited by oxygen. Bacteria are further subdivided on the basis of the Gram stain, which stains bacterial cell walls blue (gram-positive) or red (gram-negative). Some bacteria stain only with special stains such as the acid-fast stain (mycobacteria) or the Dieterle silver stain (*L. pneumophila*). Aerobic bacteria are of greatest importance clinically (Table 1.2).

Most bacterial infections are diagnosed by isolation of bacteria on appropriate culture media (Fig. 1.2). Aerobic bacteria can usually be isolated and identified in one to three days, anaerobic bacteria in three to six days, and mycobacteria in four to eight weeks. Legionnaires' disease is best diagnosed by testing for serum antibody or by direct fluorescent stain of bacteria in lung biopsy tissue.

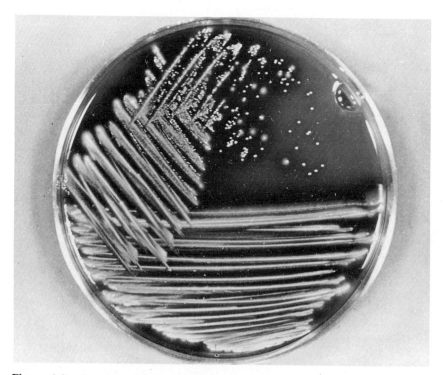

Figure 1.2.   *S. aureus*—culture on blood agar plate.

Table 1.3. Mode of Diagnosis of Fungal Infections

Organism	Mode of Diagnosis
Aspergillus	Cu
Candida	Cu
Histoplasma	Ab, Cu
Coccidioides	Ab, Cu
Cryptococcus	Ag, Cu

KEY: Cu, culture; Ab, antibody; Ag, antigen.

Fungi

Fungi are larger and more complex in structure than bacteria. They occur as single cells (yeasts) or multicellular organisms (molds). Some fungi cause endemic disease in certain areas of the country, such as histoplasmosis in the Mississippi Valley region and coccidioidomycosis in the southwestern United States. Cryptococcosis and aspergillosis occur primarily in the immunocompromised patient. *Candida* causes mucocutaneous infection, such as thrush, in the patient who is receiving antibiotics or corticosteroids.

Fungi, like mycobacteria, grow slowly in culture and usually require four to eight weeks for isolation and identification. Fungi may be seen in pathologic specimens by special staining (e.g., silver stain). Alternatively, measurement of serum antibody or antigens may be useful in the diagnosis (see Table 1.3).

Parasites

A number of parasites cause infectious diseases in humans. Protozoa are unicellular parasites; protozoa pathogenic for humans cause giardiasis, amebiasis, and malaria. Helminths or worms that infect humans vary in size from 1 mm (*Heterophyes*) to 10 m or more (*Diphyllobothrium latum*). Insects that parasitize humans include mites (scabies), lice, fleas, and ticks.

Parasitic diseases of humans are generally diagnosed by direct visualization of the parasite, either with the naked eye or with microscopic assistance. Antibody determinations are rarely helpful.

Specimen Collection

The isolation and identification of organisms from clinical specimens require that a proper specimen be obtained and delivered promptly to the microbiology laboratory. Some organisms such as anaerobic bacteria are very fragile and will not survive delays in processing. Delay also permits the overgrowth of contaminating bacteria, which can invalidate a urine or sputum culture.

Different organisms require different collection techniques or culture media. Microbiologic techniques have been described in detail for various organisms (2). Meticulous specimen collection is critical. The microbiology laboratory cannot compensate for a poorly collected sample.

Spinal fluid and blood are normally sterile. It is essential that cultures be collected aseptically, which is usually accomplished by cleansing the skin with alcohol and iodine solution prior to specimen collection. False-positive blood culture results occur most frequently with *Staphylococcus epidermidis* and *Propionibacterium acnes*, which reflects the role of these bacteria as predominant skin flora.

All sputum specimens are contaminated by oral bacteria to some extent. *Streptococcus pneumoniae* and *Hemophilus influenzae* may be respiratory pathogens or normal pharyngeal flora. A percutaneous transtracheal aspiration bypasses oral flora and is mandatory if anaerobic bacteria are sought. The throat culture is not a substitute for sputum culture in the diagnosis of pneumonia. Only group A streptococci, *Corynebacterium diphtheriae*, and *Neisseria gonorrhoeae* are of diagnostic interest when present in a throat culture.

Urine cultures are contaminated with perineal bacteria, but quantitative midstream cultures distinguish contamination from infection. Lactobacilli and *Staphylococcus epidermidis* frequently are contaminants. An improperly collected specimen is suggested by the presence of contaminants, of less than 10,000 bacteria per 1 ml of urine, or of multiple bacterial isolates.

Open wounds and decubitus ulcers are usually contaminated with cutaneous or environmental organisms. For this reason, a surface swab of the lesion is of limited value and often yields multiple bacteria. A specimen is best obtained by subcutaneous needle aspiration or wound biopsy; even a deep wound swab may be misleading. However, culture of a previously undrained abscess by needle aspiration or swab is appropriate and likely to reveal the causative organism.

Feces obviously contain large numbers of gut bacteria and should be cultured only for intestinal pathogens such as *Salmonella, Shigella,* and *Campylobacter.* Special media are required for isolation of these pathogens.

EPIDEMIOLOGY OF INFECTIOUS DISEASES

Definition of Terms in Epidemiology

Epidemiology has been defined as the dynamic study of the determinants, occurrence, and distribution of health and disease in a population

(3). There are a few background definitions and statistical calculations that are useful in the descriptive epidemiology of infections in nursing homes.

Nosocomial infections, when referring to nursing homes, are those infections that develop in the nursing home or are produced by microorganisms acquired during residence in the nursing home. When describing infections quantitatively, raw numbers are often misleading, and one prefers to describe the number of infections per unit of population per unit of time, an infection **rate** (4).

The **incidence rate** is the proportion of new cases of a disease occurring in a population in relation to the number of persons at risk for developing the disease:

$$\text{Incidence rate} = \frac{\text{number persons developing a disease}}{\text{total number at risk}} \times 100$$

Incidence rates are usually stated in terms of a definite time period, such as 1 year. For example, if 200 people resided at a nursing home during a given year, and 10 of them developed influenza during that year, then the incidence rate for influenza during that year would be $(10 \div 200) \times 100 = 5\%$.

The **attack rate** is a type of incidence rate used to describe epidemics. It is appropriate when the population is at risk for a limited time period only and the study period incorporates the entire epidemic.

The **relative risk** is the ratio of the incidence rate among those exposed to a certain factor to the incidence rate among those not exposed. The relative risk is used to quantitate the increased risk of acquiring a disease as a consequence of exposure to a particular factor. For instance, if the incidence rate of influenza in smokers is 10% and the incidence rate in nonsmokers is 2.5%, the relative risk of smoking is $10 \div 2.5 = 4.0$.

Another important epidemiologic rate is the **prevalence rate**, the proportion of persons with a disease at any given time relative to the total number of persons in the group:

$$\text{Prevalence rate} = \frac{\text{number of persons with a disease}}{\text{total number in the group}} \times 100$$

The prevalence rate provides a snapshot of a population at a certain point in time relative to a disease. If a survey of a nursing home demonstrated that 30 residents had diarrhea on a particular day and there were 200 residents in the nursing home, then the prevalance rate of diarrhea in that nursing home at that time would be $(30 \div 200) \times 100 = 15\%$.

Infectious diseases may persist at a relatively constant level in the community (**endemic**) or occur in significant excess of normal expectancy (**epidemic**). An infectious disease can be characterized by the number of existing cases in a population (prevalence), the number of new cases in a population (incidence), and the risk of transmission (contagiousness). More elaborate statistical techniques are also available to describe the epidemiology of infectious diseases (5).

Transmission of Infection

Transfer of an infectious agent may occur by either direct or indirect methods (3). Direct contact between individuals is the method of spread of staphylococcal infections and syphilis. The fecal–oral route, a common mode of spread of infectious gastroenteritis, also involves direct-contact spread. Indirect spread may involve an intermediate vehicle or vector (see Table 1.4). The list of common vehicles that have been implicated in the spread of infectious diseases is very long: Food, water, milk, blood products, intravenous fluids, drugs, medical equipment, and the hands of personnel may serve as vehicles of spread. Vector-borne spread of disease is relatively uncommon in the United States.

Airborne infectious agents may be spread on large droplets that are generated by talking and sneezing; measles, for example, is transmitted this way. Alternatively, airborne transmission may involve spread on small-droplet nuclei or dust particles that remain suspended in the air for a prolonged period of time. A defective air-handling system may then result in widespread dissemination of the organism throughout the environment. For example, Legionnaires' disease has been transmitted by defective air-conditioning systems.

The spread of infectious diseases involves the following general sequence: reservoir → means of transmission → host. The reservoir may be humans (influenza), animals (tularemia), or the environment (Legionnaires' disease).

Table 1.4. Transmission of Infection

Means of Transmission	Example
Direct contact	Staphylococci
Common vehicle	
Food	Salmonellae
Water	Hepatitis A
Contaminated equipment	*Pseudomonas*
Insect vector (mosquito)	Malaria
Airborne	Influenza

The most contagious diseases of humans are chickenpox, measles, smallpox, influenza, rubella, mumps, and pneumonic plague. The risk of acquisition of disease by a nonimmune host after exposure is over 50% for these diseases. In contrast, a number of diseases that are widely feared are not highly contagious, including leprosy, meningococcal meningitis, diphtheria, and tuberculosis.

Nosocomial Infections

Nosocomial infections are those that develop within the nursing home (or hospital). The **nosocomial infection rate** is the proportion of nosocomial infections in a given period of time relative to the number of residents at risk; the latter is best reflected by the number of residents in the nursing home during the given time period (usually one month). Alternatively, the infection rate may be more accurately calculated by using resident-days for the measurement of number at risk (denominator).

For example, if a nursing home has an average census of 200 residents during a 30-day month and 20 nosocomial infections were diagnosed in residents during that time, then the nosocomial infection rate is either

$$\frac{20 \text{ Infections}}{200 \text{ Residents}} \times 100 = 10\%$$

or

$$\frac{20 \text{ Infections}}{200 \text{ Residents} \times 30 \text{ days}} \times 1000$$
$$= 3.3 \text{ nosocomial infections per 1000 resident-days}$$

Nosocomial infection rates are discussed further in Chapter 9.

REFERENCES

1. Deal WB: Unusual manifestations of infectious diseases in the aging. *Geriatrics* 34:77–84, 1979.
2. Lennette EH: *Manual of Clinical Microbiology.* Washington, D.C. American Society for Microbiology, 1980.
3. Brachman PS: Epidemiology of nosocomial infections, in Bennett JV, Brachman PS (eds): *Hospital Infections.* Boston, Little, Brown, 1979.
4. Friedman GD: *Primer of Epidemiology,* 2nd ed. New York, McGraw-Hill, 1980.
5. Colton T: *Statistics in Medicine,* 1st ed. Boston, Little, Brown, 1974.

CHAPTER 2

IMMUNITY IN THE ELDERLY

Jane F. Potter

Immunity originally referred to the resistance of people to infection by bacteria and viruses. Immunology was then the study of immunity to those organisms. In more recent years, it had been realized that immunity plays a role in protecting the person from other disorders such as cancer. Immune reactions are not always beneficial and can, instead, result in the body reacting against its own cells (autoimmunity). Because the incidence of infection, cancer, and autoimmune phenomena increase with age, the immune system has been extensively studied for its age-related changes and as a model of cellular aging.

This chapter will examine how normal immune function protects against disease, how age-related changes in the immune system impair the body's normal defense against infectious diseases, and how other common disorders of old age predispose the aged person to infection.

THE NORMAL IMMUNE SYSTEM

The immune system is composed of a number of tissues, organs, and cells. While books have been written in explanation of this system (1–3), only a brief overview will be given here. Those aspects of immune function that show age-related changes will be the primary focus of this discussion.

The immune system is activated by exposure to an invading agent (i.e., a bacteria or virus). The body recognizes a portion of the invading agent (the **antigen**) as foreign. Once exposed to an antigen, the immune system develops specific protein molecules (**antibodies**) and sensitized lymphocytes that are capable of reacting with and destroying the invading agent. During a person's first exposure to a particular agent, it will take several days to weeks to develop an effective immune response. Considerable

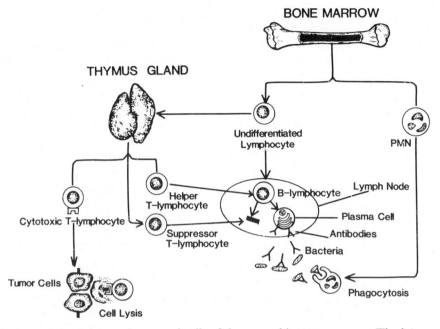

Figure 2.1. Primary tissues and cells of the normal immune system. The bone marrow is the source of undifferentiated lymphocytes, polymorphonuclear leukocytes (PMNs), and macrophages (not shown). Undifferentiated lymphocytes travel to either the thymus gland where they are transformed into T cells or to lymph tissue where they become B cells. Under stimulation by antigens, cytotoxic T lymphocytes learn to recognize tumor cells (or cells transformed by infection) that they then destroy, a process called cell lysis. When antigens are detected by B lymphocytes, these cells change into plasma cells that produce antibodies capable of recognizing the antigen on the bacterial cell. Antibodies attach to the bacteria, which are then rendered susceptible to phagocytosis by PMNs.

harm can occur during this first exposure; however, on subsequent exposure the invading organism is quickly stopped before much harm is done.

The major organs and cells of the immune system and their functions are presented diagrammatically in Figure 2.1. The cells and tissues of the immune system eliminate invading agents either by production of specific antibodies (**humoral immunity**) or through production of lymphocytes that are sensitive to the foreign substance (**cellular immunity**). The bone marrow (see Fig. 2.1) is the source of undifferentiated lymphocytes, the polymorphonuclear leukocyte (PMN), and macrophages.

Macrophages are the first line of defense in the immune system. These cells ingest a small number of bacteria or viruses and present the invading organism as an antigen to the other immune system cells. Depending on the type of organism involved, either humoral or cellular immunity may be activated.

Undifferentiated lymphocytes released from the bone marrow may travel either to the thymus gland or to the lymph nodes. Lymphocytes in the thymus gland are stimulated by hormones in the gland to become mature T lymphocytes. Mature lymphocytes are of two basic types: (1) those responsible for cell-mediated immunity, and (2) those that regulate B cells in the humoral immune response. Cytotoxic T cells are the primary mediators of cellular immunity and recognize certain kinds of antigens (T-dependent antigens) such as viruses and tuberculosis. These cytotoxic T lymphocytes recognize cells that are altered as a result of infection or cancer, travel through the bloodstream, attach to those abnormal cells, and destroy them.

The second mechanism for elimination of infectious agents from the body is production of antibodies directed specifically at those agents. B cells are stimulated by certain kinds of antigens to become plasma cells and produce antibodies. The amount of antibody produced is under the control of regulatory T cells. T helper cells stimulate production of antibodies by plasma cells. The plasma cells synthesize antibodies against the invading organisms; the antibodies are then released from the plasma cell and attach to the invading bacteria. Once the infection has been brought under control, antibody production is stopped by the action of T suppressor cells. These suppressor cells are also important in prevention of reactions against the person's own body (autoimmune reactions).

The final cellular component of the humoral immune system to be considered here is the polymorphonuclear leukocyte. These cells originate in the bone marrow and travel to sites of infection where they ingest (by a process called **phagocytosis**) bacteria to which antibodies have been attached and cells that have been damaged by the infection. Once bacteria have been phagocytosed, they are killed by the PMNs' intracellular enzymes. When PMNs engulf large numbers of bacteria and necrotic tissue, they also eventually die. After several days, a cavity is often excavated in the inflamed tissues containing varying portions of necrotic tissue and dead PMNs (**pus**).

The key tissues in the immune system are the bone marrow, lymph nodes, spleen, and thymus gland. In the adult, most cell-producing bone marrow is located in the vertebrae, sternum, and ribs.

THE EFFECTS OF AGE ON THE IMMUNE SYSTEM

Before a change in any organ system can be attributed to age, that change must be shown to occur in multiple species and in virtually all individuals of those species. Age-related changes do not affect all individuals to the same extent, and an increasing variability in performance among individuals is characteristic of aging. Changes in the immune system with age occur in multiple species and are therefore true age-related changes. There are age-related changes in both humoral and cellular immunity; however, most studies have failed to show changes in the function of either the macrophage (4) or PMN (5).

Cellular Immunity

There is a progressive involution of the thymus gland beginning after sexual maturity. Because the thymus gland is responsible for differentiation of lymphocytes into competent T cells, it is not surprising that involution of the thymus gland is followed by several important changes in the population of T cells. The population of cytotoxic T cells (see Fig. 2.1), which are responsible for cellular immunity, undergo important age-related changes. Three tests that show an age-related decline in cellular immune function are the rosette test, delayed hypersensitivity, and lymphocyte proliferation. The rosette test quantitates the number of T cells able to form clusters (rosettes) around sheep cells when the two types of cells are incubated together in a test tube. **Delayed hypersensitivity** is a reaction by T cells to an antigen injected into the skin and requires prior exposure to that antigen. Lymphocyte proliferation is a necessary part of the immune response. Normally, after exposure to an antigen, the number of T cells multiply (proliferate) in order to bring an infection under control.

When people of different ages are tested for functional activity of T cells derived from the thymus gland (using the rosette test), the percentage of T cells able to form rosettes declines markedly with age (6). It therefore seems that older people have fewer active T cells to defend against infection. Activity of T cells can also be measured by skin tests to common antigens. Active T cells are necessary for development of a positive skin test (delayed hypersensitivity). Clinical studies have shown that older people react to fewer skin test antigens (e.g., mumps, *Candida*, or purified protein derivative—PPD) than younger people (7). This suggests that a person who is exposed to, say, tuberculosis early in life and develops a positive skin test somehow loses the ability to respond to that

Table 2.1.   The Effect of Age on the Immune System

Immune System Cell or Tissue	Function	Age-Related Change
Thymus gland	Transform undifferentiated lymphocytes into T cells	Involution
B lymphocyte	Produce antibodies	Decreased antibody production
T lymphocyte	Help or suppress B cell function; cytotoxic reactions	Decreased helper cell compared to suppressor cell function
PMN	Phagocytosis	None
Macrophage	Process antigen	None

antigen as he or she grows older. Because only those people with previous exposure to an antigen would be expected to show a positive skin test, several different common antigens (a skin test battery) must be used to assess a person's capacity for delayed hypersensitivity. An alternative to the use of a skin test battery is use of an antigen to which people are not normally exposed—that is, to perform a test of primary (new exposure) delayed hypersensitivity. Dinitrochlorobenzene (DNCB) is a laboratory chemical that can be used to test primary delayed hypersensitivity. When both young and old people are given an intradermal injection of DNCB and reinjected with the antigen at a later time, fewer older people react that younger people (8). This suggests that older people are less likely to develop immunity after infection and may subsequently develop a second infection with the same organism. In addition, the ability of older people to bring an infection under control appears to be impaired. When T cells from tuberculosis patients are tested for their ability to respond to PPD, the response of the cells (cell proliferation) decreases with increasing age of the patients studied (9). This is a possible explanation for the fact that tuberculosis has become a disease of old age.

The important changes that occur in cell-mediated immunity with age are summarized in Table 2.1. The number of functional T cells declines with age, and those cells that remain are less responsive to invading organisms.

Humoral Immunity

B lymphocytes are stimulated to produce antibodies by most common pyogenic bacteria (see Fig. 2.1). Because B lymphocytes express their effects through secretion of an active humor (antibodies), the function

Table 2.2. Common Afflictions of Elderly People Associated with Impaired Local Resistance to Infection

Organ System	Condition Common in Elderly People
Gastrointestinal	Poor oral hygiene and dentition, lack of gastric acid
Skin	Skin thinning, ulceration, frequent trauma and superficial wounds
Nervous	Peripheral neuropathy, stroke
Urinary	Foley catheters, urinary retention
Respiratory	Abdominal breathing, decreased air exchange
Heart	Abnormal heart valves

of these B cells is referred to as humoral immunity. Antibodies attach to invading organisms and render them susceptible to phagocytosis by PMNs.

When older people are experimentally injected with an antigen from *Salmonella* (a common causative organism for diarrhea), antibodies are produced at a lower level than in younger people (10). Lower levels of antibody response have been seen to other antigens as well (11), which suggests that older people have impaired ability to defend themselves against infection with certain organisms.

The cause of this reduced antibody response was somewhat puzzling since the number of B cells and their conversion to plasma cells did not decrease with age. B cells are converted to plasma cells when stimulated by appropriate antigens; however, the amount of antibody produced by the plasma cells (Fig. 2.1) is under the control of helper and suppressor T cells. Helper cells appear to decrease with age in humans (12–15). It now appears that in young persons, the net effect of T cells is to stimulate antibody productivity by B cells, whereas in old persons, T cells tend to suppress antibody production. This change in T suppressor and T helper effect may account for the apparent increase in susceptibility of older persons to infection with pyogenic bacteria and their subsequent higher mortality. It now appears that age-related decline in antibody production by B cells is due to the increased activity of suppressor T cells (see Table 2.1).

Autoimmunity

Normally, the immune system only produces antibodies or sensitized lymphocytes against undesirable invaders such as bacteria or cancer cells.

The immune system recognizes normal cells and protects them from attack by T cells and antibodies. When the system for recognition of normal cells breaks down, T cells and antibodies (autoantibodies) begin to attack the body's own cells. The disorders wherein the immune system reacts against the body's own cells are called **autoimmune** phenomena. Autoantibodies directed at thyroid, gastric, and smooth muscle cells and at cell nuclei increase with age and are present in 50% of older people (16). In some cases, these autoantibodies may lead to problems, as for example when the gastric cells are destroyed and the stomach no longer produces acid, or when the thyroid gland is damaged and hypothyroidism occurs. However, more often than not, the presence of autoantibodies is asymptomatic, and studies have shown that autoantibodies do not increase mortality above that expected (11).

A disorder related to autoimmune disease is production of excessive amounts of antibodies. The extreme example of this process is the disease multiple myeloma. In this disorder, the person produces one specific portion of an antibody at very high levels and shuts off production of normal antibodies. Fortunately, multiple myeloma is rare; however, production of lesser amounts of excess antibody is quite common. This condition is not progressive, and production of normal antibodies continues. This process is of interest because it affects one in five very old people (16) and is evidence for loss of immune regulation in this age group.

Immunization

A person's first exposure to an infectious agent is the most damaging, and may result in serious injury to the infected tissue or in death for the person. On subsequent exposure to the same infectious agent, the immune system responds more quickly to control the infection. Unfortunately, many viruses (e.g., influenza) and bacteria (e.g., *Staphylococcus aureus*) come in many different strains, and the individual must be exposed to each strain in order to develop immunity.

Immunity to some infectious agents can be induced by exposing an individual to very small amounts of antigen (a vaccine), a process called **immunization**. The antigen (usually a protein from a bacteria or virus) stimulates either B or T cells in a manner similar to that seen when a person is infected with the live organism. The immunity induced by immunization is usually not as long-lasting as that resulting from active infection, and repeat immunization may be necessary.

Legitimate concern could be expressed regarding the use of vaccines in older people because of the age-related changes in immune system function. The antibody response to many antigens decreases with age, and T cell responses are generally decreased, both of which could impair the older person's ability to respond to a vaccine. Since vaccines are initially tested in young people, it is important that additional studies be done to determine if the rise in antibody titer is adequate and if older people receive protection from disease as a result of vaccination. The vaccinations of importance for the elderly are discussed in Chapter 14.

UNDERLYING DISEASES AND DISORDERS THAT PREDISPOSE TO INFECTION

Disease is not a normal part of aging, but many diseases become increasingly prevalent with age, a fact that cannot be forgotten when dealing with the older population. In this section, consideration is given to age-related changes in physiology and disorders that interact with the changes in immune function and predispose persons to development of infectious diseases in old age. The conditions of importance here are either local disorders (see Table 2.2) that lead to infection at a single site or in a single organ system or systemic factors (see Table 2.3) that increase a person's susceptibility to a variety of different infections.

Local Factors

Oral Hygiene.   Oral and dental problems are the rule rather than the exception in the elderly institutionalized population. Local infection of the gums (periodontal disease) can progress to localized abscess. Bacteria from dental infections or loose teeth may be aspirated to cause pneumonia or lung abscess. Poor oral hygiene (usually in combination with dehydration) in a debilitated patient can precipitate parotid gland

Table 2.3.   **Systemic Factors That Predispose to Infections in Elderly People**

Diabetes mellitus
Congestive heart failure
Dehydration
Malnutrition
Immobility
Hospitalization
Diminished pain sensitivity and atypical symptoms
Decreased mental status
Tumors
Drugs

infection. Measures to prevent these problems include careful oral hygiene, regular dental care, antibiotic treatment of periodontal infection, extraction of loose, nonfunctional teeth, and conscious hydration.

Gastric Acid.   The stomach is lined with cells (gastric parietal cells) that secrete acid. Acid production aids in digestion and also kills bacteria that are swallowed along with food. By 70 years of age, 30% of people have lost the ability to secrete stomach acid and, although this does not cause important problems with digestion, it allows bacteria to enter the lower part of the gut and initiate infection. As an example, *Salmonella* is a bacterium that is a common cause of epidemic diarrheal illness in institutions. In order to be infected with *Salmonella*, a person with normal stomach acid must ingest between 100,000 and 1,000,000 organisms (17). When fewer organisms are ingested, they will be killed by the stomach acid. Persons who do not produce gastric acid will be infected when exposed to far fewer organisms. For reasons that are not clear, there is an association between gastric resection and reactivation of previously inactive tuberculosis (18).

Skin Ulcers.   The rate at which the skin ages is directly related to the amount of ultraviolet light exposure. People who have worked outdoors will experience premature aging of their skin. As the skin ages, both dermal and epidermal layers become thinner, skin collagen loses strength, and skin elasticity is decreased. It is for these reasons that skin tears more easily in old age, increasing the chance for skin infection. Thinning of the skin is one reason why older people are predisposed to decubitus ulcers, which can then become a site for local or systemic spread of infection (see Chapter 7). Care must be taken to handle fragile, aged skin carefully, to keep skin lesions clean and dry, and to give tetanus toxin at appropriate intervals.

Skin ulcers also develop because of diseases in either the arteries or veins. With age, veins become less elastic and enlarge in diameter, and venous valves are less effective at preventing backflow of blood. As a consequence, blood pools in the lower extremities, tissues swell, and blistering and skin breakdown follow. Venous stasis ulcers characteristically occur on the inner aspect of the ankle and, like any ulcer, can become infected. Both treatment and prevention require regular elevation of the extremities during the day as well as at night. Atherosclerosis occurs to some extent in all older people and is sometimes considered to be a normal aging change. Severe vascular disease, however, rarely occurs in the absence of smoking or lifelong lipid disorders. Severe vascular disease leads to low blood flow, low oxygen levels in the skin, and skin breakdown (ischemic ulcers). Even minor trauma to poorly perfused tissues produces sores that heal slowly. Ischemic ulcers and slowly healing sores are readily infected because infection-fighting cells and antibodies reach these tissues in suboptimal quantities. Signs of poor blood flow are coolness of the extremity, decreased or absent pulses, lack of hair, and thick, overgrown toenails. When injury occurs to the feet or lower leg of patients with these physical findings, additional caution should be exercised, and prompt medical attention should be obtained if redness, warmth, or swelling develop, indicating the onset of infection. A final contributing factor to skin breakdown and skin infection is nervous system disease. Peripheral nerve damage occurs from a variety of toxins (e.g., alcohol abuse), vitamin deficiency (e.g., vitamin B_{12}), or diabetes mellitus. Central nervous system damage occurs most commonly due to strokes, but also from head trauma or spinal cord injury. Patients with these disorders lose sensation and are unaware of developing pressure sores. The only effective preventative measures are frequent rotation of patient and frequent observation of the affected body parts.

Urinary Tract.   The urinary tract is a very common site of infection in elderly people. A variety of conditions make the urinary tract susceptible to infections, including prostatic enlargement, urethral stricture, and neurogenic bladder. In elderly men, the prostate is most frequently at fault; this gland enlarges predictably with age, sometimes due to cancer, but much more frequently due to benign growth (hyperplasia). When the prostate reaches sufficient size, it blocks the free flow of urine and a stagnant pool of urine develops. Bacteria migrate up the urethra and enter the bladder. Because the bladder does not completely empty, the urine becomes infected. A narrowing of the blocked urethra (stricture) can develop in both men and women and cause urinary tract infection by the same mechanism as prostatic obstruction. A third problem that predisposes to incomplete bladder emptying and infection is degeneration of the nerves that produce bladder emptying (neurogenic bladder). Bladder catheters provide a direct route for spread of infection from the collection bag into the bladder. A detailed discussion of urinary tract infection is given in Chapter 6.

Pulmonary Function.   Several important age-related changes in the lungs and chest wall predispose older people to chest infections. In order to defend against infection, the lungs must take in and release air efficiently. Movement of the rib cage during inspiration draws air into the lungs, and rib cage mobility decreases as people grow older (19). The older person compensates to a degree for the loss of rib cage mobility by using abdominal muscles (20). However, when the older patient is put to bed, the abdominal muscles are no longer effective in expanding the lungs. At bedrest, the lungs do not expand well, lung secretions are not cleared from the airways, and bacteria or viruses can set up infection. Important measures to prevent pneumonia in the older patient at bedrest include elevating the head of the bed to as upright a position as possible, encouraging the patient to cough and breath deeply, and getting the patient out of bed as soon as possible.

Not only are the lungs of older people less efficient at intake of air, but they are also less efficient at air release. Movement of air out of the lungs normally occurs because elastic tissue in the lung springs back, forcing air out of the lung. There is an age-related loss of lung elastic tissue (21) that accounts for the fact that an 80-year-old person has 50% more air left in the lung at the end of expiration than a 25-year-old (22). Air trapped in the lung exchanges with inspired air very slowly and is lower in oxygen content. The increase in the amount of air trapped in the lung is a primary reason that blood oxygen decreases with age. Normally, this lower blood oxygen is well tolerated by the older person, but it does lower the reserve oxygen available should pneumonia develop. Lower blood oxygen in combination with immune system abnormalities may account for the increased mortality seen in older patients with pneumonia.

Circulation.   Certain types of heart disease occur almost exclusively in older people. Of these, calcification of the mitral and aortic heart valves are the most common (23). Calcium is deposited in the heart valves after years of wear and tear from constant opening and closing. Valves that do not move normally are further damaged, and when bacteria are present in the bloodstream (bacteremia), those damaged valves become infected (bacterial endocarditis). Calcification of the aortic and mitral valves is one reason why older people account for a high percentage of all cases of bacterial endocarditis (24).

Systemic Factors

In addition to local disorders, certain diseases, drugs, and disorders predispose older people to a variety of infections. These systemic factors interact with impaired immune function and local disorders to further increase a person's risk for infection.

Diabetes.   Diabetes mellitus is an extremely common disorder of old age. Using conservative criteria for the diagnosis of diabetes, between 6% (25) and 20% (26) of people over 65 years suffer from this disorder.

The diabetic has an increased risk of infection for a variety of reasons. The immune system cells of diabetics do not efficiently phagocytose infectious particles due to a defect in T lymphocyte function (27). In addition, high glucose levels in tissues create a rich breeding ground for microorganisms. Diabetics have an accelerated form of vascular disease and are at particular risk for infection in the lower extremities. In addition, the diabetic state is associated with infection in soft tissues, the oral cavity, sinuses, kidney, meninges, bone, joints, and a variety of other sites.

Heart Disease.   Some abnormality of the heart is found at autopsy in 75% of people over 75 years of age (28). When heart diseases progress to the point where the heart cannot pump sufficient blood to meet the needs of the body, heart failure occurs. Heart failure increases in prevalence with age (29) and affects between four and 10 times more people over 75 years than those between 45 and 65 years. People with heart failure are particularly prone to infections of the lower respiratory tract, possibly due to defects in oxygenation and perfusion of the edematous lung.

Dehydration.   The patient who becomes dehydrated is at risk for infections in any of the body's normal secretory or excretory sites. The lung's bronchial tree normally secretes a small amount of mucus that then moves upward along the bronchi to remove inspired bacteria and particles. In a similar manner, free flow of urine limits the amount of bacterial growth in a urinary tract with a low-grade infection. In the absence of obstruction, the parotid gland remains free of infection as long as adequate hydration insures a free flow of saliva. In any of these systems, dehydration decreases secretions and allows infection to develop.

Immobility.   The immobile patient is predisposed to infection because of changes induced in the skin, veins, and lungs. Perhaps the most frequent problem in such patients is development of pressure sores over bony prominences such as the buttocks, elbows, and feet. A second very common problem is stasis edema in the lower extremities. Normal venous return from the legs occurs when muscles contract and force blood upward toward the heart. Immobile muscles do not perform this important pumping action, blood pools in veins, and fluid seeps from the engorged veins into the surrounding tissues. Most immobile patients will have some degree of edema in their legs. This type of edema is not the result of an excess in total body fluid and should not be treated with diuretics. If the edema leads to skin breakdown, the primary treatment is elevation of the legs and use of elastic stockings.

Yet another problem experienced by the immobile elderly patient occurs because the lungs completely expand only when the standing position is assumed (30). Lungs that do not completely expand are prone to infection; therefore, it becomes important to have a patient stand to transfer or ambulate even for short periods of time.

Effects of Hospitalization.   Eighteen percent of people over 65 are hospitalized each year (31), and this figure is very likely higher for the more disabled residents of long-term care facilities. Hospitalization in acute care facilities predisposes to infection in several important ways. Antibiotics, which are commonly used during hospitalization, destroy the normal bacteria that live in and on the body and allow those bacteria to be replaced with antibiotic-resistant and infection-producing bacteria. Intravenous catheters and solutions become infected and seed bacteria directly into the bloodstream. Finally, proximity to other infected patients increases the possibility that infection will be transmitted to the uninfected person. As increasingly ill patients who require complex treatments are cared for in chronic care facilities, these same factors are becoming important in development and spread of infection. This problem is examined in detail in Chapter 4.

Symptoms in the Elderly.   Diminished pain sensitivity, atypical symptoms, and decreased mental status can hamper diagnosis while a disease is at an early stage and before infection develops. Although there is conflicting evidence on age-related differences in pain sensitivity (32), symptoms in the elderly people are often different than in young people, and, as a rule, symptoms in older people are less specific (33). At least one-third (34) of residents in long-term care facilities have mental disorders and therefore have some difficulty describing symptoms. Not infrequently, the only sign of illness in the resident is a further decrease in mental status. It is obviously important that the staff of long-term care facilities report such changes and obtain a medical evaluation for the patient.

Malignancy.   Sixty percent of all malignancies develop after 60 years of age, and 5% of all patients in long-term care facilities carry a diagnosis of malignancy (34). Cancer patients frequently experience abnormalities in their immune systems that involve PMNs, macrophages, T cells, and B cells (35). It is not surprising, then, that infection is the most important medical problem in these patients and a frequent cause of the patient's demise.

Nutrition.   Excluding the immune dysfunction of old age, malnutrition is probably the most common cause of impaired immunity in adults. A high percentage of hospitalized patients are malnourished, and the same is probably true of the more debilitated residents in long-term care facilities. Identification of the malnourished patient and classification as to the type of malnutrition present can be carried out by obtaining a nutritional history, body measurements, and a few simple laboratory tests. There are basically two types of malnutrition. In malnutrition with calorie deficiency but adequate protein intake (sometimes called marasmus), patients are underweight and have low fat stores, decreased muscle mass, and normal levels of serum proteins. In the second type, malnutrition with protein deficiency but adequate calorie intake (sometimes called kwashiorkor), patients have normal or even increased body weight, decreased skeletal muscle protein, and decreased serum protein levels (see Table 2.4).

Weight loss is present in both types of malnutrition. Even a small weight loss is important when it occurs over a short period of time (36). Loss of 2% of body weight over two weeks' time, or 10% over six months, leads to a malnourished state. Table 2.4 summarizes the other important measurements in the detection and classification of malnourished patients. The body mass index (BMI) is an index of body weight that has been adjusted for the fact that taller people weigh more. The body mass index is calculated by dividing the patient's weight in kilograms by the square of his height in meters (weight/height^2). There has been consid-

Table 2.4.   Detection and Classification of Malnutrition in the Elderly Patient

		Malnutrition of:	
Test	*Normal*	*Calories*	*Protein*
Body mass index (BMI)[a]			
Male	22.5–25.7	↓	→ ↓
Female	21.7–24.9		
Triceps skinfold thickness (mm)[b]			
Male	> 5.0	↓	→ ↑
Female	>12.0		
Arm muscle circumference (cm)[b]			
Male	>20.5	↓	↓
Female	>19.6		
Serum albumin (g/dl)	> 3.5	←	↓

[a]Values based on "optimal weight" for middle of the median frame according to the 1979 build and blood pressure study (40).
[b]Lower 5th percentile values for individuals 65–74 years in the 1970 U.S. DHEW health and nutrition examination survey (42).

erable discussion in the literature concerning standards for optimal body weight (37–39), and a review of this problem is beyond the scope of this chapter. Standards for optimal body weight are based on a study done in the first part of the century and published by the Metropolitan Life Insurance Company in 1959. More recent studies and analyses (37–40) have indicated that the 1959 recommendations for weight are too low. The values of BMI given in Table 2.4 reflect the fact that Metropolitan Life increased optimal weights by approximately 10%.

A second important parameter of nutritional state is the tricep skinfold thickness, which correlates fairly well with total body fat stores. This measurement, which can be done by most dieticians, is performed by measuring the thickness of the fat overlying the midpoint of the upper arm. While the tricep skinfold thickness provides an estimate of the total amount of fat in the body, the arm muscle circumference is an estimate of muscle stores of protein. This parameter is calculated by subtracting one-half the tricep's skinfold thickness from the total arm circumference (41, 42).

The patient who is consuming inadequate amounts of protein will mobilize protein from the skeletal muscle in order to maintain serum protein at normal levels. Once the skeletal muscle protein stores have been exhausted, serum protein will also fall. Skeletal protein can also be burned as energy and will be utilized during times of low caloric intake. Serum albumin is the laboratory test most commonly used to evaluate the level of serum protein. A serum albumin below 3.5 is abnormal and in the absence of liver disease usually indicates a state of protein malnutrition. The immune malfunction that occurs in malnourished patients depends on whether calories or protein are in short supply. Both calorie malnutrition and protein malnutrition reduce skin tests' reactivity (43,44), but only protein malnutrition reduces the total number of lymphocytes and the ability of those lymphocytes to become transformed by antigens into active infection-fighting cells (43). Furthermore, the ability of PMNs to kill bacteria once those bacteria have been ingested is impaired in malnourished patients (45).

Drugs.   An important factor that alters immune function in the elderly is the use of drugs. Those drugs that impinge on immune function most directly are those that are designed to do so, such as steroids and anti-cancer drugs. These drugs are powerful modulators of the immune response. Steroids cause a redistribution of lymphocytes from the circulation into other body compartments, which renders the cells less accessible to sites of infection and immune reactivity. The effects of steroids on PMNs is to prevent these cells from migrating out of the vascular system into sites of inflammation and infection. In addition to the effects on the migration of immunologically active cells, steroids also reduce the functional activity of those cells. Almost every step of the immune process is affected, including antigen processing, phagocytosis, and cytotoxic T cell function (46). Almost all cancer chemotherapeutic agents nonspecifically lower the immune response. This is accomplished by a direct attack on all immunologically active cells.

Certain drugs such as aspirin, common nonsteroidal antiinflammatory agents, theophylline, and propranolol alter laboratory tests of immune function (46). However, there is, at present, no evidence that these drugs alter the course of infectious diseases.

SUMMARY

The three major classes of immune system cells are macrophages, lymphocytes, and polymorphonuclear leukocytes (PMNs). These cells interact with one another to bring about the normal immune response. The immune system controls the first infection with a given organism and retains a memory (immunity) of that organism that prevents future infection with the same organism.

There is some decline in immune function with age, especially in antibody production and cellular immunity. Even though antibody response to vaccination is often lower in older people, sufficient levels of antibodies are generally attained to achieve protection from disease. Therefore, regular booster doses of vaccine should be given against tetanus, diphtheria, influenza, and the pneumococci.

Some age-related changes in physiology and many diseases and drugs interact with immune system alterations to further predispose the aged person to the development of infections. The physiologic changes of concern are thinning of the skin and decreased rib cage mobility. Pathologic changes that predispose to infection within the involved organ system include loss of gastric acid production, loss of normal sensory function, urinary retention, and calcification of heart valves. Diabetes mellitus, malnutrition, tumors, and drugs all interact directly with one or more of the immune system's cells to predispose the elderly person to a wide variety of infections. Either under- or overhydration predisposes to infection by impairing the normal mechanisms for clearing bacteria from the body's secretory and excretory sites. Decreased mental status is common in residents of long-term care facilities and, in combination with the atypical symptoms of many diseases in old age, impairs our ability to make a diagnosis before infection develops.

REFERENCES

1. Bach JF (ed): *Immunology*, 2nd ed. New York, Wiley, 1982.
2. McConnell I, Munro A, Waldman H: *The Immune System: A Course on the Molecular and Cellular Basis of Immunity*, 2nd edi. Oxford, Blackwell, 1981.
3. Bier OG, DaSilva WD, Gotze D, Mota I: *Fundamentals of Immunology*. New York, Springer, 1981.
4. Makinodan T, Good RA, Kay MMB: Cellular basis of immunosenescence, in Good RA, Day SB (eds): *Comprehensive Immunology*. New York, Plenum, 1977, pp 9–22.
5. Finkelstein MS, Petkin W, Citrin A: Differences in presentation of pneumococcal bacteremia based on age of patient. *Clin Res* 29:299A, 1981.
6. Singh J, Singh AK: Age related changes in human thymus. *Clin Exp Immunol* 37:507–511, 1979.
7. Makinodan T, Kay MMB: Age influence on the immune system, in Kunkel H, Dixon F (eds): *Advances in Immunology*, Vol. 29. New York, Academic Press, 1980, pp 287–330.
8. Gross L: Immunological defect in aged population and its relationship to cancer. *Cancer* 18:201–204, 1965.
9. Nilsson BS: In vitro lymphocyte reactivity to PPD and phytohaemagglutinin in relation to PPD skin reactivity and age. *Scand J Resp Dis* 52:39–47, 1971.
10. Weksler ME: The senescence of the immune system. *Hosp Pract* 16(10):53–64, 1981.
11. McKay IR, Whittingham SF, Mathews JD: The immunoepidemiology of aging, in Makinodan T, Yunis E (eds): *Immunology and Aging*. New York, Plenum, 1977, pp 35–49.
12. Antel JR, Weinrich M, Arnason BGS: Circulating suppressor cells in man as a function of age. *Clin Immunol Immunopathol* 9:134–141, 1978.
13. Gupta S, Good RA: Subpopulations of human T-lymphocytes x. alternations in T, B, third population cells and T cells with receptors for immunoglobulin M or G in aging humans. *J Immunol* 122:1214–1219, 1979.
14. Hallgren HM, Yunis EJ: Suppressor lymphocytes in young and aged humans. *J Immunol* 118:2004–2008, 1977.
15. Kishimoto S, Tomino S, Inomato K, et al: Age related changes in the subsets and functions of human T lymphocytes. *J Immunol* 121:1173–1780, 1978.
16. Hijamans W, Hollander CF: The pathogenic role of age-related immune dysfunctions, in Makinodan T, Yunis E, (eds): *Immunology and Aging*. New York, Plenum, 1977, pp 23–33.
17. Hood EW, Johnson WD: Nontyphoidal salmonellosis, in Hoeprich PD (ed): *Infectious Diseases*. New York, Harper & Row, 1972, pp 583–591.
18. Harris HW, McClement JH: Tuberculosis, in Hoeprich PD (ed): *Infectious Diseases*. New York, Harper & Row, 1972, pp 351–378.

19. Mittman C, Edelman NH, Norris, AH, et al: Relationship between chest wall and pulmonary compliance and age. *J Appl Physiol* 20:1211–1216, 1965.

20. Rizzato G, Marrazini L: Thoracoabdominal mechanics in elderly men. *J Appl Physiol* 28:457–460, 1970.

21. Turner JM, Mead J, Wohl ME: Elasticity of human lungs in relation to age. *J Appl Physiol* 25:664–671, 1968.

22. Jones RL, Overton TR, Hammerlindl DM, et al: Effects of age on regional residual volume. *J Appl Physiol: Respirat Environ Exercise Physiol* 44(2):195–199, 1978.

23. Pomerance A: Cardiac pathology in the elderly, in Noble RJ, Rathbaum DA (eds): *Geriatric Cardiology*. Philadelphia, Davis, 1981, pp 9–54.

24. Hughes P, Gauld WR: Bacterial endocarditis, a changing disease. *Q J Med* 35:511–521, 1966.

25. Andres R: Aging and diabetes. *Med Clin N Am* 55:835–846, 1971.

26. Zimmet P, Whitehouse S: The effect of age on glucose tolerance studies in a Micronesian population with a high prevalence of diabetes. *Diabetes* 28:617–623, 1979.

27. Kolterman OG, Olefsky JM, Kurahara C, et al: A defect in cell-mediated immune function in insulin-resistant diabetic and obese subject. *J Lab Clin Med* 96:535–543, 1980.

28. Noble RJ, Rothbaum DA: History and physical examination, in Noble RJ, Rothbaum DA (eds): *Geriatric Cardiology*. Philadelphia, Davis, 1981, pp 55–63.

29. Klainer LM, Gibson TC, White KL: The epidemiology of cardiac failure. *J Chronic Dis* 18:797–814, 1965.

30. Leblanc P, Ruff F, Milic-Emili J: The effects of age and body position on airway closure in man. *J Appl Physiol* 28(4):448–451, 1970.

31. *Current Estimates from the Health Interview Survey: United States, 1978*, Vital and Health Statistics Series 10, No. 130. publication No. (PHS)80-1551. US Department of Health and Human Services, Office of Health Research, Statistics, and Technology, November 1979.

32. Harkins SW, Warner MH: Age and pain, in Eisdorfer C (ed): *Annual Review of Gerontology and Geriatrics*, Vol. 1. New York, Springer, 1980, pp 121–131.

33. Hodkinson, HM: Nonspecific presentation of illness, in Hodkinson HM: *Common Symptoms of Disease in the Elderly*. Oxford, Blackwell, 1976, pp 6–20.

34. *The National Nursing Home Survey: 1977 Summary for the United States*, publication No. (PHS) 79-1794. US Department of Health, Education, and Welfare, Office of Health Research, Statistics, and Technology, July 1979, pp 31–32.

35. Armstrong D: Infectious complications of neoplastic disease: Diagnosis and management. I. *Clin Bull* 6:135–141, 1976.

36. Blackburn GL, Harvey KB: Nutritional assessment as a routine in clinical medicine. *Postgrad Med* 71:46–63, 1982.

37. Andres R: Influence of obesity on longevity in the aged, in Marois M (ed): *Aging: A Challenge to Science and Society*, Vol. I, *Biology*. London, Oxford University Press, 1981, pp 196–203.

38. Andres A: Effect of obesity on total mortality. *Int J Obesity* 4:381–386, 1980.

39. Keys A: Overweight, obesity, coronary heart disease, and mortality. *Nutr Rev* 38(9):297–307, 1980.

40. Society of Actuaries. *Build Study 1979*. Chicago, 1980.

41. Vague J, Boyer J, Jubelin J, et al: Adipomuscular ratio in human subjects, in Vague J, Denton RM (eds): *Physiopathology of Adipose Tissue*, Proceedings of the Third-International Meeting of Endocrinologists. Amsterdam, Excerpta Medica Foundation, 1969, pp 360–386.

42. *Skinfolds, Body Girths, Biacromial Diameter, and Selected Anthropometric Indices of Adults, United States, 1960–1962*, publication No. 1000, Series 11, No. 35. US Department of Health, Education, and Welfare, National Center for Health Statistics, 1970.

43. Bistrian BR, Blackburn GL, Scrimshaw NS, et al: Cellular immunity in semistarved states in hospitalized adults. *Am J Clin Nutr* 28:1148–1155, 1975.

44. Bistrian BR, Sherman M, Blackburn GL, et al: Cellular immunity in adult marasmus. *Arch Intern Med* 137:1408–1411, 1977.

45. Selvaraj RJ, Bhat KS: Metabolic and bactericidal activities of leukocytes in protein–calorie malnutrition. *Am J Clin Nutr* 25:166–174, 1972.

46. Hadden JW, Coffey RG, Spreafico D (eds): *Immunopharmacology*. New York, Plenum, 1977, pp 5–333.

CHAPTER 3

INFECTIOUS DISEASES OF THE GERIATRIC PATIENT

Ian M. Smith

GENERAL CONCEPTS

The Importance of Infections in the Elderly

The rates found in recent tables for the 10 leading causes of death for persons age 65 and over per 100,000 population are 5874 deaths from diseases of the heart, 2643 from cancer, 947 from influenza, 210 from pneumonia, and 23 from infections of the kidney. The overall figures are misleading because death certificates (only 50% accurate when checked against autopsy reports) often list sudden causes of death in the general terms of myocardial infarctions or stroke (1). Autopsy statistics show a death rate of 15% from pneumonia in nursing homes and 6% in acute care hospitals; septicemia is also a cause in 6% of the deaths in acute care hospitals. There are no autopsy figures available for this cause of death in nursing homes (2–4). By using this more accurate form of recording, it can be seen that infection is a frequent cause of death in the elderly. Autopsy studies in pneumonia suggest that another 20% of patients have pneumonia as their secondary cause of death. Single-day studies made in nursing homes find that between 2 and 15% of the patients have infections (5). The overall types of infection involved are summarized in Table 3.1. A recent study of 190 patients in a nursing home shows that 60% of the patients who had infections and did not receive antibiotics died. In contrast, only 9% of those treated with antibiotics died (6). Table 3.1 also gives a representation of the infections likely to be found in the elderly living in the community, in the acute care hospital, and elderly persons in nursing homes. Many infections such as pneumococcal pneumonia increase directly with age, as does gram-negative rod (GNR) pneumonia, particularly in men, and urinary tract infection in women. Other infections tend to be concentrated in

Table 3.1. Infections in the Home, the Nursing Home, and Acute Care Hospitals

Home	Nursing Home	Acute Care Hospital
Pneumococcal pneumonia	Infected decubiti	GNR pneumonia
Legionnaires' pneumonia	Conjunctivitis	Septicemia
Cystitis	Cystitis/pyelonephritis	Nosocomial infections
	Pneumonia	Postoperative infections
	Diarrhea	
	Influenza	

the elderly group because of anatomical or aging changes (see Chapter 2). These are represented by urinary tract infection following benign prostatic hypertrophy obstruction or vaginitis occurring on degenerated vaginal epithelium. Diabetic infections are typical in aging people. Herpes zoster and tuberculosis represent the reactivation of a latent infection acquired at an earlier age.

Fever

Fever is an exaggeration of the normal diurnal swing of temperature between a low in the early morning hours and a high at 6:00–8:00 in the evening. This difference is 2°F or 1°C. When infection occurs, therefore, the temperature spikes in the evenings. Temperature should be routinely taken in the evening and not in the morning. In addition, the response to a successfully treated bacterial infection by the use of antibiotics is best indicated by the evening temperature falling like a bouncing ball. Fever occurs after any material is phagocytosed by polymorphonuclear leukocytes, which results in the secretion of endogenous pyrogen, a proteinaceous material that interacts with the thalamus and causes fever. Approximately one-third of long, continued, and difficult infections are due to traditional bacterial infections, about one-fifth are due to collagen vascular disease, and about one-fifth are due to cancer. This is because the white cell does not identify what has been phagocytosed and can produce a fever from the engulfment of antibody antigen complexes or of dead tissue just as easily as from the engulfment of bacteria (7).

Response of the Elderly to Infection

The elderly patient's response to infection may differ because of body systems that age at a rate of approximately 0.75% per year; also, the response may differ because of an accumulation of diseases or environmental changes through treatment or institutionalization. Underlying emphysema and gram-negative rods in the throat may make an elderly patient more susceptible to pneumonia. In the gastrointestinal tract the decrease in secretion of hydrochloric acid and surface-active antigens may lead to infection. Perhaps the most important organ change in the elderly is in the loss of renal function. Degeneration in the central nervous system, particularly when it is not due to aging but is due to Alzheimer's disease, may lead to changes in hygienic habits or problems in aspiration. Both factors lead to an increase in pneumonia. Other diseases affecting the response of the elderly to infection are discussed in Chapter 2.

Among the elderly admitted to the acute care hospital, the appearance of five or six distinct diseases is not unusual. The elderly are being admitted to the acute care hospital in the 1980s at a rate approximately 35% higher than in the previous decade, compared to an overall increase in admission rate of 8%. This is leading to an increase in the diagnosis of diseases and to an increase in the use of medications that may interact or cause a decrease in response to infection. When elderly people die of disseminated infection, they die partially from the infection load and partly from underlying disease. Studies have suggested that as many as 50% of the elderly will die from exacerbation of underlying cardiac, renal, or pulmonary failure. About 5% of the elderly population are admitted to long-term care units, and about the same percentage are admitted to acute care hospitals each year. An elderly person has approximately 25% chance of being admitted to a nursing home before he or she dies. In these environments, infections tend to pass from patient to patient, particularly from patients with indwelling catheters to others with the same problem. Vaccination, isolation, and surveillance procedures need careful delineation and reinforcement to prevent the elderly person from developing an infection that can be lethal. Nosocomial infections in the nursing home are reviewed in Chapter 4.

The signs and symptoms of infection in the elderly may be modified over those in the younger age group. Fever may be absent because the autonomic nervous system has degenerated and skin vasculature does not respond to appropriate stimuli. The elderly patient may have chronic renal disease that will halve the amount of fever produced by a given infection compared with the amount appearing in the patients without renal failure. Chronic steroid therapy and possibly chronic aspirin therapy may obliterate fever. Because the fever rises in the evening and temperatures are frequently taken in the morning, the onset of fever may be missed for several days. Silent myocardial infarctions are well recorded in the medical literature. Due to the absence of pleurisy, silent pneumonia is less well recorded. In various studies of acute infection, such as pneumonia, approximately 55% of the elderly will have an abnormal white count of over 12,000. Approximately 95% of them will have a significant shift of the polymorphonuclear count to the left; therefore, a differential white blood count should always be taken (8).

The Diagnosis of Infection

An important concept to understand is the differentiation between colonization and infection. In some patients, an overwhelming exposure to a bacterium will lead to direct **infection**. With other infections a **carriage** state is first established, while later on other factors lead to the change from carriage or colonization to active infection. Colonization depends upon a dynamic interaction between the cells of the host and the bacterial cells. In addition to this, host cells can be damaged mechanically or by virus infection, which leads later to a bacterial colonization. Laboratory diagnoses greatly hinge on this concept, and in certain areas a large amount of **normal flora** is present. A sputum culture, for example, will not be "sterile" in a normal individual, but will contain normal bacterial flora of the mouth and throat. Many laboratories have adopted the policy of quantitative culture or estimating the percentage of each organism on Gram stain or culture. Another example of carriage is tuberculosis where, for example, many people are infected and carry live tubercle bacilli in the body, thereby changing their tuberculin skin test from negative to positive. In approximately 4% of these people that carriage will later develop into active tuberculosis. Almost all tuberculosis cases in the elderly come from colonized people and less commonly from direct overwhelming exposure.

The diagnosis of infection is found by answering four questions: First, is there an infection present, as demonstrated by signs and symptoms of fever and shaking chills, and a white blood count rise or change in the differential count of polymorphonuclear leukocytes? Certain signs such as ecthyma gangrenosa (a gangrenous skin lesion) indicate that *Pseudomonas aeruginosa* is growing in the endothelium of the small blood vessels; therefore, a specific microbiological diagnosis can be made at the bedside. In other cases, the ridge between normal skin and abnormal skin in erysipelas caused by the growth of streptococci in the lymphatics of the skin and its subsequent edema is characteristic. Second, what is the anatomical location of the infection? This is easy to find when there is burning and scalding from urinary tract infection or pleurisy from pneumonia, but is more difficult to locate in the presence of shaking chills only, which usually indicates a septicemia. Third, what is the etiology of the infection? It is not adequate to diagnose lobar pneumonia; rather, one must be specific and call it pneumococcal, gram-negative rod, or *Legionella* pneumonia. Fourth, how much underlying disease is present? To know this is of paramount importance because up to 85% of patients over age 65 who have pneumonia also have severe underlying disease. Approximately 50% of patients who die of infection die of underlying disease and not of the accumulation of bacteria. Accumulation of bacteria will kill when approximately 10^{13} bacteria accumulate in a 70-kg individual. This is important to know because the incision and drainage of abscesses will reduce this number of bacteria. Apart from this, patients die from the onset of cardiac, respiratory, or renal failure because their energy has been diverted from the usual support of these systems to combat the infection.

The diagnosis of a bacterial infection depends heavily on a well-equipped bacteriological laboratory (see also Chapter 1). It also depends on taking the right specimens and collecting them in the correct manner. One should know what kind of blood culture bottles and swabs to use when diagnosing an anaerobic infection. Anaerobic bacteria transported in room oxygen for 20–30 minutes will die, and the culture will have lost value because of the poor way in which it was collected. Appropriate cultures should be obtained from all visible lesions and from potentially infected fluids such as urine, blood, or cerebral spinal fluid. When in doubt, take a blood culture. In general, a single blood culture is very valuable in diagnosing pneumonia, meningitis and peritonitis. Three cultures taken two hours apart will diagnose 96% of all septicemias in patients not on antibiotics. It is also important, however, to take cultures from patients on antibiotics. When the patient on antibiotics is febrile, the organism is probably resistant to the antibiotics being administered. While three cultures are enough to diagnose 96% of all septicemias, five must be taken to diagnose endocarditis. From time to time "contaminants" are reported, such as diphtheroids or *Staphylococcus epidermidis*. One must be aware that some diphtheroids in the elderly are really *Listeria* organisms, and that although 95% of all *S. epidermidis* blood cultures represent contamination, 5% of them are potentially lethal infection. One must therefore draw another three or five sets of blood cultures (9).

SPECIFIC INFECTIONS

Skin Infections

Conjunctivitis. Many elderly persons develop acute conjunctivitis. They complain of water and irritation, often in one eye and later in two, which then goes on to redness. They will wake up in the morning with sticking of the eyelids. Examination of their eye reveals that there is hyperemia and vascular stasis, and the tarsal and epibulbar conjunctiva are reddened. There is exudate around the cilia. Occasionally, in a *Streptococcus pneumoniae* or *Hemophilus influenzae* conjunctivitis there are small petechiae. Many of these acute cases resolve spontaneously, but the *Staphylococcus aureus* and *Moraxella lacunata* cases tend to persist. Gram-stained or Giemsa-stained scrapings show a polymorphonuclear exudate and the appropriate invading organism. This disease can be treated with antibiotic eyedrops such as sodium sulfacetamide hourly or with ointment four to five times a day and at bedtime. Other physicians will treat with chloramphenicol eye ointments. Many will treat without culture, and if there is no response will discontinue the treatment and take cultures thereafter. A hyperacute syndrome is seen rarely with gonococci or meningococci with lid edema and chemosis of the conjunctiva. This is associated with copious mucopurulent discharge.

Chronic conjunctivitis is caused by a variety of organisms such as gram-negative rods, including *Proteus mirabilis, Klebsiella pneumoniae, Serratia, or Escherichia coli*, but perhaps most chronic conjunctivitis is caused by *Staphylococcus aureus*. The organisms tend to colonize a lid margin, but this in turn is a transfer from chronic nasal carriage. The patient complains of a foreign body sensation with redness and a mild to moderate mattering of the eye, particularly noticeable on awakening. The eyelids are red, inflamed and granulated. There is lid lash loss. Differential diagnosis must be made from chronic seborrheic dermatitis of the lids when greasy scales are present. Chronic conjunctivitis can lead to entropion or ectropion, two eyelid disorders. When the organisms are established chronically, one should look for a source of reinfection such as nasal carriage, and in particular when using systemic antistaphylococcal antibiotics it should be noted that the nose carriage will not be eradicated. This has to be treated separately with bacitracin ointment for two weeks, 500 units/g, twice daily inserted with the finger, and then ointment is rubbed into the hands to form a barrier cream. Eighty percent of the carriers will be cured with the first treatment, and 80% of the remainder with the second treatment.

Staphylococcal and Streptococcal Infections.   Staphylococcal infections follow nasal carriage in the patient or his attendants. Nasal carriage causes sties, boils (staphylococcal infection of a single hair follicle), or carbuncles (infection of multiple hair follicles). They can usually be controlled by antistaphylococcal antibiotics, but if the conditions are recurrent, it must be remembered that the systemic antibiotic does not reach an adequate level in the nasal secretions to eradicate carriage. Eradication can be obtained by the use of bacitracin ointment (500 units/g) applied twice daily to the anterior nares for two weeks. Occasionally, two or three courses are needed. If outbreaks of boils are occurring, the family or medical attendants may have to be examined for nasal carriage. Staphylococcal infections occur more prominently in elderly people with diabetes mellitus or renal failure than in those without these diseases (10). Wound infections are frequently staphylococcal and occur in about 5% of hospital patients. High postoperative wound rates occur in gallbladder surgery and amputations. Low rates occur in herniorrhaphy, hysterectomies and joint replacements.

Streptococcal infections, in contrast to staphylococcal, usually follow throat carriage in the patient or their attendants. The most characteristic infection here is erysipelas. This is a streptococcal infection of the lymphatics that produces swelling of the skin. There is a bright red, sharply outlined, irregular, elevated edematous lesion. Also, a firm, warm, and tender plaque with smooth, glazed, and overlying epidermis is present. Fever, headache, and malaise are caused by the toxins of the streptococci. Erysipelas occurs most commonly in the face. In very acute cases, vesicles, pustules, or bullae appear on the surface (usually in the center of the lesion). The disease can recur and may be associated with chronic lymphedema.

Either or both of these organisms can infect ischemic ulcers of the lower leg in the elderly. One has to worry, however, that these may be contaminated with multiple fecal organisms, including anaerobes.

Diabetic Skin Infections.   In diabetics who are elderly, while blood cells do not function normally (see Chapter 2), which results in an increased susceptibility to infections. Added predisposing factors are the absence of a dorsalis pedis pulse in 60%, or of a popliteal pulse in 25%, and degeneration of the peripheral nerves. This can lead to unintentional injury, which is often followed by the inoculation of fecal organisms from unwashed hands. About 10% of the diabetics with skin infections are on diet alone, about 45% are on oral antidiabetic agents, and 45% are on insulin. About one-third of the diabetics with skin infections develop osteomyelitis, and 10–20% develop gangrene; these patients usually have long-standing diabetes of 15 years or longer, and they often have complicating cardiovascular system disease, chronic renal failure, retinopathy, and peripheral vascular disease. One should be aware that if a diabetic ulcer smells putrid, this indicates superinfection with anaerobes. If anaerobes are present, clindamycin or chloramphenicol therapy is indicated (11).

Decubiti.   Decubiti (pressure sores) occur after pressure greater than 44 g/cm^2 continues for two hours or more. They can be found in about 1–5% of acute care hospital patients and in a higher percentage of chronic care institution residents. They almost always occur in patients over 50 and particularly in those over 70. Chair pressure can be as severe as bed pressure. Contributing factors are the skin shearing forces when a patient is pulled up in the bed, the presence of moisture, and immobility caused by disease or by physician-ordered tranquilizers. These decubiti eventually become infected with fecal organisms, including anaerobic flora. Preventive treatment is the use of antipressure bedding and water mattresses. Debridement by enzymes or surgery is indicated and is often done best by specially trained nursing teams. Local treatment with antibiotics may be successful and often reduces the smell. When spreading infection is present or if the patient is febrile, systemic antibiotics are indicated with clindamycin or chloramphenicol (12). Decubiti are further discussed in Chapter 7.

Herpes Zoster.   Herpes zoster is a reactivation of a varicella virus acquired in childhood. It occurs primarily in the elderly, in 1% of leukemics, and in 10% of Hodgkins' disease patients. It is a unilateral tenderness of the skin in a dermatomal pattern involving one or two dermatomes. This is associated with fever, malaise, and headache. The region involved is thoracic in 59%, trigeminal in 14%, cervical in 18%, and lumbar in 9%. In the first 12 to 24 hours, vesicles are present on top of the rash. These vesicles become pustules in 72 hours. They dry up in about seven or eight days, crust in 12 days, and fall off in 14 to 21 days. Postherpetic neuralgia occurs in 35–50% of those over 60. Patients with vesicles on the tip of the nose should be checked for corneal ulcers, and if these are present, they should be referred to an ophthalmologist. Spreading disease, which is uncommon, may be treated intravenously with acyclovir (13).

Pulmonary Infections

Influenza.   Influenza affects the elderly twice as often as the young. It usually has a sudden onset with shaking chills in 50–80%, followed by the onset of a dry, nonproductive cough associated with substernal and deep chest aching made worse by coughing. There are generalized muscle aches, particularly in the long muscles of the lower back, and patients usually complain of a severe retroorbital headache. Approximately 20% of a community can be affected at once. The attack rate in nursing homes is often even higher and can be approximately 30%. Attacks can be prevented by influenza immunization or by amantadine (see Chapter 14). The problem with influenza is that there is an antigenic shift in influenza A so that from year to year, particularly every two to four years, epidemics occur because the organism is different. Pandemics (worldwide epidemics) occur every 10 to 15 years. The main complication of influenza is the development of pneumonia, usually caused by pneumococcus, but sometimes it is due to *Staphylococcus aureus* or *Hemophilus influenzae*. This complication is mainly shown by an increase in respiratory rate, which leads the physician to order a chest x-ray. The type of organism can be differentiated by a Gram stain of the sputum, by culture, or both. The white blood count is usually normal in influenza, but in about one-half the patients who develop pneumonia the count is 12,000 or higher.

Once the diagnosis of influenza has been made in a community, a clinical diagnosis can then be made with 86% certainty in the remainder of the cases (14).

Pneumonia/influenza as a cause of death is listed as number 4 in all age groups. The incidence of these entities increases from 26 to 55 per 100,000 at ages 55–64 years, to 781 to 1138 at ages 85 and over. The lower figures are for women and the higher figures for men. Influenza is discussed further in Chapter 5.

Pneumonia.   Pneumonia (15) comes in six main categories: pneumococcal, *Legionella*, gram-negative rod, staphylococcal, mycoplasma, and aspiration pneumonias (see Chapter 5). In about 80% of the elderly, pneumonia often has a fairly sudden onset, with shaking chills and fever 102°F or higher. This is associated with the onset of productive cough, where the sputum is sometimes bloody and sometimes rusty-colored. Acute pleurisy develops, which is a stabbing pain on deep breathing or coughing in one localized area of the chest. Associated with this is an onset of a leukocytosis of 12,000 or higher and an increased respiratory rate. The latter leads to chest x-rays that will show an infiltrate in one lobe of the lung in 66% of patients and in two lobes in 25%. Pleural effusion will be present in 5% of gram-positive pneumonia and in approximately 30% of gram-negative rod pneumonias.

Pneumonias developing in the community are frequently pneumococcal or legionellal. Those occurring in the acute care hospital or in the nursing home are often due to gram-negative rods and occasionally are due to staphylococci. In Legionnaires' disease, in addition to the usual pneumonia picture, there is often evidence of disease in other systems of the body. For example, there may be diarrhea, abdominal pain, or abnormal liver function tests. There is frequently albuminuria and occasionally hematuria, which may go on to renal failure. About 30% of Legionnaires' disease patients initially have confusion, and up to 50% develop it sometime during the course of the illness (16).

The greatest concern with pneumonia in the elderly is the 15–20% of patients who present atypically. They may have no fever, or the fever may be unappreciated because their normal baseline temperature is lower than normal. One must learn to investigate patients with respiratory rates of 26 or higher or with a tachycardia of undetermined origin. The patient may not appreciate pain, and pleurisy may be totally absent. Many elderly patients may have a chronic cough, and the onset of more purulent increased sputum is not always detected. Some patients show only the end results of anoxia, which manifests itself as confusion and coma. Some elderly patients are asymptomatic and go on to develop a fulminant pneumonia that can be fatal in 48 hours. These presentations represent the problems of pneumonia in the elderly.

The objectives in the treatment of pneumonia are to reduce the total number of bacteria as quickly as possible and maintain the patient's oxygenation. Sputum cultures, blood cultures, and pleural fluid cultures are indicated. Before the time of antibiotics, blood cultures in the elderly were positive in 60%. Today they are positive in 15–30% but this provides a pure culture of the offending organism and is very important to do. In the seriously ill elderly, transtracheal aspiration or lung puncture should be considered to obtain the organism. The treatment of choice for pneumococcal pneumonia is penicillin. If the patient is allergic to penicillin, erythromycin is a suitable substitute. In *Legionella* disease the treatment of choice is erythromycin. In gram-negative rod pneumonia, a treatment with an aminoglycoside usually is indicated.

Overall, pneumococcal pneumonia is 5% fatal in adults and 8–16% fatal in the elderly. But in severely damaged elderly, the figure can approximate 30%. Bad prognostic signs are the involvement of two or more lobes, the presence of underlying emphysema, and the presence of a positive blood culture. In Legionnaires' disease, the overall fatality rate untreated is 20% and treated 5%, but figures in the elderly can be somewhat higher. In gram-negative rod pneumonia, the treated fatality rate is 8–16% but rises to 30–33% in those over age 60 (17).

Prosthetic Joint Infections

Approximately 80,000 artificial hips and perhaps half as many artificial knees are implanted annually in the United States; about 75% of these have an excellent long-term functional result. This procedure initially had a 10% infection rate, which has now fallen to less than 1%. Infection is the cause of the late loosening of prosthetic joints in 15% of cases seen. The artificial joint is an island of nonliving tissue that behaves like a sequestra. Infections can flare from this focus at any time if infection was implanted at the time of operation. In recurring infections, the same organism that caused the preceding infection usually recurs. Improved surgical technique has reduced both early and late infections because of this. Therefore, in approximately 80% of infections, *Staphylococcus aureus* and *S. epidermidis* are the causative organisms. In the remaining 20%, the appliance is seeded during the bacteremia from another focus. This is usually an abscess or an active infection somewhere else in the body. The abscesses, when incised and drained, result in 50% of patients developing temporary bacteremia that can seed a prosthetic hip. Inadequately treated pneumonia or cystitis can do the same. Catheterization of a patient with an infected urinary tract can lead to septic failure of a prosthetic joint. Therefore, all active infections in patients with prosthetic joints should be actively treated and treated for a longer period than usual. There is probably no indication for antibiotic prophylaxis in routine dental or urologic procedures (18), since these procedures would rarely cause a bacteremia that would infect a prosthetic joint.

Gastrointestinal Infections

Diarrhea occurs frequently in the elderly. In a review of nursing homes where 16% of infections were found, 1.5% were diarrheal in type. The well elderly are susceptible to traveler's diarrhea and the sick elderly to outbreaks of viral or bacterial diarrhea. Diarrhea in the elderly falls roughly into three categories: those caused by viruses, those caused by bacteria, and those caused by preformed toxins.

Viral diarrhea caused by rotavirus or parvovirus tends to be abrupt in onset and lasts only one to five days. There is usually malaise, anorexia, abdominal cramps, and voluminous, watery stools without blood or mucous. Dehydration may be a severe problem.

In contrast to this, bacterial diarrhea, typified by shigellosis, salmonellosis, or *Campylobacter* diarrhea, tends to have a rather less sharp onset with fever, diarrhea with bloody stools, or stools with occult blood and tenesmus. *Campylobacter* diarrhea causes severe abdominal pain. In each of these diseases, except *Campylobacter*, the peripheral white blood count is frequently elevated and there are many polymorphonuclear leukocytes in a Gram stain of the stool. Bacterial toxin diarrhea is best exemplified by traveler's diarrhea. About five to 15 days after arriving in a new country, the elderly traveler develops an abrupt onset of diarrhea associated with nausea, usually without abdominal pain. The stools are watery and brown and usually free of blood. Certain tropical climates witness more traveler's diarrhea than nontropical climates. It has been the habit to give these people prophylaxis with tetracycline or trimethoprim/sulfamethoxazole (TMP/SMZ), but many physicians prefer to wait until the onset of the first diarrheal stool and then treat with tetracycline, 250 mg four times daily for three to four days. A similar type of toxin-induced diarrhea can occur with the use of certain antibiotics that allow the overgrowth of *Clostridium difficile*. This happens more commonly after clindamycin, tetracycline, or erythromycin and less commonly after ampicillin or penicillin. With *Staphylococcus aureus* diarrhea an enterotoxin is involved. The only difference is that it is preformed before ingestion in food such as in ham or creampuffs contaminated by a carrier with toxogenic *S. aureus*. There is a very sudden onset of nausea and vomiting and severe, profuse, watery diarrhea. The patient may collapse due to severe dehydration.

In all these diarrheas, some thought has to be given to the community as well as the individual patient. Particularly in nursing homes, it is important to diagnose the first case exactly so that the appropriate antibiotics, where indicated, can be given to subsequent patients. It is also very important to replace fluids, and this may be done orally with a replacement fluid containing salt, sodium bicarbonate, potassium chloride, and glucose. Patients having five to 10 stools daily should drink a liter of replacement fluid daily. Ten or more stools is an indication for 2 liters daily. *Salmonella* and *Shigella* diarrhea will respond to treatment with TMP/SMZ, ampicillin, tetracycline, or chloramphenicol according to local organism sensitivities. This is probably indicated in salmonellosis only when there is a systemic reaction like fever. *Campylobacter* diarrhea will respond to erythromycin or tetracycline. Fatalities do occur after diarrhea in the elderly, and great attention must be paid to the etiology and the treatment (19,20).

Appendicitis.   Appendicitis can occur in the elderly. The symptoms are similar to those in other age groups, but the disease tends to be more severe. Chills are more frequent and the disease moves rapidly. Vomiting occurs in only 33% compared to 72% in younger people, but abdominal guarding is less frequent, as is rectal tenderness. A normal white count is found in 30% compared to 14% in the young. Because of this rapid onset and progress, perforation occurs in 46% compared to 18% and abscess in 30% compared to 10%. There may be a lapse of 72 hours or more in diagnosis in about 20% of the elderly compared to 6% in the young. All these factors result in a case fatality rate of 5–10% compared to less than 1% in young people. Postoperative complications occur in 33%, compared to 16% of younger patients. One must be particularly careful to look for underlying latent, hard-to-recognize heart failure. Considering the diagnosis and operating early are the keys to success in treatment of appendicitis in the elderly. Treatment is primarily surgical, but because of the frequency of perforation in the elderly, surgery should be combined with an antibiotic regimen likely to cover the bowel flora, and this might well be a cephalosporin with clindamycin. Peritoneal lavage may be required in addition.

Diverticulitis.   Small herniations of bowel called diverticulae occur in the sigmoid colon following increased intraluminal pressure related to dietary lack of fiber and injudicious use of laxatives. Overall, diverticulae are described in 5–20% of patients who have had a barium enema. However, the condition is found in 29% of people at 60 and 42% at age 80. These diverticulae are often asymptomatic. Diverticulitis occurs in 15% of those with diverticulae, and half of these have only a single attack without recurrence. The attack usually consists of lower abdominal tenderness and pain, usually on the left side, but occasionally on the right. This pain is associated with peritoneal irritation and muscle spasm, guarding, rebound, and tenderness. Fever and leukocytosis usually accompany this syndrome. Flatulence, nausea, and vomiting can also occur. Constipation or diarrhea or both occur, and the stool is bloody in about one-third. A mass is palpable in 25%. Complications are fistula, obstruction, bleeding, especially from the right colon, often with bright red blood, and abscess or peritonitis. A complicating myocardial infarction, congestive cardiac failure, or pulmonary embolism may occur. A good choice for antibiotic coverage is a cephalosporin with clindamycin. Patients can be treated two or three times with this medical approach, and after the third attack a partial colectomy is usually indicated. About 15–30% of patients hospitalized with diverticulitis require surgery. Elective surgery has a 2–5% fatality rate compared to 15% or higher in emergency surgery (21,22).

Hepatitis.   Many elderly people have had hepatitis, but the disease still occurs and is frequently misdiagnosed as jaundice due to some other cause. Elderly people have antibodies to hepatitis A virus in approximately 85% and to hepatitis B in 32%. There is presently no way of knowing how many have had non-A, non-B hepatitis. Various surveys of the different types of hepatitis show that the elderly comprise 5% of patients with hepatitis A, 5% of those with hepatitis B, and 8% of those with non-A, non-B hepatitis. There is some evidence that hepatitis B may be more common in psychiatric hospitals than in general elderly populations. The frequency of types of hepatitis in the elderly are approximately half due to hepatitis B, one-third to hepatitis A, and one-fifth to non-A, non-B.

The incubation period in hepatitis A is two to six weeks, in hepatitis B two to six months, and in non-A, non-B hepatitis one to six months. Hepatitis presents itself similarly in the elderly and the young, but many physicians fail to think about its occurrence. There is usually a gradual onset with anorexia and weakness. Weight loss may be prominent, even reaching 8–10 kg. Nausea and vomiting occur frequently, and vague right upper quadrant pain or discomfort is often present. In hepatitis B, the early onset may be more like serum sickness with fever, urticaria, and arthralgia. Many cases of hepatitis are asymptomatic, but most progress to a jaundice phase, with dark urine lasting approximately one to three weeks. A subdivision of the elderly has onset with mental changes such as confusion or depression. Between 60 and 90% of elderly hepatitis patients have several underlying diseases. Laboratory examination will show an SGOT and SGPT approximately eight times normal and the LDH will be two to three times normal. There will be a bilirubin in the range of 8–15 mg/dl, and the direct bilirubin will equal the indirect.

Treatment consists of providing adequate nutrition, relieving symptoms, and avoiding the use of hepatotoxic drugs. The disease is frequently serious in the elderly, particularly in elderly women, and different outbreaks have shown a death rate of 15–26%. Quite a few of these elderly people have a chronic course. Case fatality rate is increased in patients with underlying cancer and also in patients who are subjected to a laparotomy.

The use of immune serum globulin in hepatitis A and the hepatitis B vaccine are reviewed in Chapter 14. The prevention of non-A, non-B hepatitis involves eliminating paid donors from blood banks. Some degree of immunity can be given to non-A, non-B hepatitis by the higher doses of immune serum globulin. In the elderly, this disease is frequently seen in patients with cardiac operations where large numbers of transfusions are given (23).

Septicemia and Endocarditis

In different published series of patients (24–27), 40–50% of septicemias are in patients over 60, and the figure for endocarditis is 15–20%. One-quarter to one-third of the deaths occur in the elderly. If blood cultures are taken frequently in elderly people, 6% of them will be found to be positive. The correct meaning of the word **bacteremia** is a temporary one- to two-hour presence of bacteria in the bloodstream with no symptoms, which frequently follows an incision and drainage of an abscess, tooth extraction, or some relatively minor surgical procedure. **Septicemia** means the presence of positive blood cultures and signs and symptoms of systemic infection.

The patient who develops septicemia or endocarditis frequently has a significant preceding disease such as urinary tract infection, biliary tract disease, pneumonia, or surgery, particularly transurethral resection of the prostate. Localized infection elsewhere in the body is present in 15–20%. Patients who have cancer or leukemia and are treated with cytotoxic agents and have become neutropenic, particularly below the level of 1000 polymorphonuclears/ml, are especially susceptible to septicemia. Many elderly patients will present typically with shaking chills and fever, together with malaise and weakness. The difference in the endocarditis from septicemia patients is the presence of a heart murmur with evidence of embolization, as shown by petechiae and fundal, conjunctival, skin, or central nervous system embolization. Unfortunately, in about 20% of the elderly, the onset may be atypical with gradual confusion or with congestive heart failure with a mild or moderate fever. Alternatively, the fever and chills may be overshadowed by severe underlying disease, or the fever is thought to be a natural part of procedures such as bladder and intravenous catheterizations or the placement or use of a pacemaker. In some patients, the fever may be insidious, long-lasting, and associated with weight loss that directs the physician's attention to the possibility of cancer. When heart murmurs are present, a third of them are heard at the aortic area, a third in the mitral, and a third at both areas. However, no murmur is present in 30–50% of elderly patients with endocarditis. Complications occur and might be mistaken for the primary illness. These are congestive heart failure in 25%, arrhythmia in a further 25%, events such as stroke in the central nervous system in 20%, and chronic renal failure in about 60%. Because of all of these problems, the presence of septicemia may be missed in 30–50% of the elderly, and diagnosis of endocarditis missed in about 80% of the elderly. This contrasts with the misdiagnosis of 10–20% in the younger adult. The diagnosis must be distinguished from rheumatic heart disease with congestive heart failure. In patients with a severe weight loss, a cancer diagnosis may be considered. The physician's confusion may lead to consideration of a diagnosis of psychosis, or a patient's renal problems may overshadow the true illness because of hematuria and increased blood urea nitrogen (BUN) and creatinine in 30–60%.

A diagnosis must be exact; it must be attributed to a single organism. In septicemia, the most likely organisms are *Klebsiella, Enterobacter, Esch-*

erichia coli, Staphylococcus aureus, and *Bacteroides.* In contrast, in endocarditis, the most likely organisms are *S. aureus, S. epidermidis,* and viridans streptococcus. The bacterial cause must be pinpointed because the length of treatment and prognosis are different. To make a diagnosis of septicemia, three blood cultures should be taken approximately two hours apart unless the patient is very seriously ill. In contrast, in endocarditis, five blood cultures should be taken. If an organism looks like a contaminant, such as *S. epidermidis* or diphtheroids, three to five more sets of blood cultures should be taken. A complete blood count should be taken. Staphylococcal infections tend to lower the hemoglobin below 12 g and raise the white count above 15,000. In contrast to this, streptococcal organisms usually lower the hemoglobin to 12–13 g and raise the white count to 12,000 or 13,000.

Treatment involves the use of antibiotics directed against the organism for an appropriate length of time. In certain circumstances, foreign bodies, such as prosthetic heart valves or orthopedic plating, must be removed. The treatment of a minor septicemia such as pneumococcal or an uncomplicated *E. coli* is for two weeks. All other septicemias are treated for four weeks. Bacterial endocarditis on heart valves is treated for six weeks or longer. The response to treatment is often best followed by taking the evening temperature. This should begin to fall in 48 hours after the onset of treatment.

The prognosis of treated septicemia in the elderly is a case fatality rate of 31% when the organism is community-acquired (compared to 4% in younger adults). If the infection is acquired nosocomially, the case fatality rate is 56% (compared to 50% in younger adults). If septic shock develops in any situation, the fatality rate is 65% or higher. Recently, case fatality rates in endocarditis have been reduced from 75% to 35%. Rates will be higher if the organism is *Staphylococcus aureus* or a fungus and will be increased if there is any intercurrent myocardial infarction. Untreated patients have a 100% fatality rate.

Urinary Tract Infections

Urinary tract infections increase with age, are more common in women than men, and are associated with institutionalization, immobility, and incontinence (28,29). Approximately 20% of women aged 65–90 years and 43% over 90 have urinary tract infections. In men aged 65–70 the incidence is about 3%, and over 70 about 20%. The importance of noting urinary tract infections is that one-third of all septicemias are caused from this type of infection. Urinary tract infection is potentially life-threatening.

Asymptomatic bacteriuria is present in women starting at about 7% in the 20s and increasing by 1–5% per decade. At present, the consensus is that asymptomatic bacteriuria in the elderly does not require treatment. New cases of active infection will, however, come from these bacteriuric women.

Elderly patients with active urinary infection have an increased urinary frequency that may not be noticed. Frequency at night *is* noticed by most patients. Scalding of urine is infrequent, occurring in 10–20%, and incontinence occurs in 10–20%. Frequency may increase as the infection becomes more severe. Patients with upper tract infection will experience shaking chills, fever, and costovertebral angle pain. In men, one must remember that benign prostatic hypertrophy and chronic prostatitis may be causing obstruction. The latter may also be acting as a reservoir of organisms. Rarely will disease manifest itself by occurrence of septic shock, which can occur several hours after the withdrawal of an indwelling catheter.

The diagnosis is made by a positive midstream quantitative urine culture and is reinforced by a second positive culture showing 100,000 bacteria or more per ml of urine. *E. coli* is the predominant organism causing infections in women, and *Proteus* species in older males. If other organisms are present, such as *Pseudomonas*, one should suspect an underlying anatomical abnormality in the urinary tract, the presence of a renal stone, or recent instrumentation or indwelling Foley catheter.

Treatment is with ampicillin, a cephalosporin, furadantin, or TMP/ SMZ. It is always important to check local sensitivities, be it in the nursing home or hospital. Two weeks' treatment is adequate, and it is more recently known that localized bladder infections can often be treated by a single dose of 3 g of amoxacillin or a single dose of an aminoglycoside. About half the patients relapse, and a follow-up culture is important.

Figures on the prognosis of urinary tract infection are difficult to obtain, but certainly a small percentage of patients are going to develop a severe septicemia with a 50% fatality rate. Urinary tract infections are discussed in depth in Chapter 6.

THERAPEUTIC ASPECTS

Prevention of Infection

The elderly person must be protected from noxious environments. In particular, the nursing home and the hospital tend to have nosocomial parasites such as gram-negative rods that can become established in the elderly person initially as carriage of the organism and later, by iatrogenic interference, become disease. The attendants in nursing homes and hospitals should be kept healthy in order to prevent transfer of infection to the elderly. Inability to move and to take care of themselves causes some patients to be contaminated with their own secretions, particularly from fecal incontinence. General hygiene is important here. Healthy people have various barriers to infection, namely the skin and the mucociliary blanket, that prevent the penetration of organisms into the lung. These barriers can be broken down by unwise activity of the health attendants, such as the use of urinary catheters or intravenous polyethylene catheters. Surgical wounds interfere with natural protection. Various habits and diseases predispose the elderly to infection. Smoking is one obvious example. An attack of influenza will interfere with the natural protection of the lung. Patients with diabetes, chronic renal failure, congestive cardiac failure, or pulmonary failure are particularly susceptible to environmental organisms. Malnutrition often indicated by hemoglobin at 12 g/dl or less or albumin of 2.5 g/dl or less also predisposes the elderly to infection.

Certain vaccines are available to protect the elderly, such as influenza vaccine, which should be given to all patients with chronic cardiopulmonary disease or patients over 65. Influenza virus vaccine needs to be renewed every year (see Chapter 14). It's administration should be a routine procedure in nursing home patients because outbreaks can affect 20–30% of the residents. If a group of nursing home patients has not been protected against influenza when outbreak begins, it is advisable to give them amantadine and also to give them vaccine. The dose of amantadine is reduced for chronic renal failure.

One problem that the elderly should be protected against is the overuse of antibiotics (see Chapter 11). If penicillin G is used in low doses to treat pneumococcal pneumonia, there are no superinfections with invading organisms of other types. If penicillin is used in a dose of 10,000,000 units daily or more, 29% of the patients develop superinfection due to other organisms. Penicillin and streptomycin together lead to a superinfection rate of 19%, tetracycline or chloramphenicol alone to 5%, and if penicillin is used with either tetracycline or chloramphenicol, 47% of the patients develop a superinfection. This can be subclinical in many but produces a new clinically obvious pneumonia with chest x-ray infiltrates in 28%.

Lastly, a new environmental hazard for the elderly is foreign travel. Exposure in foreign countries to an enteropathogenic *E. coli* diarrhea can be treated with tetracycline, 250 mg four times a day for four days at the onset of the first diarrheal stool; malaria can be prevented by appropriate use of chloroquin or pyrimethamine/sulfadoxine; hepatitis A can be prevented with 2 ml of immune serum globulin for a short trip or 5 ml for a three-month or longer visit.

Treatment

Most infections in the healthy elderly are treatable, but many elderly people have significant underlying disease. One must learn to treat on the immediately available data backed up by confirming Gram stains and cultures. The mobile healthy elderly tend to have infections from the community, whereas the immobile institutionalized elderly have a different spectrum. Table 3.1 summarizes the types of infections to be expected in the home, the nursing home, and the acute care hospital. As

Table 3.2. Organisms Likely to Cause Infection by Area and Age

Infection/Area and Organism	Age 70+ Years	Age 30–49 Years
Septicemia		
Staphylococcus aureus	24%	13%
Polymicrobic	21	10
Streptococcus pneumoniae	15	7
Escherichia coli	10	15
Klebsiella–Enterobacter	8	18
Bacteroides	6	8
Endocarditis		
Streptococcus viridans	32	33
Staphylococcus aureus	24	15
Staphylococcus epidermidis	10	5
Other streptococci	20	11
Urinary tract infections		
Escherichia coli	62	62
Proteus	31	31
Pseudomonas	4	4
Pneumonia		
Streptococcus pneumoniae	18	44
Gram-negative rods	21	8
Legionella pneumophila	10	2
Staphylococcus aureus	6	2
Meningitis		
Streptococcus pneumoniae	46	20
Listeria	21	2
Gram-negative rods	14	4
Neisseria meningitidis	10	32
Unknown etiology	9	12

one gains experience in treating infections, one categorizes certain areas of the body as potential infection places for certain organisms. For example, bladder infections in women are almost always caused by *E. coli*; in contrast, the majority of pneumonias are caused by pneumococci. These probabilities are summarized in Table 3.2, but they should always be expanded and confirmed against the physician's own personal experience. For example, the physician must think microbiologically and categorize the disease as Legionnaires' pneumonia or *Staphylococcus aureus* endocarditis, and *not* as lobar pneumonia or bacterial endocarditis. There are useful clinical clues to back up one's assumptions regarding which organisms occur where. For example, the pus produced by *Pseudomonas* tends to be blue-green in color, particularly after exposure to sunlight, and the same organism growing in the endothelium of small blood vessels will cause ecthyma gangrenosa, which is a reliable indicator of *Pseudomonas* septicemia. Erysipelas is a beta-hemolytic streptococcal infection of the lymphatics of the skin and therefore produces swelling in a ridge between normal and abnormal skin. Unfortunately, there are all too few clinical clues, and one must use the laboratory to make exact diagnoses.

It is important to remember that bacteria kill when they have reached a certain critical number. For example, 10^{10} bacteria will kill a 30-g mouse, and the lethal number is probably 10^{13} bacteria for a 70-kg human. Treatment of infections is aimed at reducing this total population and helping the body combat it. Incision and drainage of an abscess will remove 100 ml of pus, and each milliliter usually contains 100,000 or more organisms. Therefore, the patient may be taken away from the point of death quite rapidly in comparison to use of antibiotics. Antibiotics are nonetheless very necessary.

The underlying disease in the patient must be assessed because any exacerbation of this will threaten life. In particular, chronic renal failure must be detected, and this is best done by the serum creatinine. The antibiotics that are excreted in the urine and therefore most influenced by chronic renal failure are the aminoglycosides, sulfonamides, penicillins, and cephalosporins. The carbenicillin group of antibiotics have a particularly high load of sodium attached to them; 30g of carbenicillin will deliver the amount of sodium contained in 1 liter of normal saline. Many elderly people with renal or cardiac disease cannot stand this extra sodium burden, and alternative antibiotics such as ticarcillin or pipercillin should be used.

Many elderly patients are confused by complex antibiotic treatment. In the treatment of tuberculosis, all the isoniazid and rifampin can be given in the morning at breakfast, and in the treatment of many other minor or moderate infections the antibiotics can be consolidated into a twice-daily dose. This improves patient compliance.

Table 3.3.   Antibiotics Likely to Control Infections by Designated Organisms[a]

Organism	Antibiotic
Escherichia coli	TMP/SMZ, aminoglycosides
Pseudomonas aeruginosa	Carbenicillin, aminoglycosides
Klebsiella pneumoniae	Aminoglycosides, TMP/SMZ
Enterobacter	Aminoglycosides, TMP/SMZ, chloramphenicol
Proteus mirabilis	Ampicillin, cephalosporins, TMP/SMZ
Other Proteus species	Aminoglycosides, TMP/SMZ
Hemophilus influenzae	Tetracycline, aminoglycosides, TMP/SMZ
Serratia	Aminoglycosides
Salmonella	Aminoglycosides
Staphylococcus aureus	Semisynthetic penicillins, cephalosporins, erythromycin, vancomycin
Staphylococcus epidermidis	Cephalosporins, TMP/SMZ, vancomycin
Enterococcus	Penicillin/ampicillin and an aminoglycoside
Streptococcus	Penicillin, cephalosporin, erythromycin
Pneumococcus	Penicillin, erythromycin

KEY: TMP/SMZ, Trimethoprim/sulfamethoxazole.
[a]Antibiotic sensitivities are likely to change from institution to institution.

Lastly, one must consider the route and length of treatment with antibiotics. In the severely ill patient, the intravenous route is preferred. Remember that intramuscular antibiotics are not well absorbed in the diabetic. Bactericidal antibiotics are preferred over bacteristatic antibiotics in the seriously ill patient. The bactericidal antibiotics are the penicillins, the cephalosporins, the aminoglycosides, the colistins, and vancomycin. Drug interactions and adverse reactions are increased in the elderly (see Chapter 11).

With care and laboratory backup, an accurate diagnosis can be made in the elderly when they are infected. In addition, the careful clinician will assess the extent of the infection and underlying disease. An antibiotic can be chosen on microbiological basis and confirmed by information coming from the laboratory (see Table 3.3). In general terms, minor infections should be treated for 72 hours after the last sign of trouble, whether fever, draining pus, or leukocytosis. The same length of treatment applies to pneumococcal pneumonia. Most other pneumonias require one or two weeks of treatment. Septicemia of the mild type such as E. coli or Staphylococcus aureus with an obvious removeable focus can be treated in two weeks, but most septicemias require four weeks of treatment. Endocarditis on natural heart valves requires four weeks, and on prosthetic valves, six weeks or longer. The course of treatment is best followed by the evening temperature. The antibiotic treatment of infections in the elderly is very worthwhile and quite effective in the majority of patients.

REFERENCES

1. Siegel JS: Some demographic aspects of aging in the United States, in Ostefeld AM (ed.): *Epidemiology of Aging*, publication No. NIH 77-711. Bethesda, Md. US Department of Health, Education, and Welfare, Public Health Service, 1974, pp 17–82.

2. Gerber IE: Terminal pneumonia in the aged. *Mt Sinai J Med* 47:166–167, 1980.

3. Howell TH: Terminal and subterminal infections in nonagenarians. *Gerontol Clin* 6:292–296, 1964.

4. Smith IM: Autopsy causes of death in the young and old. Presented to American Geriatrics Society, Boston, 1981.

5. Garibaldi RA, Brodine S, Matsumiya S: Infection among patients in nursing homes: Policies, prevalence, and problems. *N Engl J Med* 305:7312–7315, 1981.

6. Brown NK, Thompson DJ: Non-treatment of fever in extended-care facilities. *N Engl J Med* 300:1246–1250, 1979.

7. Smith IM: Infections in the elderly, in Issacs B (ed): *Recent Advances in Geriatric Medicine*, Vol. II. Edinburgh, Churchill, Livingstone, 1982, pp 215–239.

8. Smith IM: Infections in the elderly, in Steinberg FU (ed): *Care of the Geriatric Patient in the Tradition of E. V. Cowdry*, 6th edi. St. Louis, Mosby, 1983, pp 231–255.

9. Butler HM: *Blood Cultures and Their Significance*. London, J & H Churchill, 1937.

10. Smith IM: Staphylococcal Infections, in Spittell JA Jr (ed): *Clinical Medicine*. Philadelphia, Harper & Row, 1982, pp 1–42.

11. Smith IM: Common infections in the elderly diabetic. *Geriatrics* 35:55–58, 1980.

12. Galpin, JE, Chow AW, Bayer AS, et al: Sepsis associated with decubitus ulcers. *Am J Med* 61:346–350, 1976.

13. Miller LH: Herpes zoster in the elderly. *Cutis* 18:427–432, 1976.

14. Barker WH, Mullooly JP: Influenza vaccination of elderly persons: Reduction in pneumonia and influenza hospitalizations and deaths. *JAMA* 244:2547–2549, 1980.

15. Abright JR, Rytel MW: Bacterial pneumonia in the elderly. *J Am Geriatr Soc* 28:220–223, 1980.

16. Helms CM: Is legionnaires' disease a risk in the elderly? *Geriatrics* 35:87–94, June 1980.

17. VanMeter T: Pneumococcal pneumonia treated with antibiotics: Prognostic significance of certain findings. *N Engl J Med* 251:1048–1052, 1954.

18. Pesanti EL: Infections of prosthetic joints. *Cont Ed Fam Practit* 15:51–54, 1982.

19. Bond JH: Office base management of diarrhea. *Geriatrics* 37:52–64, 1982.

20. Dusdieker NS: Diarrhea in the elderly, in Smith IM (ed): *Medical Care for the Elderly*. New York, S. P. Medical and Scientific Books, 1982, pp 171–178.

21. Smith IM: Infections in the elderly. *Cont Ed Fam Physician* 7:18–29, 1977.

22. Yusuf MF, Dunn E: Appendicitis in the elderly: Learn to discern the untypical picture. *Geriatrics* 34:73–79, 1979.

23. Fenster LF: Viral hepatitis in the elderly: An analysis of 23 patients over 65 years of age. *Gastroenterology* 49:262–271, 1965.

24. McGowan JE Jr, Barns MW, Finland M: Bacteremia at the Boston City Hospital: Occurrence and mortality during 12 selected years (1935–1972) with special reference to hospital acquired cases. *J Infec Dis* 132:316–335, 1975.

25. Esposito AL, Gleckman RA, Cram S, et al: Community acquired bacteremia in the elderly: Analysis of 100 consecutive episodes. *J Am Geriatr Soc* 28:315–319, 1980.

26. Robbins N, DeMaria A, Miller MH: Infective endocarditis in the elderly. *So Med J* 73:1335–1338, 1980.

27. Habte-Gabr E, January LE, Smith IM: Bacterial endocarditis: The need for early diagnosis. *Geriatrics* 28:164–170, 1973.

28. Kaye D: Urinary tract infections in the elderly. *Bull NY Acad Med* 56:209–220, 1980.

29. Platt R: Diagnosis and management of urinary tract infections. *Infec Dis Prac* 3:1–6, 1980.

SECTION 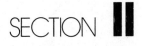 II

NURSING HOME INFECTIONS

CHAPTER 4

NOSOCOMIAL INFECTIONS IN NURSING HOMES

Philip W. Smith

OVERVIEW OF NOSOCOMIAL INFECTIONS

The term *nosocomial* derives from the Greek *nosos* meaning disease and *komeo* meaning to care for. It has generally been applied to hospitals, in which context nosocomial infections are those infections that develop within a hospital or are produced by microorganisms acquired during hospitalization (1). The term may also be applied to infections that develop in a nursing home.

Hospitals and nursing homes share a number of similar factors that predispose patients to nosocomial infections. In both settings, patients with weakened defenses against infection are clustered together, and contact with potential pathogens is frequent. There is a chain of infection consisting of the three interlocking elements necessary for a nosocomial infection: a reservoir of pathogenic organisms, a means of transmission and a susceptible host (see Fig. 4.1).

Two types of nosocomial infections may develop. The organisms that cause an **endogenous** infection are part of the patient's own normal bacterial flora, such as *Escherichia coli, Klebsiella, Proteus,* and group D streptococci in the gut, *Staphylococcus aureus* in the nares, and *Staphylococcus epidermidis* on the skin. In an **exogenous** infection, the causative organisms are not part of the patient's normal flora, but spread from the external environment. For example, *Pseudomonas* may originate from water or equipment, and *Salmonella typhi* or the hepatitis B virus may spread from sick patients.

The presence of nosocomial infection does not necessarily imply that the hospital or the nursing home was in any way negligent. Although nosocomial infections can be minimized by a good infection control program, a certain number of nosocomial infections are inevitable. Nosocomial infections may be either **endemic**, occurring at a relatively constant

59

DEVELOPMENT OF NOSOCOMIAL INFECTION

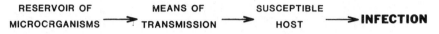

RESERVOIR OF MICROORGANISMS → MEANS OF TRANSMISSION → SUSCEPTIBLE HOST → **INFECTION**

Figure 4.1. Development of nursing home nosocomial infections.

level, or **epidemic**, occurring at greater than expected frequency. Most infections in hospitals and nursing homes are endemic, although epidemics attract a great deal of attention (see Chapter 10). Geographic or temporal clustering of infections suggests an epidemic.

Hospital-Associated Infections

Nosocomial or hospital-associated infection develops in 5–10% of all hospitalized patients. In the United States as a whole, this results in about two to three million cases per year. The consequences of nosocomial infection are serious in terms of morbidity, mortality, and cost. The mortality of nosocomial infections is approximately 1%, and the morbidity, as reflected by prolongation of hospital stay, is very significant (2,3).

The first link in the chain of infection is the organism. *Staphylococcus aureus, E. coli, Pseudomonas aeruginosa*, enterococci, *Klebsiella* spp. and *Proteus* spp. are the leading causes of nosocomial infection in hospitals (4). In addition to these bacteria, a number of new organisms have been found to be nosocomial pathogens, including *Legionella pneumophila* (the agent causing Legionnaires' disease), *Clostridium difficile* (which causes antibiotic-associated enterocolitis), and atypical mycobacteria (5). Gram-negative bacteria and fungi have steadily increased in importance since the early 1970s as nosocomial pathogens. In recent years, multiply antibiotic-resistant gram-negative bacteria have caused severe outbreaks of infection in hospitals. The hospital abounds with microorganisms that may cause nosocomial infection. The patient himself serves as a reservoir of endogenous bacteria; the environment and hospital personnel are reservoirs of exogenous organisms.

The second link in the chain of infection is a means of transmission. Endogenous bacteria do not require a vehicle of transmission to the patient. Exogenous infections may be spread by personnel or equipment. Spread from patient to patient, personnel to patient, or equipment to patient is most often via the hands as a final common pathway. This process is largely preventable and emphasizes the importance of hand-washing in the hospital setting. In general, gram-positive infections are transmitted by contact. Personnel with dermatitis or boils may serve as the source of epidemics of streptococcal or staphylococcal infections. Many such outbreaks have been described (6). Gram-negative infections, on the other hand, are often associated with the hospital environment. Almost anything in the environment may serve as the reservoir or the agent for transmission of gram-negative bacteria. Well-documented examples include intravenous fluid, intravenous catheters, respiratory therapy equipment, room humidifiers, hand lotion, prosthetic implants, sinks, foods, surgical instruments, endoscopes, air-conditioning systems, scales, thermometers, and flowers.

The final link in the chain of infection is the susceptible host. What determines if the patient will be infected with an organism or merely colonized? The patient in the hospital is much less able to defend himself against pathogens than the healthy individual in the community. A variety of treatments breach local defenses, the body's first line of defense against infection. Intravenous cannulas, urinary catheters, nasotracheal tubes, endotracheal tubes, endoscopy, and surgery bypass local defenses of the skin, urinary tract, intestine, or respiratory tract. Antibiotics inhibit the normal bacterial flora of the skin, mouth, gut, and vagina, predisposing patients to colonization and infection. In addition, many of the diseases that afflict hospitalized patients impair host defenses against infection (see Chapter 2).

To determine which organ systems are most often involved in nosocomial infections in the hospital one must consider the predisposing factors. The urinary tract is the leading site of hospital-associated infection, accounting for about 40% of all nosocomial infections (4). Some 60–90% of nosocomial urinary tract infections follow urinary tract instrumentation or catheterization. Nosocomial pneumonia is a very serious infection that occurs primarily in patients who have nasotracheal or endotracheal tubes in place, are receiving assisted ventilation, are immunosuppressed, have underlying chronic obstructive pulmonary disease, reside in intensive care units, or have undergone surgery. Surgical wound infections cause significant morbidity and mortality in hospitalized patients.

Most epidemic nosocomial infections involve the gastrointestinal tract, skin, or bloodstream. Urinary tract infections, wound infections, and pneumonias are generally endemic or sporadic. *E. coli*, enterococci, *Staphylococcus aureus, Pseudomonas, Proteus,* and *Klebsiella* cause most endemic nosocomial infections. The leading causes of epidemic infections are *S. aureus, Salmonella*, hepatitis B, and *E. coli* (7). Multiple cases of bacteremia, gastroenteritis, or hepatitis due to the same agent should raise the question of an epidemic. Most investigated epidemics are traced to a contaminated common vehicle, although infection due to cross-contamination is very important. Airborne outbreaks are rare. Several comprehensive reviews of hospital nosocomial infections are available to the reader (1,8).

One needs to keep in mind that a knowledge of infection patterns in hospitals is important to the nursing home practitioner because there is a dynamic equilibrium between the reservoir of infectious agents in nursing homes and in hospitals due to transfer of patients between these institutions. Many nursing home admissions are transferred from hospitals, and a significant number of nursing home infections, especially those that occur shortly after admission to the nursing home, are associated with pathogens that more closely reflect usual hospital bacteria rather than nursing home flora (9). Nursing home bacterial flora consists of organisms that are less antibiotic-resistant than hospital bacteria. Resistant *Pseudomonas,* for example, is a relatively common cause of nosocomial infection in hospitals, but unusual in nursing homes.

Causes of Nursing Home-Associated Infections

There are many similarities between hospital and nursing home nosocomial infections in terms of risk factors and types of infections acquired, but several major differences exist. First of all, hospitals and nursing homes have different high-risk areas: in the hospital, the patients at greatest risk are immunosuppressed patients (e.g., cancer patients, renal transplant recipients), postoperative and burned patients, and those receiving ventilatory support. Infections are increased by drug or radiation therapy, intravenous catheters, and invasive procedures. In the nursing home, the population is elderly, but less acutely ill. They are impaired by a variety of underlying diseases, immobilization, and urinary catheterization.

Secondly, the focus of hospitals and nursing homes is different. The hospital orientation is toward acute care, emphasizing early discharge. Usually, effort is made to evaluate and treat the patient to the limit of modern technology. There is a general urgency about the patient stay that is not noted in the nursing home setting. The nursing home, on the other hand, is geared to long-term care, with a greater emphasis being placed on the social and psychological aspects of care. The nursing home room, unlike the temporary hospital bed, is a living arrangement for the resident that he views as a home.

Thirdly, ancillary and support services differ greatly between the two types of institutions. Nursing homes have lower nurse-to-patient ratios, less physician availability, and less elaborate laboratory and support services.

Reservoirs of Infection. In nursing homes, as in hospitals, there is a chain of events that leads to nosocomial infection (see Fig. 4.1). The first element is a **reservoir** of infection. Residents themselves can be reservoirs of infection; many are colonized or infected with potentially pathogenic organisms. Decubitus ulcers and urinary catheters, for example, are often colonized with bacteria. Colonization of the resident with potentially pathogenic bacteria may occur, such as *Staphylococcus aureus* nasopharyngeal colonization or *Pseudomonas* colonization of the perineum. Antibiotic therapy may encourage colonization with multiply antibiotic-resistant bacteria. Finally, an infected resident may serve as a reservoir of infectious organisms (e.g., *S. aureus* in a boil, or *Salmonella* in the stool).

Organisms may also be found in the environment. Almost any part of the nursing home environment may serve as a reservoir of pathogenic organisms. Common reservoirs include food, air-conditioning systems, thermometers, bathtubs, humidifiers, linen, dust, and even nursing home employees. Bacteria are the most significant microorganisms in the nursing home reservoir. As a general rule, gram-negative bacteria, such as *E. coli, Proteus, Pseudomonas,* and *Serratia,* are the most important organisms in the inanimate environmental reservoir. Gram-positive staphylococci and streptococci are found in personnel. The nursing home reservoir is discussed in Chapter 15.

Means of Transmission. The second step in the development of infection is a **means of transmission.** Physicians, nurses, and other personnel go from room to room, thereby serving as potential transmitters of infectious diseases. Hands are the most important pathway for spread of infection in the hospital and certainly play a similar role in the nursing home. In nursing homes, as in hospitals, people are in close proximity, which makes transmission more likely. Resident factors encouraging transmission of infection include incontinence and shared activities. Parts of the environment that contact multiple residents may spread organisms (e.g., personnel, food, bathtubs, bedpans, and other equipment).

Spread of organisms may be encouraged by improper handling of food, poor aseptic technique with resident care, or lack of educational and training programs for the health care worker (10). Nursing homes frequently lack rooms specifically designed for isolation and sinks that are located in close proximity to the rooms, thereby discouraging handwashing (11). Other factors that contribute to the spread of infection in some nursing homes include the high percentage of nonprofessional staff, high resident/staff ratios, inconsistent immunization practices, work policies that penalize staff for taking sick leave, rapid turnover of employees, and lack of uniform policies and procedures relating to infection control (12).

Cross-infection in the nursing home setting is most dramatically exemplified by outbreaks of infection. In Garibaldi's study, clustering of infections according to site was frequently observed and accounted for more than 20% of all infections identified. Clusters of upper respiratory tract infections, diarrhea, conjunctivitis, and urinary tract infections were found, which suggested that epidemics of infection occurred frequently (12). Nursing home epidemics are discussed in Chapter 10 and measures to control transmission in Chapter 16.

Host Factors.   The third link in the chain of infection is host resistance to infection. Not all persons who have contact with a potentially pathogenic organism become infected. The body resists infection with the help of immune defenses. The elderly have impaired resistance to infection because of deficiencies in immune defenses that occur with aging and because of other medical problems that afflict them (see Chapter 2).

A nursing home resident may have additional host defense problems. The majority of residents in nursing homes have multiple underlying chronic diseases (12,13), and many have indwelling urinary catheters or decubitus ulcers that breach local defenses. Therapeutic drugs that residents receive may contribute to the problem. Antibiotics impair the protective function of normal bacterial flora, sedatives depress the cough reflex, and anticholinergics dry respiratory secretions and decrease bladder contractility. These effects in turn predispose to respiratory and genitourinary tract infections. Immobilization and incontinence predispose to decubitus ulcers and urinary tract infections. Host factors are discussed in Chapter 14.

General Factors.   A number of factors inherent in the nursing home care delivery system impact nosocomial infections. There is evidence to suggest that physicians spend proportionately less time on aging patients, and medical students tend to have stereotyped negative images of elderly patients (14). Inadequacy of physician visits to residents in skilled nursing and intermediate care facilities is cited by facility staff as being one of the major and continuing problems in provision of long-term care (15) and is a major concern of health planners (16). There are a significant number of errors made by physicians in the admission diagnoses of nursing home residents that contribute to subsequent confusion in their care (17).

Many nursing homes do not provide services required by the physician to give optimal medical care to the resident. Services such as urinalysis, chest x-ray, or common blood studies (18) are often beyond the financial scope of nursing homes. There is a wide variation in incidence of urinary catheterization and in approach to such problems as removal of catheters through policies and procedures (19). Finally, very few nursing homes perform systematic surveillance for infection, routinely monitor resident care practices, or conduct training programs in infection control techniques on a regular basis (12). When a nursing home does designate an infection control practitioner, she frequently has other responsibilities as well.

The above features of nursing home care may contribute to delays in the diagnosis and treatment of individual infections in residents. They may also affect prevention of infection in the nursing home community.

Prevalence of Nursing Home-Associated Infections

There is a relative scarcity of information about the prevalence of nursing home nosocomial infections (20). The studies available, however, suggest that nosocomial infections are as prevalent in nursing homes as in hospitals. A discussion of the methods used to gather data on nosocomial infections in nursing homes can be found in Chapter 9.

In a 1964 survey of infections in nursing homes, 14.4% of the 2147 patients examined by public health nurses in 101 nursing homes had evidence of infection (21). Both nosocomial (nursing home-acquired) and community-acquired (present on admission) infections were counted and were roughly equal in number. Skin infections, especially infected decubiti, were the most common type encountered, with genitourinary tract infections a distant second. Emphasis in this survey was placed on direct observation of infections.

Cohen et al. found an infection rate of only 2.7% in a one-day prevalence survey of 31 skilled nursing homes in Connecticut (13). Infections of the urinary tract were the most common, followed by skin and respiratory tract infections. Surveillance was limited to these three sites, and only nosocomial infections were counted. The low infection rate in this study may be explained by the fact that medical records provided the only source for infection data. While this technique is standard in hospitals, the nursing home medical record is felt to be much less complete and accurate (17,19).

Magnussen et al. collected incidence data on nosocomial infections for two months in a single 400-bed long-term care facility associated with a Veterans Administration hospital in Pennsylvania (11). In their study, they relied not only on the medical record but also on laboratory slips, x-ray reports, antimicrobial drug usage, and nurse inquiries. The total nosocomial infection rate was 18.2%, of which 72% were urinary tract infections, 14% respiratory tract infections, 11% skin infections, and 3% bacteremias. The predominant pathogens in patients with urinary tract infections were *Proteus mirabilis* and *Providencia stuartii*. Eighty-three percent of the 58 residents with urinary tract infections used some type of catheter, which in one-third was an indwelling catheter. The infection rate was based on the unit average daily census for a month. The mean age of infected residents was 70.5 years.

A very thorough one-day prevalence study of nursing home infections was undertaken by Garibaldi et al. in Utah (12). They identified infections in residents when diagnosed by the attending physician or nurse, when antibiotics had been prescribed, or when the signs or symptoms on examination suggested the diagnosis to a member of the study team. In this study, as in Magnussen's, the diagnosis of infection was always compatible with the guidelines established by the Centers for Disease Control (22). The median age of those infected was 81 years. Fifty-eight percent of their residents were ambulatory, 10% were receiving systemic antimicrobials, and 12% had indwelling urinary catheters. They found a total nosocomial infection rate of 16.2%, with the leading sites of infection being infected decubitus ulcers (33%), conjunctivitis (19%), symptomatic urinary tract infection (14%), lower respiratory tract infection (11%), upper respiratory tract infection (8%), and diarrhea (7%). Skin infections were significantly more common in residents who were nonambulatory, fecally incontinent, or diabetic. The most common urinary tract isolates were enterococci, *Proteus,* and *E. coli.* They noticed frequent clustering of cases of upper respiratory tract infection, diarrhea, conjunctivitis, and antibiotic-resistant urinary tract bacteria, suggesting nosocomial spread of infection in outbreaks.

In spite of the variation in methodology and findings in the above studies, it is clear that nosocomial infections in nursing homes occur with a frequency comparable to that of hospitals. Infected decubitus ulcers and urinary tract infections are the most common nosocomial infections, but many other sites are involved (see Table 4.1). The overall nosocomial infection rate has varied from 3–16% in several studies, and is probably similar to the hospital rate of 5–10%.

A majority of nursing home-acquired infections arise endogenously from the resident's own bacteria, which become pathogenic because of indwelling urinary catheters, abraded skin, or depressed immunity. This situation parallels that occurring in the hospital. A significant percentage of infections occur by cross-infection; epidemic infections accounted for over 20% of nosocomial infections in nursing homes in the Utah survey (12).

Table 4.1. Leading Nosocomial Infections

Nursing Homes	Hospitals
Urinary tract infection	Urinary tract infection
Infected decubitus ulcer	Wound infection
Pneumonia/influenza	Pneumonia
Diarrhea	Bacteremia
Conjunctivitis	

The importance of nursing home nosocomial infections lies not just in their frequency. Nosocomial infections cause symptomatic complications ranging from fever to septic shock and death. The morbidity of nosocomial infections may profoundly affect the resident. Anyone who has cared for a person with an infected decubitus ulcer, for instance, is impressed with the pain, the tissue destruction, and the chronicity of this nosocomial infection. Finally, nosocomial infections threaten not just the afflicted resident, but also other residents and nursing home personnel. The potential for spread is always present.

SPECIFIC INFECTIONS OF IMPORTANCE IN NURSING HOMES

In this section, the most important infections that occur in nursing home residents will be identified, with emphasis on epidemiology, diagnosis, prevention, and treatment. The most important infections in nursing homes (urinary tract infection, infected decubitus ulcers, and pulmonary infections) are reviewed in depth in the following three chapters.

Urinary Tract Infection

Urinary tract infection is probably the leading nosocomial infection seen in nursing homes (9,11). By far the most important predisposing factor to urinary tract infection in the institutionalized elderly is the presence of an indwelling urinary catheter. Hence, control measures should be directed toward prevention of contamination of the catheter system.

Urinary tract infections occur predominately with gram-negative aerobic bacteria, many of which are normal gut flora (*E. coli, Proteus, Klebsiella,* and *Enterobacter*). Even though endogenous bacteria account for the majority of cases, cross-infection is also a risk in nursing homes. The urinary tract is also a major site of epidemic, gram-negative antibiotic-resistant infections (23).

Table 4.2.   Cutaneous Infections in the Nursing Home

Infected decubitus ulcers
Erysipelas
Cellulitis
Cutaneous abscesses
Herpesvirus infections
Scabies

Control measures for prevention of urinary tract infection in the nursing home are directed at any or all of the three links in the chain of infection. The reservoir may be controlled (e.g., by minimizing urinary catheterization); transmission of organisms may be blocked (e.g., by isolation and good handwashing between care of catheterized residents); or steps may be taken to prevent disease from developing in the host (e.g., minimizing antibiotic usage in the catheterized resident and minimizing urethral trauma from catheter manipulation). A full discussion of urinary tract infection is presented in Chapter 6.

Skin and Soft Tissue Infections

Skin infection has been a major nosocomial infection in all nursing home surveys (see Table 4.2). Infected decubitus ulcers comprise the bulk of cutaneous infections in that setting.

Infected Decubitus Ulcers.   Those at greatest risk of developing pressure sores are the elderly, those with altered mental status, the incontinent, and residents who are unable to ambulate without assistance (24). The majority of organisms that colonize the ulcer and cause secondary complicating infections of soft tissue or bone are endogenous bacteria, such as enteric gram-negative bacilli, anaerobic gut bacteria, and *Staphylococcus aureus* (25).

The best way to prevent infected decubitus ulcers is to prevent formation of the ulcers themselves by frequent changes in position, use of air mattresses, and debridement of established ulcers. A decubitus ulcer that is draining a large amount of purulent material or contains *S. aureus* or group A streptococci requires isolation (26). A complete discussion of decubitus ulcers is found in Chapter 7.

Bacterial Skin and Soft Tissue Infections.   Most uncomplicated infections of skin and soft tissues are caused by gram-positive cocci, specifically group A streptococci and *S. aureus*.

Streptococci are chain-forming cocci that produce disease in man on the basis of invasiveness and toxin production. **Erysipelas** is a rapidly spreading superficial infection caused by group A streptococci. The patient is usually febrile. Physical examination reveals lymphangitis and a painful, advancing, red raised area of dermal inflammation. Prompt therapy is important, especially for facial infections. Penicillin is the drug of choice.

Cellulitis, infection of the skin that extends deeper than erysipelas to involve subcutaneous tissues, is almost always caused by group A streptococci or *S. aureus.* Local heat, swelling, and tenderness are seen. Streptococcal cellulitis is rapidly progressive. Antibiotic therapy of cellulitis, usually with a penicillin derivative, is important.

Staphylococci appear as clusters of gram-positive cocci when viewed microscopically (see Chapter 1, Fig. 1.1). *S. aureus* is a virulent bacteria capable of producing a variety of extracellular toxins and enzymes. It may be carried in the moist areas of the skin (nares, axilla, rectum) without causing disease, but the skin and soft tissues are frequent sites of staphylococcal infection. *S. aureus* is the leading cause of furuncles, carbuncles, cellulitis, and wound infections. A **furuncle,** or **boil,** is a localized cutaneous infection that begins as an infection of a hair follicle and evolves to a pustule. A **carbuncle** is a deeper and more destructive abscess that extends into the subcutaneous tissue. Furuncles generally resolve without therapy, but carbuncles and abscesses require surgical drainage. Antibiotic therapy is required for cellulitis and extensive abscesses.

The diagnosis of specific infectious skin lesions is by culture. Both staphylococci and streptococci grow readily on standard bacterial media (see Chapter 1, Fig. 1.2). A swab of involved skin, however, seldom provides useful information; the correct diagnostic approach involves aspiration of fluid or pus for culture. Streptococci remain extremely sensitive to penicillin, whereas most staphylococci encountered in the nursing home are resistant to penicillin. Antistaphylococcal penicillins, such as methicillin, oxacillin, or nafcillin, are the antibiotics of choice for serious staphylococcal infection. Cephalosporins are alternatives for the penicillin-allergic patient.

Preventive aspects must be addressed. Cellulitis usually poses little hazard for cross-contamination in the nursing home. However, an infected wound or decubitus ulcer that drains pus containing *S. aureus* or group A streptococci poses a serious threat and requires contact isolation. In spite of the technical difficulties in isolating residents in some nursing homes, the value of isolation in preventing the spread of staphylococcal infection in nursing homes is quite clear (27).

The institutional reservoir of staphylococcal and streptococcal bacteria is people. This can be either an infected resident, an infected staff member, or a person who is an asymptomatic carrier of the potentially hazardous organism (28,29). The approach to the carrier state in personnel is discussed in Chapter 15.

A rare but serious problem is necrotizing soft tissue infection or gas gangrene. This is more likely to occur in the elderly, the diabetic, and the resident with impaired circulation (30,31). Because of the high incidence of tetanus-prone wounds in the elderly, especially those in nursing homes, it has been argued that tetanus immunization needs to be current in the nursing home resident (32).

Other Cutaneous Infections

Herpesvirus Infections.   Herpesviruses are DNA viruses that tend to persist in the host and produce recurrent infections. The two most important viruses in this group are herpes simplex virus and varicella–zoster virus. Herpesviruses are spread by direct contact. Herpes simplex type 1 involves disease above the waist, primarily the mouth and lips, and is generally acquired during the first decades of life. Herpes simplex type 2 involves areas below the waist, primarily genital sites, and is usually transmitted venereally. The varicella–zoster virus causes chickenpox in children. The virus survives in dorsal nerves and reactivates years later to produce herpes zoster (shingles).

Herpes simplex vesicles (blisters) are characteristically painful and evolve from vesicles to ulcers. Herpes simplex type 1 virus is responsible for ulcerative gingivostomatitis (cold sores). Herpetic vesicles or ulcers occur most frequently on the lips, but may be seen anywhere on the skin. Herpes lesions tend to recur. Recurrences may be spontaneous or may follow stress. Primary infections are more severe than recurrent infections; fever and lymphadenopathy are typical clinical manifestations. Extensive, widespread skin lesions occasionally develop in persons with atopic dermatitis, eczema, or abnormal immunity.

The incidence of herpes zoster peaks at ages 50–80. The vesicles resemble chickenpox, evolving from macules to papules to vesicles, but occur in a dermatomal distribution. Herpes zoster is usually unilateral and most commonly affects the thoracic dermatomes. Local paresthesias or pain may precede the rash. Severe, long-lasting pain (postherpetic neuralgia) is seen most commonly in the elderly.

The diagnosis of cold sores and herpes zoster is primarily clinical, since herpesviruses cannot be routinely cultured and antibody studies are not helpful. There is no reliable cure for herpes simplex or herpes zoster cutaneous lesions at the present time. Corticosteroid therapy should be avoided. The lesions should be kept dry and clean to prevent secondary bacterial infection.

Nosocomial transmission of herpesviruses requires direct contact and is relatively uncommon. A special nosocomial hazard is herpetic whitlow, a herpes simplex infection of the digit that occurs primarily in medical personnel (33). The cutaneous lesions of herpes simplex or herpes zoster remain infectious until the lesions are dry and crusted. Most authorities recommend secretion precautions for patients with localized herpes simplex and for patients with localized herpes zoster. Strict isolation is suggested for disseminated herpes infection because of the possibility of airborne transmission (26,34).

Scabies.   Scabies, a disease of the skin produced by the mite *Sarcoptes scabiei,* can be a problem in the nursing home (35,36). The mite burrows into the skin, deposits its eggs, and causes a characteristic pruritic skin eruption. A symmetrical eruption is seen most commonly in the axillary region, around the waist, between the fingers, on the inner thighs, and on the backs of the arms and legs. In the nursing home resident, scabies may be limited to sites in contact with the sheets. The disease is spread by contact or through objects such as bedding and clothing. Outbreaks often involve both residents and staff because of the extensive hands-on care in nursing homes. If a number of residents and staff members in a nursing home complain of a pruritic eruption, scabies is a likely diagnosis.

The diagnosis is made by placing a drop of a mineral oil on the lesion and scraping with a sharp scalpel blade. The mite or its eggs may be seen under low-power microscopy. Because there are a number of conditions that mimic the itching dermatitis of scabies, making a specific diagnosis by scraping is imperative.

Infected individuals should be treated with gamma benzene hexachloride, 1% lindane (Kwell) lotion, which is applied to the entire body from the neck down and thoroughly washed off 24 hours later. Alternative drugs are crotamiton (Eurax) and 6% sulfur in petrolatum, which must be applied topically for two and three successive days, respectively. Treatment will generally make the patient noninfectious in 24 hours. A thorough cleaning of the environment is also indicated; laundering and heat drying of clothing and bedding is usually sufficient to kill mites in exfoliated scales.

Respiratory Infections

A number of respiratory infections are of importance in the nursing home (see Table 4.3). Pneumonia, tuberculosis, and influenza are discussed in depth in Chapter 5.

Table 4.3. Respiratory Infections in the Nursing Home

Bacterial pneumonia (e.g., pneumococcal)

Tuberculosis

Influenza

Respiratory tract infections

   Rhinovirus

   Parainfluenza

   Respiratory syncytial virus

Pneumonia.   Pneumococcal pneumonia is the leading cause of pneumonia in the elderly. Nursing home residents more frequently have pneumonia associated with a high mortality rate (e.g., *Klebsiella* or staphylococcal pneumonia) than patients with community-acquired pneumonia (37).

Control measures for pneumonia include administration of pneumococcal vaccine to high-risk residents, discontinuation of smoking, minimizing antibiotic usage, and avoiding aspiration with elevation of the head of the bed, especially after tube feeding. Isolation is indicated for pneumonia in those instances where cross-infection is considered a risk. The nursing home should minimize colonization of the elderly resident by proper cleaning of inhalation therapy equipment. Room humidifiers may be a source of nosocomial infection and should be avoided if possible (38).

Tuberculosis.   Outbreaks of tuberculosis in nursing homes are common (39–42). Both residents and personnel may be involved in such outbreaks, and the infection may cause serious morbidity or even death. Control measures include adequate screening of personnel and residents for tuberculosis (43,44). In addition, since tuberculosis is spread by the airborne route, it is important to institute appropriate isolation measures for residents who have active disease. Residents who are receiving appropriate antituberculous chemotherapy become noninfectious within several weeks, although prolonged therapy is recommended for cure.

Influenza.   Influenza is a very contagious disease spread from person to person by respiratory aerosol. The virus causes epidemics of respiratory disease. Influenza deaths occur predominantly among the elderly and the chronically ill.

Influenza outbreaks in nursing homes are not uncommon (45–50) and may have a significant impact on a nursing home population (see Table 4.4). In the outbreak described by Goodman (45), 25% of the residents

Table 4.4. Influenza Outbreaks in Nursing Homes

Influenza Type	No. of Residents Ill (Attack Rate)	No. of Deaths	Reference
?	161	4	47
B	195 (37%)	26	48
B	129 (36%)	1	46
A	30 (25%)	9	45
A	49 (60%)	4	50

developed influenza and the case fatality ratio was 30%. Attack rates as high as 60% may be seen in nursing homes (49). Influenza outbreaks in nursing homes are analyzed in more depth in Chapter 10.

A number of measures have been suggested to prevent or terminate an outbreak of influenza. Spread from the community to the nursing home may be prevented by barring admission of residents with influenza during a community outbreak and restricting visitors to high-risk residents during an outbreak. Individuals may be immunized by influenza vaccination or temporarily protected by antiviral prophylaxis (amantadine).

Spread within the nursing home may be blocked by several means: *(1)* Contact between residents may be diminished by temporarily discontinuing social activities and restricting acutely ill residents to the floor. *(2)* Residents with confirmed or suspected influenza, especially if they are seen within the first five days of the illness, should be cohorted (separated from residents who have not had influenza). *(3)* During an influenza outbreak, staff members should leave work as soon as they develop the first signs of influenza, such as fever, cough, myalgias, malaise, or headache, and not return until they have recovered. *(4)* Residents should be considered infectious from two days before until three to five days after the onset of symptoms. Although isolation has been recommended for influenza, by the time the diagnosis is made most residents are no longer infectious (51). *(5)* For the protection of personnel, only those who have recovered from influenza (and are immune) or who have been vaccinated should care for residents with influenza. *(6)* Residents and staff alike should emphasize covering the mouth and nose with sneezing and coughing.

Viral Respiratory Tract Infections. A number of viral respiratory tract infections are important in nursing homes. Upper respiratory infection (URI), especially the common cold, is the most common infectious human disease. The illness is quite contagious, with peak incidence in the winter months. Nasal congestion, rhinorrhea, headache, and low-grade fever are the primary symptoms. URIs are caused by many viruses, especially rhinoviruses. Antibiotics have no place in the treatment of this self-limited viral illness. There is evidence to suggest that transmission of rhinovirus infection is as efficient by hand contact as it is by the aerosol route (52). Good handwashing is most important in preventing spread of URIs. Aqueous 2% iodine applied to the fingers has been shown to block transmission of certain viruses that cause URI (53).

Outbreaks of respiratory syncytial virus (RSV) and parainfluenza respiratory disease have been reported in nursing homes (54,55). RSV, which is primarily a pathogen of infants and children, caused an outbreak of URI and pneumonia in a nursing home in Missouri (56). The disease appears to be spread by the aerosol route. Most residents have fever, cough, and rhinorrhea; pneumonia may occasionally develop.

Parainfluenza is a virus that may cause URI, bronchitis, and occasionally pneumonia. In nursing home outbreaks, case clustering in living units and dining areas suggested person-to-person spread. The illness occurred in both employees and residents, suggesting that employees may be an important transmission line (57,58). Close contact may be more important than the airborne route in transmission of this virus. Diagnosis of these viral illnesses can be made by measuring a rise in serum antibody level.

Gastroenteritis

Classification.   Large numbers of organisms enter the gastrointestinal tract by way of the mouth, but most are killed by gastric acid. The normal bacterial flora of the intestine is protective; it competes with potential invaders for space and nutrients. Once an infection develops, diarrhea serves as a protective mechanism by increasing clearance of pathogens or toxins. Achlorhydria, gastric surgery, and antacids lower gastric acidity and thereby predispose to bacterial and parasitic infections of the gut. Disturbance of normal gut flora by antibiotics lowers the dose of *Salmonella* needed to cause infection. Opiates and anticholinergics decrease intestinal motility and may increase the severity of infectious gastroenteritis.

The agents causing infectious diarrhea in the nursing home may be classified epidemiologically or pathologically. Epidemiologically, infectious agents causing diarrhea have a **reservoir** that is either humans or food/water. Organisms in the latter category are often pathogens of animals spread to humans by ingestion of contaminated food, whereas organisms carried by people are spread from person to person by the fecal–oral route (see Table 4.5). *Staphylococcus aureus* resides in humans but is spread by contaminated food.

Table 4.5. Epidemiologic Classification of Gastrointestinal Pathogens

Reservoir = Man	*Reservoir = Food/Water*
Salmonella typhi	Nontyphoid *Salmonella*[a]
Viral gastroenteritis[a]	Clostridium perfringens[a]
Shigella[a]	Clostridium botulinum
Staphylococcus aureus	Yersinia enterocolitica
Amoebae	Campylobacter
Escherichia coli	
Giardia	

[a]Significant pathogen in nursing homes.

Outbreaks of food poisoning (epidemic **common-vehicle** gastroenter-itis related to food or water contamination) are quite common in the nursing home setting. Alternatively, epidemics of gastroenteritis in the nursing home may be spread from **person to person** by the fecal–oral route (see Chapter 10). *Salmonella* is the leading cause of confirmed foodborne outbreaks in the United States, accounting for about 20% of such outbreaks reported to the Centers for Disease Control (59). Other common causes of foodborne outbreaks are *Staphylococcus aureus, Clostridium perfringens, C. botulinum,* and *Shigella.* Outbreaks may be traced to a variety of foods that serve as the common source. Factors that con-tribute to outbreaks include improper holding temperatures for food, inadequate cooking of food, contaminated equipment, and poor personal hygiene of food preparers.

Pathologic organisms can conveniently be classified into two groups: those that produce disease by **invasion** of the intestine and those that produce disease by means of a **toxin** (see Table 4.6). In general, invasive pathogens cause fever and frequent small stools containing mucus and blood. The incubation period is 12 to 72 hours. Toxin-mediated diseases have shorter incubation periods; nausea, vomiting, and diarrhea develop 1 to 36 hours after ingestion. Stool cultures are of no value in the di-agnosis of toxin-related diarrhea. Diagnosis depends on history and cul-ture of the suspected food.

Table 4.6. Pathologic Classification of Gastrointestinal Pathogens

Invasive Organisms	*Toxin-Producing Organisms*
Shigella	Clostridium botulinum
Salmonella	Clostridium perfringens
Amoebae	Staphylococcus aureus
Giardia	Escherichia coli
Yersinia enterocolitica	Vibrio cholerae
Campylobacter jejuni	

Toxin-Mediated Gastroenteritis. *Staphylococcus aureus* and *Clostridium perfringens* are the leading causes of toxin-mediated foodborne outbreaks. Staphylococcal enterotoxin is acid-stable. Nausea and vomiting begin one to six hours after ingestion of precooked food, often custard products. *C. perfringens* has an incubation period of 10 to 24 hours and is often associated with ingestion of gravy or beef products. Botulism is associated with home-canned foods. Toxigenic *E. coli* is a common cause of "traveler's diarrhea." Antibiotic therapy is not helpful, but toxin-mediated gastroenteritis due to *E. coli*, *C. perfringens*, and *S. aureus* is self-limited.

C. perfringens and *S. aureus* cause outbreaks of toxin-mediated gastroenteritis in the nursing home or hospital setting (60). In institutional outbreaks, most episodes were traced to preheated meat and poultry dishes that had been cooked one day earlier and inadequately cooked or stored before serving the following day. The incriminated foods were stews, pies, meats, and chicken dishes. Precooked foods, particularly baked goods, may become contaminated with *S. aureus*. Three percent of *C. perfringens* outbreaks occur in nursing homes (61).

Salmonella Infections. Typhoid fever, the best known type of *Salmonella* infection, is relatively uncommon in the United States compared to other strains of nontyphoid *Salmonella*. Even a single case of typhoid fever in a nursing home should be viewed with great concern and prompt a search for a human carrier.

Nontyphoid salmonellosis may occur with a variety of different strains and is known to be a very important problem in nursing homes (60,62–65). The leading serotypes of nontyphoid *Salmonella* isolated from humans in the Unites States are *Salmonella typhimurium*, *S. enteritidis*, *S. newport*, and *S. heidelberg* (65). Salmonellosis tends to be unusually severe in nursing homes, where the mortality for outbreaks can be as high as 8.7% (66). Most outbreaks in nursing homes are common-source outbreaks associated with contaminated food, where an explosive cluster of cases is seen 12 to 48 hours after exposure. Epidemics may be continued or propagated by a secondary person-to-person or hand-to-mouth contact. The most common vehicles are poultry and egg products. *Salmonella* epidemics are discussed in Chapter 10.

Residents with salmonellosis manifest fever, abdominal pain, and diarrhea. Bacteremia, common with *Salmonella typhi,* is an unusual complication in nontyphoid salmonellosis. The diagnosis is made by stool culture. Antibiotic therapy is generally not necessary for nontyphoid *Salmonella,* and antibiotics may actually prolong fecal excretion of the organism (64). Enteric precautions should be employed for all infected individuals. This basically means a private room if the resident is incontinent or regular room if the resident is continent of stool, with good handwashing and wearing of gloves by persons having direct contact with the resident or articles contaminated with fecal material. In large outbreaks, it may be necessary to cohort infected residents. Good food-handling practices should be followed, with periodic review of principles of hygiene for dietary employees (see Chapter 15). Outbreaks may involve both residents and staff (62).

Shigella **Infections.** Shigellosis, like salmonellosis, presents with fever, cramping, abdominal pain, and diarrhea after an incubation period of 36 to 72 hours. Occasionally severe or bloody diarrhea may be seen. The diagnosis is made by stool culture. In the United States, the most common species isolated are *Shigella sonnei* and *S. flexneri;* 0.9% of outbreaks in the United States in 1981 were in institutions, where *S. flexneri* was the leading isolate (67).

Although *Shigella* generally causes outbreaks by person-to-person transmission, occasional common-source outbreaks of foodborne illness may be seen. When these outbreaks occur, they can almost always be traced to contamination of food by an infected food handler (68). Antibiotics are indicated for residents with significant diarrhea, and enteric precautions must be enforced to prevent further spread of the organism.

Yersinia **and** *Campylobacter.* *Yersinia enterocolitica* and *Campylobacter jejuni* cause diarrhea in the community. Both have animal reservoirs. *Y. enterocolitica* can cause foodborne gastroenteritis outbreaks (69). *Campylobacter* enteritis usually is spread by contaminated food or water (70).

Parasitic Gastroenteritis. Two parasites may cause gastroenteritis in the institutional setting. Institutional outbreaks of amebiasis have been reported in the United States (71,72). The diagnosis is made by finding *Entamoeba histolytica* trophozoites or cysts in the stool. Symptoms range from severe diarrhea to asymptomic passage of cysts. Spread of this organism is person-to-person. *Giardia lamblia* is a parasite that causes mild diarrhea, abdominal cramps, and bloating. It has caused communitywide waterborne and foodborne outbreaks, but person-to-person transmission may occur, especially in institutions (73). This disease is also diagnosed by stool examination. Both of these parasitic diseases require antibiotic therapy of infected residents, and both require enteric precautions to prevent spread of the infection, especially to those who have direct contact with feces.

Viral Gastroenteritis. Viral gastroenteritis is a very common, usually self-limited infectious disease that causes diarrhea and occasionally low-grade fever. The diagnosis depends on obtaining paired serum antibody levels that demonstrate a rise in titer. Rotavirus, Norwalk virus, and enteroviruses are the usual causes of viral gastroenteritis. Antibiotic therapy is of no benefit. Norwalk virus has caused a number of nursing home outbreaks (74). Outbreaks are spread primarily by person-to-person transmission. The characteristic duration of outbreaks is five to nine days. Rotavirus infections are also generally mild, although they may be more severe in the elderly population. In nursing homes, outbreaks have been reported with mortality rates ranging from 0 to 10% (75–77). Enteric precautions are advisable for residents with viral gastroenteritis; this involves careful handwashing and proper disposal of feces.

Viral Hepatitis

Etiology and Epidemiology. Viral hepatitis is a syndrome that can be caused by a number of viral agents, including hepatitis A virus, hepatitis B virus, cytomegalovirus (CMV) and Epstein–Barr virus (EBV). A significant number of cases of viral hepatitis are not caused by one of these four viruses. These cases, termed non-A, non-B hepatitis, resemble hepatitis B clinically. Most cases of viral hepatitis are caused by hepatitis A virus or hepatitis B virus. Old terminology referred to hepatitis A as infectious hepatitis and to hepatitis B as serum hepatitis. Many patients with hepatitis are asymptomatic, but fever, anorexia, nausea, and right upper quadrant pain may occur. Laboratory tests demonstrate liver injury with elevation of serum transaminases and bilirubin.

Hepatitis A has an incubation period of two to six weeks and tends to occur in epidemics. Spread is from person to person by the fecal–oral route. Shellfish, contaminated water, and infected food handlers have been responsible for outbreaks. The virus is found in the stool two weeks prior to the onset of symptoms and remains until liver function tests begin to return to normal. Some 20–60% of the population in the United States has hepatitis A antibodies, implying past infection.

Hepatitis B, which is less common than hepatitis A, has a much longer incubation period of one to six months. The virus can be found in blood and body secretions. Transmission of the virus is usually by the parenteral route. Blood transfusion, hemodialysis, and drug abuse are significant risk factors. Health care personnel, especially those who have close contact with blood or blood products, are at increased risk.

Hepatitis A has a very good prognosis. Symptoms usually resolve within several weeks, and chronic liver disease does not develop. Hepatitis B, on the other hand, leads to chronic active hepatitis in as many as 10% of cases. Cirrhosis, or scarring of the liver, may eventually result. Non-A, non-B hepatitis may also lead to chronic liver disease.

Diagnosis. A number of specific diagnostic tests are now available. Hepatitis A IgG antibody is present for years after infection and is associated with immunity, whereas the presence of IgM antibody suggests recent infection. A variety of particles relating to the hepatitis B virus have been identified, including hepatitis B surface antigen (HBsAg), hepatitis B core antigen, and e antigen. These particles or the antibodies produced against them have been used to diagnose hepatitis B. The hepatitis B surface antigen and the e antigen correlate well with infectiousness. Most patients eliminate hepatitis B surface antigen from their blood in several months and develop protective anti-HBsAg antibody, although 5–10% become chronic HBsAg carriers.

Prevention—Hepatitis A. There is no specific therapy for hepatitis, although a number of preventive measures are available. Pooled immune serum globulin (ISG) confers significant protection against hepatitis A when given within two weeks of exposure. It is 80–90% effective. It is indicated for household contacts of hepatitis A cases at a dose of 0.02 ml/kg by the intramuscular route.

Institutional outbreaks of hepatitis A are not uncommon (78,79). A resident with hepatitis A, particularly one with vomiting, diarrhea, and fecal incontinence, poses a hazard to other residents and nursing home personnel. In one outbreak, 10% of susceptible exposed employees acquired hepatitis A from an incontinent patient with hepatitis A (80). Enteric precautions are appropriate measures for hepatitis A or hepatitis of unknown type (81). There is no vaccine for hepatitis A.

Prevention—Hepatitis B. While standard ISG does not reliably protect against hepatitis B, special high-titer hepatitis B immune globulin (HBIG) may offer some protection, especially following accidental needle stick. The recommended dose is 0.06 ml/kg intramuscularly within one week of exposure, followed by a second dose one month later.

Hepatitis B vaccine consists of surface antigen of the virus. Three injections are recommended—the primary inoculation and booster doses at one and six months. Vaccine is recommended for high-risk groups, including certain health care workers, renal dialysis patients, and institutionalized patients (82). Both HBIG and hepatitis B vaccine are relatively expensive. The institutional use of hepatitis B vaccine applies primarily to patients and staff of mental institutions. Its use in nursing homes is not indicated on a routine basis unless an epidemic of hepatitis B occurs. One outbreak in a nursing home involved six of 59 residents and was felt to be related to the use of bath brushes on multiple residents (83). Blood precautions are appropriate for the resident with hepatitis B and for HBsAg carriers (84).

Miscellaneous Nosocomial Infections in the Nursing Home

Conjunctivitis.   Conjunctivitis was found in 3.4% of the patients surveyed by Garibaldi (12). Clustering of cases suggested cross-infection or epidemics of conjunctivitis. Persons with conjunctivitis classically have a red and painful eye associated with a scratchy foreign body sensation. Most epidemic conjunctivitis is viral in origin. Nosocomial outbreaks have occurred with a number of viruses, especially adenovirus and Coxsackievirus (85,86). Transmission is usually person-to-person, although transmission of adenovirus has been associated with medical instruments (87).

Conjunctivitis may involve both residents and staff at a nursing home. Secretion precautions are recommended for residents with conjunctivitis. The resident is not required to be in a private room, but the staff should practice careful handwashing and special handling of infected secretions and dressings (26). Others have recommended sterilization of instruments between uses, heating instruments in a bath at 75°C for 10 minutes, or immersing instruments in a 1–2% solution of sodium hypochlorite (88).

Helminthic Infections.   A number of helminthic infections are occasionally seen, notably the intestinal nematodes *Trichuris trichiura, Ascaris lumbricoides,* and hookworm. These infections are diagnosed by finding helminth eggs in the stool. No isolation is necessary because of the minimal risk of transmission. Appropriate antihelminthic drugs are available.

Enterobius vermicularis, pinworm, is contagious, and patients who have this infection need excretion precautions. The worm lives in the cecum of humans; the major symptom is perianal pruritus, and spread is by hand-to-mouth contact. Diagnosis is made by seeing eggs on microscopic examination after gummed transparent tape has been applied to the perianal area. Appropriate drugs are available for therapy.

Bacteremia.   Nosocomial bacteremia is relatively uncommon in nursing homes compared to hospitals, but has been found in surveys (11). Gram-negative bacilli are now the most common cause of bacteremia in the hospital. Gram-negative bacteremia has a high mortality rate.

Bacteremias may be primary, in which case they generally originate from contaminated intravascular devices, or they may be secondary to other infections such as wound infection, intraabdominal infection, urinary tract infection, or pneumonia. Bacteria causing infusion-related bacteremia may originate from the patient's skin, the hands of personnel, or the intravenous fluid or apparatus.

Guidelines have been published for minimizing intravenous-related nosocomial infections (89), including minimizing intravenous catheter use, changing the intravenous catheter frequently, inserting the intravenous catheter with proper aseptic technique, changing the infusion apparatus every 48 hours, changing intravenous bottles at least every 24 hours, and suspecting that the intravenous catheter may be the source of infection in any patient with such a catheter who develops fever.

REFERENCES

1. Brachman PS: Epidemiology of nosocomial infections, in Bennett JV, Brachman PS (eds): *Hospital Infections*. Boston, Little, Brown, 1979.

2. Freeman J, Rosner BA, McGowan, JG Jr: Adverse effects of nosocomial infection. *J Infect Dis* 140:732–740, 1979.

3. Green MS, Rubinstein E, Amit P: Estimating the effects of nosocomial infections on length of hospitalization. *J Infect Dis 145:667–672, 1982.*

4. *Reported Nosocomial Infections, 1979*, National Nosocomial Infections Study (NNIS). Atlanta, Center for Disease Control, 1979.

5. Fraser DW: Bacteria newly recognized as nosocomial pathogens. *Am J Med* 70:432–437, 1982.

6. Walter CW: The physician's role in cross infections. *RI Med J* 60:534–548, 1977.

7. Stamm WE, Weinstein RA, Dixon RE: Comparison of endemic and epidemic nosocomial infections. *Am J Med* 70:393–397, 1981.

8. Wenzel RP (ed): *Handbook of Hospital Acquired Infections*. CRC Press, Boca Raton, Fl., 1979.

9. Sherman FT, Tucci V, Libow LS, Isenberg HD: Nosocomial urinary-tract infections in a skilled nursing facility. *J Am Geriatr Soc* 28:456–461, 1980.

10. Campbell DG: Prevention of infections in extended care facilities. *Nurs Clin N Am* 15:857–868, 1980.

11. Magnussen MH, Robb SS: Nosocomial infections in a long-term care facility. *Am J Infect Control* 8:12–17, 1980.

12. Garibaldi RA, Brodine S, Matsumiya S: Infections among patients in nursing homes: Policies, prevalence, and problems. *N Engl J Med* 308:731–735, 1981.

13. Cohen ED, Hierholzer WJ Jr, Schilling CR, et al: Nosocomial infection in skilled nursing facilities: A preliminary survey. *Publ Health Rep* 94:162–166, 1979.

14. Nixon SA: The family physician's role in the care of the elderly. *J Am Geriatr Soc* 30:417–420, 1982.

15. Solon JA, Greenawalt LF: Physician's participation in nursing homes. *Med Care* 12:486–495, 1974.

16. Rango N: Nursing-home care in the United States: Prevailing condition and policy implications. *N Engl J Med* 307:883–889, 1982.

17. Miller MB, Elliott DF: Errors and omissions in diagnostic records on admission of patients to a nursing home. *J Am Geriatr Soc* 34:108–116, 1976.

18. Brown MN, Cornwell J, and Weist JK: Reducing the risks to the institutionalized elderly: I. Depersonalization, negative relocation effects, and medical care deficiencies. *J Gerontol Nurs* 7:401–404, July 1981.

19. Zimmer JG: Medical care evaluation studies in long-term care facilities. *J Am Geriatr Soc* 27:62–72, 1979.

20. Schneider EL: Infectious diseases in the elderly. *Ann Intern Med* 98:395–400, 1983.

21. Lester MR: Looking inside 101 nursing homes. *Am J Nurs* 64:111–116, 1964.

22. *Outline for Surveillance and Control of Nosocomial Infections.* Atlanta, Center for Disease Control, 1976.

23. Weinstein RA, Nathan C, Gruensfelder R, et al: Endemic aminoglycoside resistance in gram-negative bacilli: Epidemiology and mechanisms. *J Infect Dis* 141:338–345, 1980.

24. Reuler JB, Cooney TG: The pressure sore: Pathophysiology and principles of management. *Ann Intern Med* 94:661–666, 1981.

25. Galpin JE, Chow AW, Bayer AS, et al: Sepsis associated with decubitus ulcers. *Am J Med* 61:346–350, 1976.

26. Centers for Disease Control: Guideline for isolation precautions in hospitals. *Infect Control* July/Aug 1983.

27. Kunin C: Staphylococcal infection control in long-term facility. *JAMA* 245:2352, 1981.

28. Schaffner W, Lefkowitz LB Jr, Goodman JS, et al: Hospital outbreak of infections with group A streptococci traced to an asymptomatic anal carrier. *N Engl J Med* 280:1224–1225, 1969.

29. St. Leger AS: Nasal carriage of *Staphylococcus aureus* among patients on a general surgical ward. *J Hosp Infect* 1:333–339, 1980.

30. Dellinger EP: Severe necrotizing soft tissue infections: Multiple disease entities requiring a common approach. *JAMA* 246:1717–1721, 1981.

31. Caplan ES, Cluge RM: Gas gangrene: A review of 34 cases. *Arch Intern Med* 136:789–791, 1976.

32. Irvine P, Crossley K: Tetanus and the institutionalized elderly. *JAMA* 244:2159–2160, 1980.

33. Rosato FE, Rosato CF, and Plotkin SA: Herpetic paronychia: An occupational hazard of medical personnel. *N Engl J Med* 283:804–805, 1970.

34. Valenti WM, Betts RF, Hall CB, et al: Nosocomial viral infections: II. Guidelines for prevention and control or respiratory viruses, herpes viruses, and hepatitis viruses. *Infect Control* 1:165–177, 1981.

35. Scabies in institutions. *J Iowa Med Soc* 71:78–78, 1981.

36. Burkhart CG: Scabies: An epidemiologic reassessment. *Ann Intern Med* 98:498–503, 1983.

37. Garb JL, Brown RB, Garb JR, et al: Differences in etiology of pneumonias in nursing home and community patients. *JAMA* 240:2169–2172, 1978.
38. Smith PW, Massanari RM: Room humidifiers as the source of *Acinetobacter* infections. *JAMA* 237:795–797, 1977.
39. Stead WW: Tuberculosis among elderly patients: An outbreak in a nursing home. *Ann Intern Med* 94:606–610, 1981.
40. Center for Disease Control: Tuberculosis in a nursing home—Oklahoma. *Morbid Mortal Weekly Rep* 29:465–467, 1980.
41. Center for Disease Control: Tuberculosis—North Dakota. *Morbid Mortal Weekly Rep* 27:523–525, 1979.
42. Birss JW: Tuberculosis in nursing homes. *N Engl J Med* 279:347–348, 1968.
43. Stead WW: Control of tuberculosis in institutions. *Chest* 76 (suppl): 797–800, 1979.
44. Kent DC, Atkinson ML, Eckmann BH, et al: *Screening for Pulmonary Tuberculosis in Institutions*, official statement of the American Thoracic Society. February 1977.
45. Goodman RA, Orenstein WA, Munro TF, et al: Impact of influenza A in a nursing home. *JAMA* 247:1451–1453, 1982.
46. Hall WN, Goodman RA, Noble GR, et al: An outbreak of influenza B in an elderly population. *J Infec Dis* 144:297–302, 1981.
47. Genesove LJ, Riddiford M: Influenza in a nursing home. *CMA J* 118:1202, 1978.
48. Silverstone FA, Libow LS, Duthie E, et al: Outbreak of influenza B, 1980 in a geriatric long term care facility. *Gerontologist* 20 (Part 2):200, 1980.
49. Centers for Disease Control: Update: Influenza in nursing homes—Michigan, Minnesota. *Morbid Mortal Weekly Rep* 32:18, 1983.
50. Centers for Disease Control: Impact of influenza on a nursing home population—New York. *Morbid Mortal Weekly Rep* 32:32–34, 1983.
51. Hoffman PC, Dixon RE: Control of influenza in the hospital. *Ann Intern Med* 87:725–728, 1977.
52. Gwaltney JM, Moskalski PB, and Hendley JO: Hand to hand transmission of rhinovirus cold. *Ann Intern Med* 88:463–467, 1978.
53. Gwaltney JM, Moskalski PB, and Hendley JO: Interruption of experimental rhinovirus transmission. *J Infect Dis* 142:811–815, 1980.
54. Mathur U, Bentley DW, Hall CB: concurrent respiratory syncytial virus and influenza A infections in the institutionalized elderly and chronically ill. *Ann Intern Med* 93 (Part I):49–52, 1980.
55. Garvie DG, Gray J: Outbreak of respiratory syncytial virus infection in the elderly. *Br Med J* 281:1253–1254, 1980.
56. Center for Disease Control: Respiratory syncytial virus—Missouri. *Morbid Mortal Weekly Rep* 26:351, 1977.
57. Center for Disease Control: Parainfluenza outbreaks in extended care facilities—United States. *Morbid Mortal Weekly Rep* 27:475–476, 1978.

58. Dixon R: Parainfluenza 3 spread linked to direct contact. *Hosp Infect Control* 7:16, 1980.

59. *Foodborne Disease Surveillance*, annual summary. Atlanta, Center for Disease Control, 1980.

60. Sharp JCM, Collier PW: Food poisoning in hospitals in Scotland. *J Hyg Camb* 83:231–236, 1979.

61. Shandera WX, Tacket CO, and Blake PA: Food poisoning due to *Clostridium perfringens* in the United States. *J Infect Dis* 147:167–170, 1983.

62. Anand CM, Finlayson MC, Garson JZ, et al: An institutional outbreak of salmonellosis due to a lactose fermenting *Salmonella newport*. *Am J Clin Path* 74:657–660, 1980.

63. Gotoff SP, Broing JR, Lepper MH: An epidemic of *Salmonella St. Paul* infections in a convalescent home. *Am J Med Sci* 58:16–22, 1966.

64. Schroeder SA, Aserkoff B, Brachman PS: Epidemic salmonellosis in hospitals and institutions. *N Engl J Med* 279:674–678, 1968.

65. Centers for Disease Control: Human *Salmonella* isolates—United States, 1981. *Morbid Mortal Weekly Rep* 31:613–615, 1982.

66. Baine WB, Gangarosa EJ, Bennett JV, et al: Institutional salmonellosis. *J Infect Dis* 128:357–360, 1973.

67. Centers for Disease Control: Shigellosis—United States, 1981. *Morbid Mortal Weekly Rep* 31:681–682, 1982.

68. Center for Disease Control: Shigellosis in a Children's Hospital—Pennsylvania. *Morbid Mortal Weekly Rep* 28:498–499, 1979.

69. Centers for Disease Control: Outbreak of *Yersinia enterocolitica*—Washington State. *Morbid Mortal Weekly Rep* 31:562–564, 1982.

70. Blaser MJ, Reller LB: *Campylobacter* enteritis. *N Engl J Med* 305:1444–1451, 1981.

71. Sexton DJ: Amebiasis in a mental institution: Serologic and epidemiologic studies. *Am J Epidemiol* 100:414–423, 1974.

72. Krogstad DJ, Spencer HC Jr, Healy GR, et al: Amebiasis: Epidemiologic studies in the United States, 1971–1974. *Ann Intern Med* 88:89–97, 1978.

73. Thacker SB, Simpson S, Gordon TJ, et al: Parasitic disease control in a residential facility for the mentally retarded. *Am J Pub Health* 69:1279–1281, 1979.

74. Kaplan JE, Gary GW, Baron RC, et al: Epidemiology of Norwalk gastroenteritis and the role of Norwalk virus in outbreaks of acute nonbacterial gastroenteritis. *Ann Intern Med* 96 (Part I):756–761, 1982.

75. Marie TJ, Lee SHS, Faulkner RS, et al: Rotavirus infection in a geriatric population. *Arch Intern Med* 142:313–316, 1982.

76. Cubitt WD, Holzel H: an outbreak of rotavirus infection in a long-stay ward of a geriatric hospital. *J Clin Pathol* 33:306–308, 1980.

77. Halvorsrud J. Orstavik I: An epidemic of rotavirus-associated gastroenteritis in a nursing home for the elderly. *Scand J Infect Dis* 12:161–164, 1980.

78. Dienstag JL, Szmuness W, Stevens CE, et al: Hepatitis A virus: New insights from sero-epidemiologic studies. *J Infect Dis* 137:328–339, 1978.
79. Matthew, EB, Dietzman DE, Madden DL, et al: A major epidemic of infectious hepatitis in an institution for the mentally retarded. *Am J Epidemiol* 98:199–215, 1973.
80. Goodman RA, Carder CC, Allen JR, et al: Nosocomial hepatitis A transmission by an adult patient with diarrhea. *Am J Med* 73:220–226, 1982.
81. Favero MS, Maynard JE, Leger RT, et al: Guidelines for the care of patients hospitalized with viral hepatitis. *Ann Intern Med* 91:872–876, 1979.
82. Centers for Disease Control: Inactiviated hepatitis B virus vaccine. *Morbid Mortal Weekly Rep* 31:317–328, 1982.
83. Braconier JH, Nordenfelt E: Serum hepatitis at a home for the aged. *Scand J Infect Dis* 4:79–82, 1972.
84. Maynerd JE: Nosocomial viral hepatitis. *Am J Med* 70:439–444, 1981.
85. Center for Disease Control: Nosocomial outbreak of phayrngoconjunctival fever due to adenovirus, type 4—New York. *Morbid Mortal Weekly Rep* 27:49, 1978.
86. Christopher S, Theogaraj S. Godbole S, et al: An epidemic of acute hemorrhagic conjunctivitis due to coxsackievirus A-24. *J Infect Dis* 146:16–19, 1982.
87. Sprague JB, Hierholzer JC, Currier RW II, et al: Epidemic keratoconjunctivitis. *N Engl J Med* 189:1341–1346, 1973.
88. Keenlyside RA, Hierholzer JC, D'Angelo LJ: Keratoconjunctivitis associated with adenovirus type 37: An extended outbreak in an ophthalmologist's office *J Infect dis* 147:191–198, 1983.
89. *Guidelines for Prevention of Intravenous Therapy-Related infections*, Atlanta, Centers for Disease Control, October 1981.

CHAPTER 5

PULMONARY INFECTIONS: PNEUMONIA, INFLUENZA, AND TUBERCULOSIS

Robert G. Penn

Pneumonia is an inflammatory process in the lung parenchyma. The principle infectious causes of pneumonia in the aged are bacteria, viruses, and tubercle bacilli. Although there is increased susceptibility of all major organ systems to infection in the aged, the respiratory tract appears to be especially vulnerable. Pneumonia and influenza together are the fourth most common cause of death and the leading infectious cause of death among the elderly (1). Prevalence surveys performed by Garibaldi (2) in skilled care nursing homes found pneumonia or lower respiratory tract infections to be present in 2.1% of all residents. Pneumonia was fourth in frequency behind infected decubitus ulcers, conjunctivitis, and symptomatic urinary tract infections. Residents of nursing homes who are hospitalized because of pneumonia have been found to be infected with more resistant bacteria. Moreover, the mortality rate of nursing home–acquired pneumonia is twice the rate found in a comparable elderly group admitted with community-acquired pneumonia (3).

Although pneumonia has been described as "the friend of the aged," this appears to be far from the truth in the nursing home setting. In addition to cutting life short, pneumonia may worsen an underlying disease, such as chronic obstructive pulmonary disease, complicating and increasing the level of care required for an individual resident. Thus, a relatively productive life might be reduced to a bedridden state after an episode of pneumonia.

The discussion on bacterial pneumonia, influenza, and tuberculosis will emphasize the following:

1. It is important for all nursing home personnel to be aware of the special threat of pneumonia in the elderly. The more subtle pre-

sentation of pneumonia in this age group must be recognized, so that early treatment can be given.

2. Preventive measures, especially immunization, should be incorporated into nursing home policies and procedures.

3. The nursing home infection control program should include careful monitoring of the tuberculosis status of both residents and employees.

ETIOLOGY OF PNEUMONIA

The important etiologic agents of pneumonia in the elderly are outlined in Table 5.1. Bacterial causes of pneumonia are determined by examination and culture of an expectorated sputum or blood cultures. The bacterial cause of pneumonia may not be documented in up to 50% of cases. However, with adequate sputum samples and with prompt culture of specimens, the yield of the sputum culture may be as high as 90–100% for bacterial pneumonia. The etiologic agent for viral pneumonia can also be determined by culture of respiratory secretions but requires special culture methods. Likewise, an examination and culture of expectorated sputum can document tuberculosis but requires special staining and culture methods.

The major cause of viral pneumonia in the elderly is influenza. In addition, influenza is an important predisposing factor to bacterial pneumonia.

Another important pulmonary infection in the aged is tuberculosis. In Western countries, tuberculosis is known to reach its peak incidence

Table 5.1. Etiology of Pneumonia

Bacteria
 Streptococcus pneumoniae
 Staphylococcus aureus
 Hemophilus influenzae
 Anaerobes
 Enterobacteriaceae (e.g., *Escherichia coli*, *Klebsiella pneumoniae*)
 Pseudomonas aeruginosa
 Legionella pneumophila
Viruses
 Influenza A and B
Mycobacteria
 Mycobacterium tuberculosis

in those 65 years of age or older. This appears to arise largely from recrudescence of infection acquired at an earlier age. Thus, not unexpectedly, outbreaks of tuberculosis have been reported in nursing homes (4,5). Such outbreaks of tuberculosis pose a threat to fellow residents, employees, and volunteers.

Although most pneumonia in the elderly will be caused by one of these etiologic agents alone, polymicrobial etiology (e.g., *Klebsiella* and anaerobes) is not uncommon in the more seriously ill patient.

BACTERIAL PNEUMONIA

Agents Causing Pneumonia

Streptococcus pneumoniae (the pneumococcus) is recognized as the most common bacterial cause of pneumonia for all age groups. In adults, the incidence increases with age. Increased susceptibility is associated with underlying diseases such as chronic lung or heart disorders, diabetes mellitus, or chronic alcoholism with cirrhosis. The pneumococcus is carried in the upper respiratory tract of 5–70% of normal people, depending on the season. Pneumonia usually develops after aspiration of organisms from the oropharynx. Pneumococcal pneumonia occurs predominantly during the winter and early spring, presumably because of increased crowding of people in an enclosed environment. Person-to-person transmission of the pneumococcus by contact with respiratory droplets is undoubtedly common, but true epidemics of pneumococcal pneumonia are rare. This is true even in closed populations such as nursing homes.

Pneumococcal pneumonia occurs more commonly in men than women. The incidence is three to four times greater in patients over 40 years of age than those under 30 years. Increased mortality is also associated with bacteremia, chronic underlying disease, immune deficiency states (splenectomy, multiple myeloma, and sickle cell disease), and increased age. Even with penicillin therapy, the mortality of bacteremic pneumococcal pneumonia approaches 30–40% in those 50 to 69 years of age and 55–60% in those 70 years or older. This is in contrast to a mortality rate under 10% in those less than 30 years of age (6).

Pneumonia caused by *Staphylococcus aureus* (staphylococcal pneumonia) is generally considered an unusual infection that seldom occurs as a primary disease. However, Garb et al. (3) found that the incidence of staphylococcal pneumonia in those older than 65 years of age from nursing homes who were hospitalized with pneumonia was equal to the incidence of pneumococcal pneumonia (see Table 5.2). Being a resident in a nursing

Table 5.2 **Microbial Agents of Pneumonia in Community and Nursing Home Patients**

Isolate	Community Patients No. (%) (N = 35)	Nursing Home Patients No. (%) (N = 35)
Streptococcus pneumoniae	15 (42.9)	9 (25.7)
Staphylococcus aureus	5 (14.3)	9 (25.7)
Hemophilus influenzae	7 (20.0)	2 (5.7)
Enterobacteriaceae	12 (34.3)	28 (80.0)
Pseudomonas aeruginosa	1 (2.9)	2 (5.7)
Other	3 (8.6)	0 (0.0)
Total number of isolates	43	50

Source: Adapted from Garb JL et al: Differences in Etiology of pneumonias in nursing home and community patients. JAMA 240:2169–2172, 1978. Copyright © 1978 the American Medical Association. Used with permission.

home was the only factor identified that contributed to a higher incidence of staphylococcal pneumonia. The main reservoir for *S. aureus* is the human nose—specifically, colonization on the anterior nasal mucosa. Fifty percent or more of individuals will be nasal carriers of *S. aureus* at any given time. In serial studies on hospital personnel, it has been found that 36% were persistent carriers and 15% were consistently negative. A staphylococcal carrier can serve as a disseminator or reservoir for epidemic staphylococcal disease. Other than being associated with epidemic staphylococcal disease, the characteristics of a disseminator are not clearly defined. However, the risk of transmission is increased in the presence of active staphylococcal disease, such as a boil, paronychia, or sty. The mode of transmission of *S. aureus* is primarily direct or indirect contact. Transmission via hands of personnel is especially important.

Staphylococcal pneumonia in adults is characteristically associated with prior viral respiratory tract infection, especially influenza. Approximately 12–36% of all postinfluenza pneumonia is caused by staphylococci. The influenza virus alters host defenses by destroying the ciliated surface epithelium of the respiratory tract. This destroys the normal clearance mechanism and allows for bacterial invasion. Mortality for postinfluenza staphylococcal pneumonia is reported to be 30–50% (7).

Hemophilus influenzae appears to be a relatively uncommon cause of pneumonia in nursing home patients who are hospitalized with pneumonia (Table 5.2). However, in general, *H. influenzae* is becoming an increasingly recognized cause of bacterial pneumonia in adults. This, in part, is related to declining immunity as well as improved bacteriologic methods. *H. influenzae* can be recovered from the nasopharynx in up to 80% of healthy people. The majority of these isolates are unencapsulated and nontypeable. The capsulated, typeable strains are found less commonly (0.4–6%) in the upper respiratory tract of healthy adults. The latter is a more invasive form of the organism associated with childhood meningitis, acute epiglottitis, and bacteremia. *H. influenzae* is present in the sputum of 50–60% of patients with chronic bronchitis and is associated with acute exacerbations of bronchitis and pneumonia in these patients (8). Among elderly adults, those with primary lung disease or alcoholism are prone to develop pneumonia with *H. influenzae* (9). Increased susceptibility is also associated with sickle cell disease, splenectomy, agammaglobulinemia, and treated Hodgkin's disease. Mortality in *H. influenzae* pneumonia ranges from 6 to 57%. The high mortality rate is associated with bacteremia and the presence of serious underlying disease in patients over the age of 50 years.

Pneumonia due to gram-negative bacilli *(Enterobacteriaceae* and *Pseudomonas)* is becoming an increasingly important problem in the institutionalized elderly. Gram-negative bacillary pneumonia becomes increasingly more common with age (10). Sullivan et al. (11) noted that 59% of cases of gram-negative bacillary pneumonia in patients admitted to a large municipal hospital occurred in residents living in private nursing homes and public facilities. Garb et al. (3) found significantly increased occurrence of gram-negative bacillary pneumonia in comparing 35 elderly patients hospitalized with pneumonia acquired in nursing homes and 35 elderly patients hospitalized with community-acquired pneumonia (Table 5.2). *Klebsiella pneumoniae* was isolated in 14 (40%) of the nursing home patients but in only 3 (8.6%) of the community patients. A significant factor associated with the isolation of *K. pneumoniae* in the sputum of nursing home patients was the prior administration of antibiotics. In patients who had received prior antibiotics, 56.3% had pneumonia associated with *K. pneumoniae*. Antibiotics alter the respiratory tract flora and allow for colonization or superinfection by resistant gram-negative organisms. Those at greatest risk for antibiotic-induced colonization or superinfection are those older than 50 years and those with underlying chronic disease. Other factors associated with gram-negative bacillary pneumonia include alcoholism, chronic pulmonary disease, and diabetes mellitus. There is a 50% mortality rate associated with gram-negative pneumonia (12).

Pneumonia caused by anaerobes (anaerobic pneumonia) characteristically occurs in patients with altered consciousness or dysphagia, both of which predispose to aspiration. Infection caused by anaerobic bacteria is among the most destructive lung infections. Infection ranges from simple pneumonia to necrotizing pneumonia, lung abscess, and empyema. In adults, oropharyngeal secretions contain approximately 10^8 anaerobic bacteria per milliliter. Although there are wide differences in their susceptibility to oxygen, anaerobes thrive only in selected areas of the upper respiratory tract such as crevices around the teeth or tonsillar crypts. The presence of mixed bacterial flora, including aerobic as well as anaerobic organisms, is often necessary for survival. Thus, they are often associated with mixed or polymicrobial infections, including other anaerobes and aerobes. The number of anaerobes in oral secretions increase in the presence of infection such as chronic sinusitis or pyorrhea. Their numbers are decreased but not absent in the oral secretions of edentulous patients. Thus, the bedridden elderly patient with poor dental hygiene and obtundation would be particularly prone to develop pneumonia with an anaerobic component (13).

Classically, anaerobic pleuropulmonary infections are included as one of the three aspiration syndromes. The two noninfectious ones are aspiration of gastric contents and aspiration of foreign bodies. Both may lead to secondary bacterial pneumonia. The clinical course of gastric content aspiration is dependent on the pH of the aspirated material as well as the presence of food particles and bacteria. Acidic fluid alone may be widely disseminated in the lung to produce prompt, diffuse hemorrhage and pulmonary edema. Aspiration of foreign bodies may produce acute airway obstruction. This may present as atelectasis or an asthmalike illness (14). Both noninfectious aspiration syndromes compromise host respiratory defenses, predisposing to bacterial pneumonia. Finally, oropharyngeal secretions containing aerobic or anaerobic bacteria may be aspirated to cause pneumonia. The outcome is dependent on bacteria–bacteria interactions and bacteria–host interactions. Since the aerobic bacteria of the normal mouth and throat flora are usually nonpathogenic, the anaerobes frequently emerge as pathogens in this setting. However, colonization or the presence of *Streptococcus pneumoniae, Staphylococcus aureus, H. influenzae, Enterobacteriaceae,* or *Pseudomonas* in the throat may allow one of these to emerge as the primary pathogen or "coexist" with the anaerobes in aspiration pneumonia. Conditions predisposing to the aspiration syndromes are outlined in Table 5.3.

Legionella pneumophila is a gram-negative bacillus that causes a pneumonia called Legionnaires' disease. *Legionella* is commonly found in soil and water. Humans are infected by airborne spread when *L. pneumophila* is aerosolized by various mechanisms. In the nursing home setting this could include water supply systems, humidifiers, water faucets, shower heads, construction, or contamination of ventilating systems (often by cooling towers). No person-to-person transmission has been documented. Legionnaires' disease occurs sporadically or in epidemic clusters and may be a fatal illness. The incidence of Legionnaires' disease in the United

Table 5.3.   Conditions That Predispose to Aspiration in the Elderly

Altered consciousness
  Sedatives
  Alcoholism
  Seizure disorder
  Cerebrovascular accident
  General anesthesia

Abnormal gag and swallowing reflexes
  Neurologic deficit
  Esophageal motility disorders
  Esophageal reflux
  Oral cancer

Mechanical disruption of host defenses
  Nasogastric intubation
  Tracheostomy
  Endotracheal intubation

States is unknown. Most cases of Legionnaires' disease have occurred in middle-aged or older adults; the mean age in many outbreaks has been 50–60 years. Important risk factors include cigarette smoking, alcohol consumption, and compromised immune function. The bacteria cannot be readily cultured from sputum. In most cases, the diagnosis of Legionnaires' disease is confirmed serologically by obtaining a blood test in the acute phase of the disease and then again in the convalescent phase. Seroconversion may take six weeks. Mortality rates have ranged from 5% to 24% (15).

Pathogenesis of Bacterial Pneumonia

Bacteria may reach the parenchyma of the lungs by one of three routes: the bloodstream, inhalation of contaminated aerosols, or aspiration of oropharyngeal secretions. The first, and least common, is associated with a distant focus of infection, (e.g., pyelonephritis) that causes bacteremia, leading to secondary pneumonia. However, no distant focus of infection can be identified in the majority of patients with pneumonia. Second, bacteria can be aerosolized into the lungs by breathing or inhalation therapy equipment that incorporate reservoir nebulizers. Finally, pneumonia may develop after aspiration of secretions containing bacteria from the oropharynx. Most bacterial pneumonias appear to develop by the latter route. Aspiration of oropharyngeal contents has been shown to occur commonly in normal subjects during deep sleep and even more frequently in patients with pathologically depressed consciousness. Normally, aspirated bacteria are cleared effectively. However, in patients with impaired pulmonary defenses, pneumonia may result. For the elderly, a number of factors are known to interfere with normal host defenses of the respiratory tract (16). These include alterations in the level of consciousness that can compromise epiglottic closure (e.g., stroke and parkinsonism). Compromised abdominal and diaphragmatic muscle function may result in an impaired cough reflex and inadequate removal of tracheobronchial secretions. Retained secretions then enhance bacterial growth. Cigarette smoking disrupts mucociliary clearance activity in the airways so that particles trapped in mucus are not carried proximally to the throat. Poor serum antibody response to antigen and impaired cell-mediated immunity may also decrease resistance to infection in the elderly. In addition, underlying malnutrition and immunosuppressive drugs may increase susceptibility.

For bacteria to be aspirated and initiate pneumonia, they must first colonize the oropharynx or throat area. Factors involved in this colonization have been reviewed (17). Of special importance in the elderly is the breakdown of the normal local throat defenses preventing colonization with gram-negative bacteria. Valenti et al. (18) studied the factors responsible for oropharyngeal colonization with gram-negative bacteria among elderly persons in institutions. Colonization increased with level of care from 9% in independent residents of apartments to 60% in patients in an acute hospital ward, where all had multisystem diseases and many were moribund. *Klebsiella* species were found in 41% of those colonized. Associated with colonization were bladder incontinence, deteriorating or terminal clinical status, inability to walk without assistance, difficulty performing activities of daily living, and incapacitation due to neoplastic, respiratory, or cardiac disease. Those factors contributing most to colonization were the presence of respiratory disease and being bedridden. Other factors that can predispose to colonization by gram-negative bacteria include antibiotics, alcoholism, and diabetes mellitus. Although the exact mechanism for breakdown in local defenses is unknown, this appears to be related to increasing the availability of receptor sites on the throat epithelial cells for gram-negative bacteria and alteration of bacterial interference normally found in the throat (17).

Clinical Features of Bacterial Pneumonia

Bacterial pneumonia is often incompletely expressed in elderly patients. The onset may be insidious with tiredness and mental confusion as the only early signs. Pneumonia in patients older than 65 years of age frequently does not result in copious, purulent sputum, and coughing may be mild and nonproductive. Occasionally, pneumonia first manifests itself by sudden worsening of congestive heart failure, acute respiratory failure in patients with chronic obstructive pulmonary disease, marked prostration, or shock. In other patients typical symptoms of fever, productive cough, and chest pain appear abruptly and overwhelm the patient in several days. Fever may be absent or delayed, especially in patients with gram-negative pneumonia taking steroids or in shock. Two key physical signs are increased respiratory and pulse rates.

Pneumococcal pneumonia is characteristically associated with a single shaking chill and greenish, bloody, or rusty sputum. Variable but not uncommonly stormy courses are associated with *Staphylococcus aureus, H. influenzae,* and gram-negative bacilli. Anaerobic infections tend to be more insidious. Legionnaires' disease generally has a subacute onset. Frequent manifestations of Legionnaires' disease include malaise, fever and chills, cough, dyspnea, headache, myalgias, prostration, and delirium. Fever with recurrent chills, relative bradycardia, and nonproductive cough are characteristic.

After treating bacterial pneumonia for several days, persistence of high fever and appearing ill should suggest a complication. These include empyema, endobronchial obstruction, abscess formation, superinfection, or pericarditis. In addition, metastatic spread via the bloodstream may have occurred, resulting in arthritis, meningitis, or endocarditis.

Diagnostic Aspects

Chest roentgenograms are important in diagnosing all suspected pulmonary infections (see Fig. 5.1). With increased age, more cases of pneumonia have mottled rather than homogeneous consolidation, especially in patients with underlying emphysema. Involvement of two or more lobes is a poor prognostic sign.

Identification of the etiologic agent should be attempted by sampling the patient's sputum for microscopic examination and culture. Obtaining a satisfactory sputum specimen in the elderly is often difficult. Individuals should be instructed to bring up sputum by deep coughing. Consultation with a respiratory therapist, pulmonologist, or specialist in infectious diseases may be of value in establishing a protocol for collection of sputum specimens. Rapid processing of sputum specimens will also be critical in optimizing recovery of a potential pathogen. A positive culture is found in approximately 30% of patients with pneumococcal pneumonia. Blood cultures will occasionally be positive when a sputum sample is negative or difficult to obtain.

Ideally, the choice of antibiotic therapy is determined by identification of the responsible organism. Initial and empiric therapy is usually in-

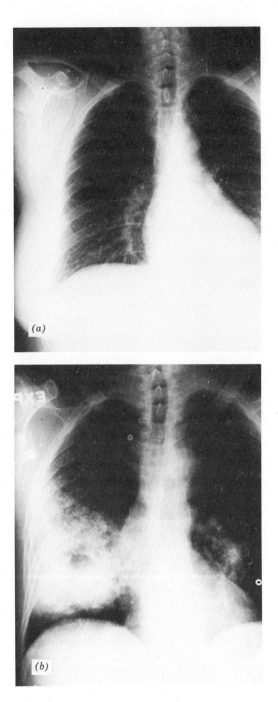

Figure 5.1. (a) Normal chest x-ray. (b) *Streptococcus pneumoniae* lobar pneumonia, right lung.

dicated based on the Gram-stain of the sputum and the clinical picture. One is referred to a standard infectious disease textbook for antibiotics of choice for bacterial pneumonia.

Prevention of Bacterial Pneumonia

The major morbidity and mortality associated with bacterial pneumonia in the elderly obligate each nursing home to develop a program of prevention. This program should be designed around the individual needs of the residents. Larger facilities that admit individuals with more advanced, debilitating diseases will need to develop more complex programs. The initial step, especially for larger-care facilities, is to gather information on "how much" and "what kind" of pneumonia is occurring in the given nursing home. This is done by establishing an infection control program (see Chapter 8) and performing surveillance (see Chapter 9). Criteria are established to define bacterial pneumonia (19). The ongoing surveillance program then defines the endemic pneumonia problems for a given nursing home. This will help set priorities in developing the prevention program and make adjustments as problems arise.

The next step is to identify the control measures to prevent bacterial pneumonia in the elderly. Some of the measures recommended by the Centers for Disease Control for prevention of nosocomial pneumonia are applicable to the nursing home setting (20). These guidelines are centered around preventing colonization, preventing aspiration, and enhancing host defenses.

Since most bacterial pneumonias are caused by bacteria that have colonized the oropharynx, control of this initial phase of infection might prove beneficial. At present, general infection control measures are available to control or halt transmission of potential colonizing bacteria. These measures include review and update of all aseptic techniques and eradicating all potential reservoirs and sources of pathogenic bacteria. Bathroom and sink facilities should be disinfected on a regular basis. If nebulizers and humidifiers are used, the fluids should be kept sterile. Unused fluid should be discarded within 24 hours.

Transmission of potential pathogenic bacteria can be interrupted by proper handwashing techniques. Hands should be washed before and after significant contact with any resident. The Centers for Disease Control guidelines should be followed for disinfection and maintenance of any respiratory therapy equipment used (21). Aseptic techniques should be used for nasotracheal suctioning and in the care of tracheostomies (22). Finally, appropriate isolation procedures should be instituted for residents with active pulmonary or other infections as discussed in Chapter 16. In general, residents with bacterial pneumonia need to be approached with respiratory secretion precautions. Gloves are desirable when handling respiratory secretions or articles contaminated with respiratory secretions. Articles contaminated with respiratory secretions should be either disinfected or discarded. More seriously ill residents infected with organisms such as *Staphylococcus aureus,* for whom strict isolation would be indicated, will usually require hospitalization.

Measures to enhance local host defenses of the oropharynx to prevent colonization are limited at this time. In part, this relates to poor understanding of the local host defenses as well as the fact that serious illness in itself predisposes to colonization of the oropharynx with gram-negative bacteria. The one measure that may be of value is assuring the judicious use of antibiotics to help minimize superinfection. Justification for each antibiotic used should be well documented.

Prevention of aspiration is centered around general supportive care measures. A program of pulmonary hygiene may be indicated for some residents. This would include residents who are unable to take deep breaths unless they are encouraged to do so. Residents can be encouraged to take deep breaths and expand their lungs by efforts to stimulate coughing, turning in bed, and walking. The incentive spirometer is a device that helps encourage periodic, voluntary expansion of the lung. Respiratory-assist devices probably are of limited value in the nursing home setting. If a resident is having trouble with retained secretions that are not removed by coughing, chest physical therapy may be indicated. This would include breathing exercises, postural drainage, and percussion. All these measures would be designed to assist residents in expectorating sputum.

Prevention of pneumonia in aspiration-prone residents may be difficult. All efforts should be made to minimize depression of level of consciousness. This would include ongoing activities of resident stimulation and reducing dosage or discontinuing sedative drugs. A program of intravenous hyperalimentation or a gastrostomy tube might be preferrable to a nasogastric tube. Alternatively, a resident that requires nasogastric tube feedings could be turned on his side rather than on his back and receive small, frequent feedings rather than large ones.

Enhancing host defenses can be accomplished through vaccination. At present, the only vaccine available for bacterial pneumonia is a polyvalent pneumococcal polysaccharide vaccine, which is discussed in Chapter 14.

INFLUENZA

Influenza is an acute and usually self-limited febrile illness caused by infection with influenza type A or B virus. This infection occurs in outbreaks of varying severity almost every winter. The most characteristic clinical manifestations are fever, myalgias, and cough. The two most important features of influenza are its epidemic nature and the mortality that results primarily from its pulmonary complications.

Influenza virus infection is acquired by person-to-person transmission. Large amounts of virus are present in respiratory secretions of infected persons at the time of illness and are dispersed by small particle aerosols created by sneezing, coughing, and talking. It appears that a single infected person can transmit the virus to a large number of susceptible persons. Small-particle aerosols generated can travel a considerable distance. The incubation period of influenza is 18–72 hours. Characteristically, the onset of influenza is abrupt with myalgias. The most troublesome symptoms, fever and chills, may be striking. Upper respiratory symptoms begin to become more prominent as systemic symptoms diminish. Cough is a common respiratory complaint and may be accompanied by substernal discomfort or burning. Cough may persist up to two or more weeks. The two major pulmonary complications of influenza are primary influenza virus pneumonia and secondary bacterial infection. The former is associated with rapid progression of fever, cough, dyspnea, and cyanosis. The mortality is high. Secondary bacterial pneumonia is a complication most often found in the elderly or those who have chronic pulmonary, cardiac, or metabolic disease. This often develops after a period of improvement of one to four days following the classical influenza illness. Recurrent fever occurs, associated with symptoms and signs of bacterial pneumonia such as cough and purulent sputum production. The bacteria involved are usually the pneumococcus, *Staphylococcus aureus* or *H. influenzae.*

The mainstay for prevention of influenza is the inactivated virus vaccine. Yearly revaccination is required because of the unique and remarkable feature of influenza virus to change its surface structure or its antigenicity. Annual vaccination of elderly or chronically ill persons against influenza is recommended (see Chapter 14).

A supplementary measure to vaccination in helping prevent influenza A is amantadine hydrochloride, an oral antiviral drug. It is not a substitute for the vaccine but may be useful for persons who need protection but have not been vaccinated. Amantadine is approximately 70% effective in the prevention of influenza A, not influenza B. It must be taken orally each day for the duration of an epidemic (usually 6–8 weeks) or until active immunity can be expected to develop from vaccination, about 10–14 days. Precautions must be taken for residents with certain chronic conditions. Also, there are sometimes mild but occasionally troublesome side effects—for example, insomnia, especially among older persons. Amantadine, a prescription drug, must be ordered and monitored by a physician. Details of dosage, precautions, and other information on use are specified in the drug insert.

During influenza epidemics, deaths occur primarily in persons older than 65 years and in persons with certain chronic illnesses. Investigations of nursing home influenza A outbreaks, although limited in numbers, have shown substantial mortality (see Chapter 10). Goodman (23) found 30 (25%) of 120 residents had onset of influenzalike illness during a nursing home outbreak. Thirteen persons were hospitalized and nine died (case/fatality ratio, 30%). These authors emphasized that health care providers for the institutionalized elderly should be aware of preventive measures for influenza. A program should be instituted to ensure that as high a proportion as possible of high-risk residents are appropriately vaccinated. Outbreaks of acute, febrile respiratory disease should be promptly investigated, especially during the influenza season. Rapid confirmation· of influenza A by throat culture may be helpful in guiding selection of control measures. In addition to vaccination and amantadine, control measures include restricting high-risk residents' visitors during community outbreaks and close monitoring of personnel for influenza infection.

TUBERCULOSIS

Pathogenesis

Tuberculosis is a communicable disease resulting from infection with the tubercle bacillus, *Mycobacterium tuberculosis*. Humans are the main reservoir of tubercle bacilli. Infection in humans is generally acquired by inhalation of droplet nuclei that contain tubercle bacilli. Droplet nuclei are expelled in aerosols from talking, coughing, sneezing, or singing by persons with pulmonary tuberculosis. They can be dispersed throughout the environment and inhaled by a susceptible host. After inhalation, the droplet nuclei pass through the mucociliary airway defenses into the alveoli. The tubercle bacilli multiply slowly, at a rate of about one multiplication every 24 hours. During the next 3 to 10 weeks, while a cellular immune response is developing in the human host, bacilli may be transported from the lymphatic channels to the regional hilar lymph nodes

Table 5.4.   Classification of Tuberculosis

0. *No tuberculosis, not infected* (no history of exposure, negative to tuberculin skin test)

I. *Tuberculosis exposure, no evidence of infection* (history of exposure, negative tuberculin skin test)

II. *Tuberculous infection, without disease* (positive tuberculin skin test, negative bacteriologic study, if done; no roentgenographic findings compatible with tuberculosis, no symptoms due to tuberculosis.)
Define chemotherapy status (preventive therapy).

III. *Tuberculosis: infected, with disease*
Define location of disease listing predominant sites and other sites if significant.
Define bacteriological status.
Define chemotherapy status.
Define roentgenogram findings.

Tuberculosis suspect: May be used until diagnostic procedures are complete, but not for more than three months.

Source: Adapted from American Thoracic Society, Medical Section of American Lung Association: *Diagnostic Standards and Classification of Tuberculosis and Other Mycobacterial Diseases,* 1981. Used with permission.

and then into the bloodstream. The bacilli are seeded throughout the entire body via the bloodstream. Early hematogenous spread is generally asymptomatic. This initial spread may lead to generalized or "miliary" tuberculosis. However, it is usually controlled by activated host defenses, and a host–parasite relationship is established. Some organisms are slowly destroyed as lesions heal, but significant numbers of bacilli retain their viability in a dormant condition. About 5–15% of those infected with *M. tuberculosis* will develop clinically apparent tuberculosis within five years. Another 3–5% will develop the disease later in life. Dormant bacilli begin to multiply or "reactivate" with resulting progressive disease (24). Thus, tuberculosis occurs in two stages, the infection and the disease.

The classification of tuberculosis is shown in Table 5.4. This reflects the lifelong interaction of the host and tubercle bacilli. All persons can be classified into one of these categories. Most people are class 0. Exposure to tuberculosis makes a subject class I. A positive tuberculin skin test separates the infected subject, or class II, from the Class I person. A chest roentgenogram will usually determine the presence of disease, or class III.

Epidemiology

The largest reservoir of tuberculous infection is in the elderly. An elderly person with dormant infection can potentially develop active tuberculosis at any time. Signs and symptoms of pulmonary tuberculosis can range from the entirely asymptomatic patient to the very ill patient with fever,

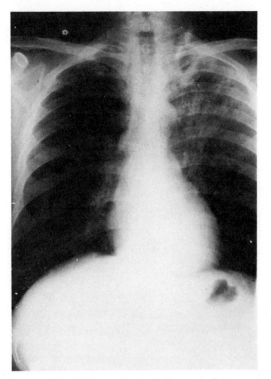

Figure 5.2. Tuberculosis—left upper lobe cavity.

sweating, weight loss, productive cough, hemoptysis, and extensive infiltrates with cavitation in the lung on chest roentgenogram (see Fig.
5.2). There are a large number of potential complications of tuberculosis.
These include pleuritis, pericarditis, peritonitis, enteritis, meningitis, and
infection of the kidneys, bones, and joints. Also, the generalized form
of tuberculosis, or miliary tuberculosis, can develop at any time, but usually is associated with chronic disease or drugs (especially steroids) that
compromise immunity.

Tuberculosis is not a highly contagious disease. Relatively prolonged
or frequent association with an infectious source is generally required
for infection to be transmitted. The greatest hazard of infection is borne
by persons who share the same enclosed environment with an infectious,
but unsuspected, case of tuberculosis. Risk factors include the size of the
tubercle bacilli population in the source case, the efficiency with which
the bacilli are being excreted, the adequacy of ventilation in the environment, and the susceptibility of the individual who inhales the infectious nuclei (26). An outbreak or epidemic of tuberculosis may exist,

undetected, for several years in the nursing home setting. This relates to the frequent insidious nature of the disease, the turnover of persons in the populations, and the lack of information on the tuberculin status of the residents. Stead (4) has suggested that new tuberculous infections may be more common in elderly residents in nursing homes than is generally realized. Tuberculosis in this setting may produce serious disease and even death. One reported outbreak involved a 240-bed nursing home. This outbreak was caused by the presence of a highly infectious patient who was a gregarious 72-year-old man who had lived in the home for three years. He had had a chest roentgenogram read as "probably bronchogenic carcinoma." The patient had refused diagnostic studies and was returned to the nursing home. A persistent cough and weight loss were attributed to the "bronchogenic carcinoma." He moved about freely in the home and took part in the meals and social activities in the dining room. One year after his original hospitalization, he was rehospitalized with hemoptysis. A chest roentgenogram showed a cavitary infiltrate. Sputum smears showed many acid-fast bacilli, later confirmed to be *M. tuberculosis*. His unconfirmed "cancer" had, in fact, been active tuberculosis. During this period, 49 (30%) of 161 previous tuberculin-negative residents with a mean age of 73.5 years became infected. Eight (17%) developed progressive primary tuberculosis, including one who died. In addition, 21 (15%) of 138 tuberculin negative employees were infected, with one developing clinical tuberculosis. In addition to recognizing the index case, this epidemic was finally stopped by giving preventive treatment with isoniazid to all convertors despite their advanced ages.

Preventive Aspects

Control of tuberculosis in the nursing home should include a program for both residents and personnel (27). Identification of residents who harbor infection at the time of admission is important because it is among them that reactivation of old infection may occur. Both a tuberculin skin test and a chest roentgenogram should be included in preadmission screening.

TB Skin Testing. The standard tuberculin skin test is the Mantoux test. This test is recommended for screening and diagnosis of tuberculosis in the nursing home setting. The test is based on the principle that individuals infected with the tubercle bacillus develop a delayed hypersensitivity or cellular immunity. Five tuberculin units (TU) of polysorbate-80 stabilized purified protein derivative (PPD) is used; 0.1 ml is injected intracutaneously, usually in the volar aspect of the forearm. Most infected

Table 5.5. Patients for Whom Chemoprophylaxis with Isoniazid Is Recommended

1. Household members and other close associates of persons with recently diagnosed tuberculous disease
2. Positive tuberculin reactors with findings on the chest roentgenogram consistent with nonprogressive tuberculous disease, in whom there are neither positive bacteriologic findings nor a history of adequate chemotherapy
3. Newly infected persons
4. Positive tuberculin reactors in the following special clinical situations:
   a. Prolonged therapy with adrenocorticoids
   b. Immunosuppressive therapy
   c. Some hematologic reticuloendothelial diseases, such as leukemia or Hodgkin's disease
   d. Diabetes mellitus
   e. Silicosis
   f. After gastrectomy
5. Reactors without special risk factors, under the age of 35 years

Source: American Thoracic Society: Preventive therapy of tuberculous infection. *Am Rev Resp Dis* 110:371–374, 1974. Used with permission.

persons will respond to a 5-TU PPD test with 10 mm or more induration in 48 to 72 hours. It takes two to ten weeks after initial infection for the test to become positive. It usually remains positive throughout life. However, increased age is associated with waning of sensitivity and a false-negative test. A two-step skin test is recommended in the elderly who have not been skin-tested for years. The elderly, with a negative initial Mantoux test, should be retested using the same test in one to two weeks. The second test then may be positive because the first test "boosted" sensitivity to tuberculin. But this second test may also be "falsely negative" in the elderly because of an anergic state (suppression of delayed hypersensitivity). Anergy is associated with chronic diseases and drugs that suppress immunity (29). Both are frequently present in the elderly admitted to nursing homes. Thus, the chest roentgenogram remains an important tool for preadmission screening of tuberculosis in the elderly.

On admission, each resident should receive a tuberculosis classification (see Table 5.4). A history, tuberculin skin test, and chest roentgenogram will provide the data for this. Certain residents will be candidates to receive prophylactic therapy (chemoprophylaxis) based on these findings (Table 5.5).

Prophylaxis of Tuberculosis. Prophylactic therapy consists of administration of a one-year course of isoniazid 300 mg daily for adults. This is highly effective in preventing patients with tuberculous infection (class II) from developing pulmonary and extrapulmonary tuberculosis (class III). The guidelines for using isoniazid have been balanced against the potential for hepatotoxicity of the drug. This one major toxic side effect is a form of hepatitis that can cause death. The risk of this side effect increases with age, up to the age of 64. Case rates of hepatitis based on age have ranged as follows: less than 20 years = 0%, 20–34 = 0.3%, 35–49 = 1.2%, and 50–65 = 2.3%. (28). However, clinical monitoring for the prodromal symptoms of hepatitis (malaise, weakness, anorexia, nausea, and vomiting) will usually avert any serious side effects from isoniazid. Periodic laboratory tests may be indicated in high-risk persons—for example, the middle-aged alcoholic. If the laboratory tests reveal significant abnormalities in liver function, isoniazid therapy should usually be discontinued.

Individuals with positive skin tests who are not treated should have a notation made on the front of their chart. Whenever a nontreated reactor develops pulmonary symptoms, such as a persistent cough, he or she should be examined by chest roentgenogram and a sputum specimen submitted for culture of tuberculosis. Also, any unexplained fever or weight loss should also raise suspicion of recrudescence of the dormant infection.

Control of Tuberculosis in the Nursing Home.   The major risk to personnel is in contracting infection from inadvertent exposure to un-detected tuberculosis among residents (4). Each new employee should be tested with a tuberculin skin test and a record kept. Healthy reactors should also be considered for prophylactic therapy according to the guidelines in Table 5.5. Nonreactors should be skin-tested annually, and converters should be treated prophylactically with isoniazid if the chest roentgenogram shows no disease. If disease is present, two drugs are indicated for treatment. Converters not receiving prophylactic therapy should be examined by chest roentgenogram yearly and whenever pul-monary symptoms or loss of weight develop.

Careful epidemiologic investigation should be conducted when there is an inadvertent exposure to a "potential transmitter." Tuberculin skin tests should be immediately provided to those persons previously having a negative reaction to a skin test. Those who remain negative should be retested 6 to 10 weeks from the time of exposure. Preventive therapy may be necessary for some negative reactions if they have had heavy exposure (30).

Accurate records should always be kept on all skin tests performed on both residents and employees. This will help in monitoring infection rates and determining risks. Records should include the date of each tuberculin skin test and the method used. The measurement of the skin test reaction in millimeters of induration should be recorded. Those with a positive skin test should have dates and results of chest roentgenograms recorded. The dates of initiation and completion of preventive therapy should be documented. Also, the dates of diagnosis, initiation, and completion of any treatment for active tuberculosis should be recorded.

Reevaluation of the tuberculosis control program should be done annually by reviewing data of skin test results on residents and personnel. The best indication of effectiveness of an infection control program is the absence of new tuberculous infections.

REFERENCES

1. Kovar MG: Health of the elderly and use of health services. *Public Health Rep* 92:9–19, 1977.

2. Garibaldi RA, Brodine S, Matsumiya S: Infections among patients in nursing homes: Polices, prevalence, and problems. *N Engl J Med* 305:731–735, 1981.

3. Garb, JL, Brown RB, Garb JR, et al: Differences in etiology of pneumonias in nursing home and community patients. *JAMA* 240:2169–2172, 1978.

4. Stead WW: Tuberculosis among elderly persons: An outbreak in a nursing home. *Ann Intern Med* 94:606–610, 1981.

5. Center for Disease Control. Tuberculosis—North Dakota. *Morbid Mortal Weekly Rep* 29:465–467, 1980.

6. Austrian R, Gold J: Pneumococcal bacteremia with a special reference to bacteremic pneumococcal pneumonia. *Ann Intern Med* 60:759–776, 1964.

7. MillerWR, Jay AR: Staphylococcal pneumonia in influenza. *Arch Intern Med* 109:276–286, 1962.

8. Schreiner A, Bjerkestrand G, Digranes A, et al: Bacteriological findings in the transtracheal aspirate from patients with acute exacerbation of chronic bronchitis. *Infection* 6:54–56, 1978.

9. Wallace, RJ, Musher, DM, Martin RR: *Hemophilus influenzae* pneumonia in adults. *Am J Med* 64:87–93, 1978.

10. Ebright, JR, Rytel, MW: Bacterial pneumonia in the elderly. *J AM Geriatr Soc* 28:220–223, 1980.

11. Sullivan, AJ, Jr, Dowdle WR, Marihe WM, et al,: Adult pneumonia in a general hospital: Etiology and risk factors, *Arch Intern Med* 129:935–942, 1972.

12. Pierce, AK, Sanford, JP: Aerobic gram-negative bacillary pneumonias. *Am Rev Resp Dis* 110:647–658, 1974.

13. Bartlett, JR, Finegold, SM: Anaerobic infections of the lung and pleural space. *Am Rev. Resp Dis* 110:56–77, 1974.

14. Bartlett, JG, Gorbach, SL: The triple threat of aspiration pneumonia. *Chest* 68:560–566, 1975.

15. Meyer RD, Finegold SM: Legionnaires' disease. *Ann Rev Med* 31:219–232, 1980.

16. Dhar, S, Shastri, SR, Lenora RAK: Aging and the respiratory system. *Med Clin N AM* 60:1121–1139, 1976.

17. Penn RG, Sanders WE, Jr, Sanders CC: Colonization of the oropharynx with gram-negative bacilli: A major antecedent to nosocomial pneumonia. *Am J Infect Control* 9:25–34, 1981.

18. Valenti WM, Trudell RG, Bentley DW: Factors predisposing to oropharyngeal colonization with gram-negative bacilli in the aged. *N Engl J Med* 298:1108–1111, 1978.

19. Sanford, JP, and Pierce AK: Lower respiratory tract infections, in Bennett JV and Brachman PS (ed): *Hospital Infections*. Boston, Little, Brown, 1979, pp 255–286.

20. Simmons BP, Wong ES: Guidelines for prevention of nosocomial pneumonia. *Infect Control* 3:327–333, 1982.

21. *Recommendations for the Disinfection and Maintenance of Respiratory Therapy Equipment*. Atlanta, Hospital Infections Branch and Hospital Infections Laboratory Section, Epidemic Investigations Branch, Bacterial Diseases Division, Bureau of Epidemiology, Center for Disease Control, 1977, pp 1–12.

22. *The Control of Pulmonary Infections Associated with Tracheostomy*. Atlanta, Hospital Infections and Microbiologic Control Branches, Bacterial Diseases Division, Bureau of Epidemiology, Center for Disease Control, 1979, pp 1–3.

23. Goodman RA, Orenstein WA, Munro TF, et al: Impact of influenza A in a nursing home. *JAMA* 247:1451–1453, 1982.

24. Johnston RF, and Wildrick KH: "State of the art" review: The impact of chemotherapy on the care of patients with tuberculosis. *Am Rev Resp Dis* 109:636–660, 1974.

25. Ad Hoc Committee to Revise Diagnostic Standards, American Thoracic Society, Scientific Assembly on Tuberculosis: *Diagnostic Standards and Classification of Tuberculosis and Other Mycobacterial Diseases*. New York, American Lung Association, 1981.

26. Leff, A, and Geppect, EF: Public health and preventive aspects of pulmonary tuberculosis. Infectiousness, epidemiology, risk factors, classification and preventive therapy. *Arch Intern Med* 139:1405–1410, 1979.

27. American Thoracic Society: Screening for pulmonary tuberculosis in institutions. *Am Rev Resp Dis* 115:901–906, 1977.

28. American Thoracic Society: Preventive therapy of tuberculous infection. *Am Rev Resp Dis* 110:371–374, 1974.

29. Reichman LB: Tuberculin skin testing: The state of the art. *Chest* 76 (suppl.): 764–770, 1979.

30. American Thoracic Society: Guidelines for the investigation and management of tuberculosis contacts. *Am Rev Resp Dis* 114:459–463, 1976.

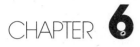
URINARY TRACT INFECTION

Philip W. Smith

CLINICAL ASPECTS OF URINARY TRACT INFECTION

The term *urinary tract infection* (UTI) includes urethritis, cystitis (bladder infection), and pyelonephritis (kidney infection), but most commonly refers to bacterial cystitis (see Figure 6.1).

Host Defenses

The most important host defense against urinary tract infection is mechanical: The normal unidirectional flow of urine prevents perineal bacteria from ascending up the urethra to the bladder. In addition, antibodies are secreted in the urine.

Neurogenic bladder, urethroceles, ureterovesical reflux, and bladder diverticuli impair the rapid and complete emptying of the bladder. Diabetic visceral neuropathy frequently results in abnormal bladder contractility and incomplete emptying. Urinary tract stricture and prostatic hypertrophy result in functional obstruction to urinary flow. All the above disorders predispose to UTI because of decreased bacterial clearance and because residual urine provides a good growth medium for bacteria. Urinary catheterization and cystoscopy predispose to urinary tract infection by introducing bacteria upstream into the normally sterile bladder.

Few lower urinary tract infections develop into pyelonephritis because of the downstream flow of urine from the kidney to the bladder and because of host defenses. Upper tract obstruction, diabetes mellitus, and renal calculi predispose to ascending infection and pyelonephritis by interfering with urine flow or providing a nidus for infection.

Epidemiology

As might be expected, the leading causes of bacterial UTIs are the bacteria that comprise bowel and perineal flora. Periurethral colonization

URINARY TRACT

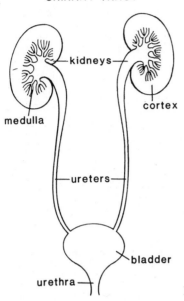

Figure 6.1.   The urinary tract.

with pathogenic organisms frequently precedes urinary tract infection (1). The bacteria most often responsible for UTIs are gram-negative bacilli: *Escherichia coli, Klebsiella, Proteus, Enterobacter,* and *Pseudomonas. E. coli* accounts for 90% of UTIs, particularly in the community. Enterococcal streptococci, *Staphylococcus aureus, S. epidermidis,* and *Candida albicans* are occasional pathogens.

Urinary tract infection is much more common in women because of the shorter female urethra and the correspondingly greater chance of ascent by perineal bacteria. In females ages 15–35 years, UTI is particularly common, reflecting the effects of sexual activity and pregnancy on local urinary defenses. Prostatitis is the leading antecedent to urinary tract infection in males; the infected prostate provides a focus of infection that spreads to the bladder.

Manifestations

Dysuria, urgency, and frequency signal a UTI, but the patient may be asymptomatic. Fever, flank pain, and costovertebral angle tenderness are classically associated with pyelonephritis. However, symptoms may mislead the physician about localization of a UTI.

In the patient without anatomic or functional abnormalities of the urinary tract, the vast majority of UTIs, whether treated or not, will resolve without complications. Bacteremia is not common unless urinary tract instrumentation has taken place; metastatic infection, perinephric abscess, and intrarenal abscess are rare but serious sequelae of pyelonephritis. It is most unusual for even recurrent UTIs to result in chronic renal failure. Most cases of chronic pyelonephritis are associated with obvious structural defects of the urinary tract.

Diagnosis

The vast majority of patients with urinary tract infection have significant numbers of white blood cells in the urine on urinalysis (pyuria). White blood cell casts are suggestive of pyelonephritis. The urinalysis, then, will provide rapid evidence of a urinary tract infection long before final urine culture results are available. The isolation and identification of the bacteria responsible for urinary tract infection generally takes 24 to 48 hours.

The urine culture is the cornerstone of the diagnosis. The urine culture should be obtained prior to institution of antibiotic therapy, since even a single dose of an antibiotic may interfere with the growth of bacteria on culture. The periurethral area must be cleansed prior to collection of the specimen because the terminal urethra and periurethral skin are colonized with bacteria, particularly in the female and uncircumcised male. Even clean-catch, midstream urine cultures are contaminated by some bacteria. As a result, quantitative urine cultures are employed, with a level of 100,000 bacteria per milliliter of urine separating infection from contamination.

Less than 1000 bacteria per milliliter, multiple bacterial isolates, or the presence of common contaminants (e.g., lactobacilli) suggests an improperly collected specimen or the absence of infection. Catheterization of the bladder to obtain a urine culture will facilitate collection of a proper sample, particularly in an uncooperative patient. However, this procedure does not circumvent the problem of perineal contamination, and carries a small (1–3%) risk of introducing urinary pathogens. Occasionally, a suprapubic bladder aspiration for culture will be needed to confirm an infection.

There are a number of pitfalls in the cultural diagnosis of urinary tract infection. The specimen should be processed within two hours of the time it is obtained or overgrowth of bacterial contaminants may result (2). Refrigeration of urine will slow the growth of bacteria and is advisable if delays in processing are unavoidable.

In addition, female patients in particular need to be explicitly instructed in obtaining a good midstream, clean-catch specimen. Useful instructions for patients have been outlined (3). Some of the key points stressed in the ambulatory female include comfortable positioning on an appropriate seat, washing of hands, spreading of the labia with one hand, washing of urethral area with soaped sponges, and obtaining a midstream specimen. In the bedridden patient, the nurse must cleanse the perineum, separate the labia, and obtain the midstream specimen herself; the nurse should, of course, wear gloves during the procedure. When urethral catheterization is employed, aseptic technique should be used. The technician should wash hands and wear gloves, the meatus should be thoroughly cleansed, and the catheter should be lubricated. Suprapubic needle aspiration should be performed by a physician with appropriate skin preparation.

Therapy

Outpatients with lower tract infection are almost always infected with *E. coli*. Because of the sensitivity of most *E. coli* to antibiotics and the high urinary levels achieved by many antibiotics, eradication of infection is usually readily accomplished. A sulfonamide is the initial agent of choice; nalidixic acid, nitrofurantoin, ampicillin, trimethoprim, trimethoprim/ sulfamethoxazole, and oral cephalosporins are good alternatives. Nursing home–associated urinary tract infections are more likely to be caused by more resistant bacteria such as *Proteus mirabilis*. Therapy with ampicillin, a cephalosporin, or trimethoprim/sulfamethoxazole may be useful in this setting. Hospital-acquired urinary tract infection is often caused by even more resistant organisms, such as *Pseudomonas aeruginosa*, and parenteral therapy with aminoglycosides (gentamicin, tobramycin, or amikacin) is often required. Liberal fluid intake is also advisable. In addition to bacterial washout, it may improve the immunologic response of the kidney.

The recommended duration of therapy is generally 5–7 days for cystitis and 10–14 days for pyelonephritis. There has been a tendency toward shorter duration of therapy for lower urinary tract infections. In fact, single-dose therapy with a variety of antimicrobial agents has been shown to be effective in certain settings (4). Complicated or persistent urinary tract infections require prolonged therapy for 4–6 weeks.

Antibiotics used in the treatment of urinary tract infections are excreted by the kidneys. In the presence of renal insufficiency, a number of these drugs, particularly sulfonamides, aminoglycosides, tetracycline, nitrofurantoin, and nalidixic acid should be either avoided entirely or used in significantly reduced dosage.

Most patients who have repeated urinary tract infections will be found to have recurrences of UTIs with different bacteria. These patients will generally be young women between the ages of 15–35. Occasionally, repeat infection will be shown to be due to the same bacterial strain (relapse), in which case a longer trial of an appropriate antibiotic is indicated.

Bacteriuria

Bacteriuria, defined as 100,000 or more bacteria per milliliter of a properly collected urine specimen, is commonly seen in urinary tract infections. The patient often has symptoms, such as fever or dysuria, and the urinalysis reveals pyuria. However, bacteriuria may occur without other signs or symptoms of infection (asymptomatic bacteriuria). In this context, bacteriuria may not indicate a true infection, with invasion of the genitourinary tract mucosa, but rather colonization of the genitourinary tract without evidence of disease production.

Like urinary tract infection, bacteriuria is much more common in women than in men. The overall prevalence of bacteriuria in an unselected population was 3.5%, increasing with age in a linear fashion (5). The significance of asymptomatic bacteriuria in the general population is controversial. Asymptomatic bacteriuria does not usually require therapy.

Urinary Tract Infection in the Elderly

A number of factors contribute to the increased risk of UTI in the elderly. First, the elderly are more likely to have underlying diseases that predispose to UTI, such as diabetic visceral neuropathy, prostatitis, and kidney stones. Secondly, urethral flora changes with advancing age (6), and in the elderly gram-negative bacilli such as *E. coli* and *Proteus* are often found (7). Finally, a major determinant of urinary tract infection in the elderly is the progressively increasing risk of urinary tract instrumentation and catheterization with advancing age.

NURSING HOME URINARY TRACT INFECTIONS

Epidemiology

Surveys of infections acquired in nursing homes have demonstrated the importance of UTIs in long-term care facilities. In two surveys, UTIs were the leading nosocomial infection in nursing homes. Magnussen found a nosocomial infection rate of 18.2%, with UTIs accounting for

Table 6.1.   Nursing Home Urinary Tract Infections: Risk Factors

Indwelling bladder catheter
Urinary tract instrumentation
Urinary tract pathology (e.g., kidney stones)
Prostatitis
Systemic diseases (e.g., diabetes)
Dehydration
Incontinence

72% of the infections (8). Of these residents, 48% had indwelling or suprapubic catheters. A survey at a skilled nursing facility found UTIs comprising 82% of infections, 43% occurring in catheterized residents (9).

The most important risk factor for UTIs in the nursing home is the presence of an indwelling bladder catheter (see Figure 6.2). The catheter predisposes not only to asymptomatic and symptomatic urinary tract infection, but also to complications of UTI, such as bacterial sepsis. In Garibaldi's prevalence study of nursing homes, 85% of residents with indwelling catheters had asymptomatic bacteriuria (10). Gleckman studied 13 elderly patients admitted to the hospital with catheter-related urosepsis, most of them from nursing homes. In these patients, he uniformly found an identifiable traumatic event that appeared to initiate the acute septic episode, such as catheter obstruction, catheter manipulation, or removal of an inflated indwelling bladder catheter within 72 hours before hospital admission (11).

Urinary incontinence is frequent in nursing home residents and was identified in 50% of elderly nursing home residents in a survey of seven nursing homes (12). Urinary incontinence was important because of its association with fecal incontinence and other complications, although urinary tract infection and skin breakdown were significantly more common in catheterized residents than in catheter-free, incontinent residents. Other predisposing factors for nursing home UTIs can be identified (see Table 6.1).

Etiology

Gram-negative bacteria cause the vast majority of UTIs (see Table 6.2). Nursing home UTIs generally occupy a place intermediate between community-acquired and hospital-acquired UTIs in terms of bacterial antibiotic resistance. Community-acquired UTIs are most often caused by *E. coli,* and testing usually reveals sensitivity to all commonly used oral antibiotics.

Table 6.2.   Nursing Home Urinary Tract Infections: Leading Organisms

Proteus spp.
Enterococci
Escherichia coli
Providencia spp.
Klebsiella spp.
Pseudomonas aeruginosa

In the nursing home, the leading isolates in UTIs have been *Proteus* spp. (9,11). *Proteus,* other gram-negative bacilli, and enterococci are more prevalent than *E. coli.* Compared to community-acquired UTIs, nursing home UTIs are more likely to be polymicrobic (10) and are more likely to be resistant to the oral antibiotics commonly used for urinary tract infections, such as ampicillin, cephalothin, tetracycline, and trimethoprim/sulfamethoxazole. These findings underscore the importance of proper culture of urine before therapy of nursing home-acquired urinary tract infections, and the need for reliance upon aminoglycoside therapy when the resident is critically ill with suspected urinary tract–related sepsis.

In planning therapy, it is also important to consider the immediate prior medical history of the resident. Sherman found that 63% of nursing home–associated urinary tract infections were acquired in the nursing facility, while 37% were acquired during a preceding stay in a general hospital (9). The infections acquired in the hospital were still more antibiotic-resistant than those acquired in the nursing home, with *Pseudomonas aeruginosa* being the single most common urinary tract isolate.

The urinary tract is the leading site of nosocomial infection in hospitals. In the hospital setting, urinary tract infection is responsible for about 40% of all nosocomial infections, and the majority of these patients have undergone prior urinary tract instrumentation or catheterization. Interestingly, urinary catheterization appears to be a more frequent predisposing factor in hospital-acquired urinary tract infections than in nursing home–acquired infections.

Pathogenesis of Urinary Tract Infections

Residents without urinary catheters acquire bacteriuria by intraluminal ascent of fecal bacteria that normally contaminate the distal urethra. In catheterized residents, bacteria ascend up the urethra either around the catheter or inside the catheter. The former mechanism is probably of greater importance in view of the association between positive meatal cultures and subsequent acquisition of bacteriuria (13).

The risk of UTI following catheterization is proportional to the length of time the catheter remains in place. With an "in-and-out" catheterization, the risk of UTI is approximately 1–2%, but if the catheter is allowed to remain in place as an indwelling catheter, the risk of UTI increases progressively. Another important determinant of infection is the type of system used. The risk of bacteriuria is approximately 90–95% after three to four days with use of an open drainage system. With use of a sterile, properly inserted closed drainage system, the risk of bacteriuria is about one-third this, although eventually bacteriuria is nearly universal (14).

Prolonged urinary catheterization not only increases the risk of urinary tract infection, but also increases the likelihood of developing infection with a more resistant bacteria. *E coli* and *Proteus* cause a smaller percentage of urinary tract infections as the period of catheterization lengthens, whereas *Serratia, Pseudomonas,* and *Klebsiella* increase in relative incidence (15). This is due to the elimination of sensitive organisms by antibiotics and colonization with more resistant institutional flora.

In most instances, the bacteria that cause urinary tract infection originate from the resident's own perineal flora. Cross-contamination of urinary catheters or transmission of bacteria from patient to patient by the hands of personnel occurs less frequently (10–15%), but is still an extremely important mode of spread of organisms (15).

Epidemic Urinary Tract Infections

Hospital epidemics of urinary tract infections have been traced to urometers, urine measuring devices (16,17) and even bedpans (18). While the greatest epidemic potential is associated with colonization of patients who have indwelling bladder catheters, even patients with condom catheter drainage systems may serve as reservoirs of gram-negative bacteria (19). Epidemics may also be traced to the movement of a patient who is colonized with an epidemic strain from one ward to another (20). The final common pathway, however, for most epidemics of urinary tract infection is the hands of personnel caring for patients (21).

Similar factors predispose to UTIs in the nursing home. In addition, clustering of urinary tract infections suggesting an epidemic is not rare in nursing homes (11).

One of the most hazardous aspects of outbreaks of nosocomial urinary tract infections is the fact that they are generally caused by gram-negative bacteria that are resistant to many antibiotics (see Chapter 11). Outbreaks of multiply antibiotic-resistant bacteria causing hospital UTIs are very common, and have been reported with *Klebsiella, Serratia, Proteus, Pseudomonas, Providencia,* and other gram-negative bacilli. Factors that contribute to these outbreaks include previous antibiotic therapy, urinary catheterization, and inadequate handwashing by personnel (21–23). Resistance to multiple antibiotics appears to be significantly more frequent in epidemic than in sporadic cases of nosocomial UTI (23).

PREVENTION AND CONTROL OF URINARY TRACT INFECTIONS IN THE NURSING HOME

Antibiotic Suppressive Therapy

The use of antibiotics is frequently associated with the emergence of multiply antibiotic-resistant bacteria that have the potential for causing outbreaks of nosocomial UTIs. Many studies have confirmed both the potential hazards and the lack of effectiveness of antibiotics in the prevention of nosocomial UTIs, especially in the catheterized person (24–26). Antibiotics do not prevent infection of the catheterized resident, but select out resistant strains of bacteria, which in turn may cause infection. Similarly, antibiotic irrigation in catheterized residents is ineffective and should not be used (27,28). Any theoretical advantage of instilling an antibacterial substance into the bladder appears to be outweighed by the hazards of breaking the closed catheter system, with the attendant risk of introducing institutional bacteria.

Control of Epidemic Urinary Tract Infections

As discussed above, an important percentage of institutionally acquired urinary tract infections occur in epidemics. The reservoir for the bacteria that cause epidemic UTIs is often a catheterized resident, and the organisms are spread by cross-infection.

The key to epidemic control is early detection of outbreaks by an effective surveillance system (see Chapter 9). Vigilance for potential epidemics must be maintained, especially in high-risk groups such as residents with indwelling bladder catheters or underlying diseases of the urinary tract that predispose to UTIs.

Recognition of clinical and asymptomatic urinary tract infections requires criteria for the diagnosis of urinary tract infection, an ongoing surveillance system of some type, and the ability to culture the urine in residents suspected of having a UTI. Confirmation of an outbreak of antibiotic-resistant bacteria causing UTIs also requires antibiotic susceptibility testing of bacterial isolates. An epidemic is suggested by a significant increase in the incidence of UTI in a nursing home or an increase in the number of urinary tract isolates of a particular bacteria, especially if it is a somewhat unusual organism such as *Providentia stuartii* or *Serratia marcescens*.

An outbreak of multiply resistant gram-negative bacilli causing epidemic urinary tract infections is heralded by the presence of bacteria with an identical antibiotic resistance pattern. Since resistance factors may be passed from one genus of bacteria to another, an identical resistance pattern may emerge in several different bacterial strains.

The evaluation and control of an epidemic is discussed further in Chapter 10. These are some specific measures for interrupting a UTI epidemic:

1. Handwashing procedures should be reviewed and emphasized. This is especially important in view of the fact that most epidemics can be traced to hand carriage of bacteria by personnel.

2. Residents with urine culture positive for the epidemic strain, especially if it is a multiply resistant strain, should be placed in some type of isolation. At a minimum, it is recommended that residents be placed in a separate room and that gloves be worn during all perineal care and urinary catheter manipulation (see Fig. 11.2, Chapter 11). Such isolation precautions have been shown to interrupt epidemics (21,23,29).

3. Residents with indwelling urinary catheters, whether or not they are infected, should be separated from one another. At a minimum, this means separate rooms. The rationale for this measure is the observation that catheterized individuals have the highest risk of acquiring epidemic strains and subsequently developing infection (23).

4. During an outbreak, all relevant bacterial isolates should be saved by the microbiology laboratory or reference laboratory in the event that future studies, such as serotyping or quantitative antibiotic sensitivity testing, become desirable later in the course of the investigation.

5. Careful records should be kept on all the residents involved in the epidemic, including name, age, room, culture results, and antibiotic administration information.

6. Special care should be taken in the disposal of urine, since urometers, urine collection devices, and bedpans may serve as vectors for transmitting infection.

7. Antibiotics should be used very judiciously to avoid the selection of antibiotic-resistant bacteria.

8. Policies and procedures for cleaning or disinfection of equipment that comes in contact with the resident should be reviewed. In one outbreak, it was demonstrated that urinals were used to empty the urine drainage bags of catheterized patients and then randomly redistributed, resulting in exchange of urinals among patients and rooms. This was felt to contribute to the outbreak (19).

9. It has been recommended that residents newly admitted to a long-term care facility from a general hospital who have a confirmed UTI should be separated for one week from catheterized residents already in the institution to minimize the chance of introduction of an epidemic strain from a hospital, a problem that may be common (9).

General Preventive Measures

Prevention of UTIs in the nursing home involves controlling the major risk factors (see Table 6.3). Measures include minimizing urinary tract instrumentation and catheterization, correcting treatable host problems (such as urinary tract obstruction, diabetes mellitus, and prostatitis) as much as possible, maintaining adequate hydration, evaluating incontinence, and minimizing antibiotic usage.

Up to 50% of the elderly in institutions have a problem with incontinence. The risk of UTI is significantly less in catheter-free incontinent residents than in catheterized nursing home residents (12). Diapers, while inconvenient, are preferred to an indwelling bladder catheter. Ouslander, in a survey of seven nursing homes, noted that many residents had not been evaluated for treatable causes of incontinence, and many were receiving drugs that could affect continence, such as psychotropic drugs, autonomic drugs, or diuretics (12).

Table 6.3. Nosocomial Urinary Tract Infection Prevention

General measures
1. Treat underlying diseases (e.g., prostatitis, diabetes).
2. Maintain adequate hydration.
3. Evaluate incontinence.
4. Detect epidemics of UTIs promptly.

Measures relating to catheterization
1. Minimize indwelling catheters.
2. Insert catheters aseptically.
3. Use closed systems.
4. Maintain good urinary flow.

URINARY CATHETER SYSTEM

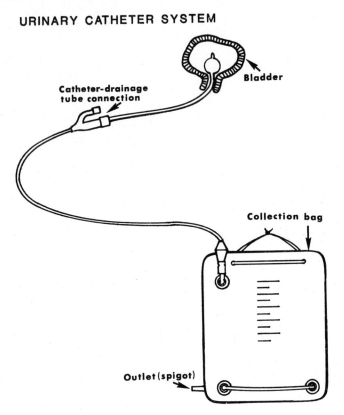

Figure 6.2. A urinary drainage system.

Proper Use of Urinary Catheters

The best way to prevent UTIs is to minimize the use of indwelling urinary catheters (see Figure 6.2). Catheters should be used only for legitimate indications (urinary tract obstruction, urinary retention, or obtaining accurate measurements of urinary output in critically ill residents) and not for the convenience of nursing home personnel or physicians.

Condom catheters appear to be safer than indwelling Foley catheters but require meticulous nursing care in order to avoid local complications such as skin maceration. In addition, there are some infectious risks associated with the condom catheter itself (20,30). In some individuals, especially women, a suprapubic catheter has the theoretical advantage of avoiding perineal flora. For certain types of bladder-emptying dysfunction, such as spinal cord injuries, intermittent catheterization is commonly employed. In spite of the theoretical risks of urethral trauma, this technique may in fact result in fewer UTIs than a permanent indwelling bladder catheter, although rigorous studies are lacking (31).

The Closed System.   When residents do require an indwelling urethral catheter, a closed system should be used. A number of features are now used to decrease the need for opening the drainage system, thereby minimizing the chance of contamination. These include the addition of a urine-sampling port in the drainage tubing, the preconnected catheter/collecting tube system, and the insertion of airvents, drip chambers, or one-way valves designed to prevent reflux of contaminated urine.

It has been shown that strict adherence to care of closed drainage systems can be expected to reduce rates of catheter-associated infections. Garibaldi noted common errors in the management of closed drainage systems, such as the frequent opening of the drainage system (which often resulted in bag contamination), improper positioning of drainage bag, and unclamped outflow spigots (26). High rates of drainage bag contamination followed catheter manipulation, and acquisition of bacteriuria often followed bag contamination when catheters were cared for improperly.

Irrigation of catheters with antibiotics does not prevent infection and should be avoided. Any benefits of the irrigation are outweighed by the opening of the system (27,28). When irrigation is necessary (e.g., to prevent obstruction due to bleeding), intermittent irrigation is preferred to continuous irrigation (32).

In order to preserve the closed system, urine samples should be obtained properly, preferably through the distal sampling port after cleansing with a disinfectant, or obtained aseptically from the drainage bag.

Catheter Insertion.   The catheter should be inserted aseptically by experienced personnel. There is evidence that the risk of acquiring bacteriuria increases with the inexperience of the person inserting the catheter (26). The risk of acquiring bacteriuria within 48 hours was 10% for patients catheterized by a physician, 21% for patients catheterized by a R.N., and 34% for those catheterized by an L.P.N.

Catheter insertion should thus be performed by experienced personnel using aseptic technique and sterile equipment. Gloves, drapes, sponges, an appropriate antiseptic solution for periurethral cleansing, and a single-use packet of lubricant jelly are needed for insertion. The smallest catheter possible should be selected, and an indwelling catheter should be properly secured after insertion. In the female a catheter about size 14

French is used, while in the male a catheter of size 16 or 18 F is recommended (3).

Catheter Care. Important elements of catheter care include maintaining unobstructed urine flow, providing adequate fluid intake for residents, handwashing by personnel before and after catheter manipulation (to prevent cross-infection), avoiding prophylactic antibiotics in the catheterized resident, and securing the catheter.

Collecting bags should be emptied regularly and positioned correctly. If the bag is not below the level of the bladder, reflux may occur. The bag should, however, not be allowed to fall onto the floor, where contamination may occur. Condom catheters should be changed on a regular basis (e.g., daily).

Catheters should not be changed on a regular schedule, but rather when malfunctioning or contaminated (26). Frequent changes may result in urethral trauma. Hand restraints should be used to avoid trauma to the urethra for agitated or confused residents who tug at their catheters.

The role of meatal care is controversial. Cleansing of the meatus at the meatal–catheter junction has traditionally been performed once or twice per day with soap and water, or povidone–iodine solution, since meatal colonization by gram-negative bacteria may occur before urinary tract infection (13). However, this method has not been scientifically proven, and recent studies suggest that it is not useful. In the well-controlled study by Burke (33), the risk of bacteriuria was actually higher in the group treated with povidone–iodine solution and ointment or with a nonantiseptic solution of green soap and water than in the control group that was not given special meatal care. At the present time, meatal care regimens are not recommended (32).

One final issue to be addressed is the question of efficacy of installation of hydrogen peroxide in the urinary catheter drainage bag. In one study, 30 ml of 3% hydrogen peroxide were instilled into urinary catheter bags in patients with Foley catheter systems. In small numbers of patients, this was demonstrated to decrease bacterial contamination of the drainage bag and also to reduce drainage bag bacteriuria (34). However, this study has been criticized (35). In addition, there is a theoretical objection to this practice, since the majority of urinary tract infections appear to occur by ascent of bacteria around the outside of the catheter (13) and not from the bag up through the inside of the catheter. Thus, it does not appear that hydrogen peroxide installation will have a great impact on catheter-associated UTIs.

Detailed techniques have been described for catheter care, aspiration of urine specimens, irrigation methods, self-catheterization, application external catheters in the male, and comparison of various catheter systems (3). Each nursing home should develop its own policies and procedure that will minimize the risk of UTIs in its residents.

REFERENCES

1. Kunin CM, Polyak F, Postel E: Periurethral bacterial flora in women: Prolonged intermittent colonization with *Escherichia coli. JAMA* 243:134–139, 1980.
2. Hindman R, Tronic B, Bartlett R: Effect of delay on culture of urine. *J Clin Micro* 4:102–103, 1976.
3. Kunin CM: *Detection, Prevention, and Management of Urinary Tract Infections* 3rd ed Philadelphia, Lea & Febiger, 1979.
4. Souney P, Polk BF: Single-dose antimicrobial therapy for urinary tract infections in women. *Rev Infect Dis* 4:29–34, 1982.
5. Evans DA, Williams DN, Laughlin LW, et al: Bacteriuria in a population-based cohort of women, *J Infect Dis* 138:768–773, 1978.
6. Marrie TJ, Swantree CA, Hartlen M: Aerobic and anaerobic urethral flora of healthy females in various physiological age groups and of females with urinary tract infections. *J Clin Micro* 11:654–659, 1980.
7. Alling B, Brandberg A, Seeberg S, et al: Aerobic and anaerobic microbial flora in the urinary tract of geriatric patients during long-term care. *J Infect Dis* 127:34–39, 1973.
8. Magnussen MH, Robb SS: Nosocomial infections in a long-term care facility. *Am J Infect Control* 8:12–17, 1980.
9. Sherman FT, Tucci V, Libow LS, et al: Nosocomial urinary tract infections in a skilled nursing facility. *J Am Geriatr Soc* 28:456–461, 1980.
10. Garibaldi RA, Brodine S, Matsumiya S: Infections among patients in nursing homes: Policies, prevalence, and problems. *N Engl J Med* 305:731–735, 1981.
11. Gleckman R, Blagg N, Hibert D, et al: Catheter-related urosepsis in the elderly: A prospective study of community-acquired infections. *J Am Geriatr Soc* 30:255–257, 1982.
12. Ouslander JG, Kane RL, Abrass IB: Urinary incontinence in elderly nursing home patients. *JAMA* 248:1194–1198, 1982.
13. Garibaldi RA, Burke JP, Britt MR, et al: Meatal colonization and catheter-associated bacteriuria. *N Engl J Med* 303:316–318, 1980.
14. Fass RJ, Klainer AS, Perkins RL: Urinary tract infection: Practical aspects of diagnosis and treatment. *JAMA* 225:1509–1513, 1973.
15. Turck M, Stamm W: Nosocomial infections of the urinary tract. *Am J Med* 70:651–654, 1981.

16. Rutala WA, Kennedy VA, Loflin HB, et al: *Serratia marcescens* nosocomial infections of the urinary tract associated with urine measuring containers and urinometers. *Am J Med* 70:659–663, 1981.

17. Kocka FE, Roemisch E, Causey WA, et al: The urometer as a reservoir of infectious organisms. *Am J Clin Path* 67:106–107, 1977.

18. McLeod DW: The hospital urine bottle and bedpan as reservoirs of infection by *Pseudomonas pyocyanea. Lancet* 1:394–397, 1958.

19. Fierer J, Ekstrom M: An outbreak of *Providentia stuartii* urinary tract infections: Patients with condom catheters are a reservoir of the bacteria. *JAMA* 245:1553–1555, 1981.

20. Whiteley GR, Penner JL, Stewart IO, et al: Nosocomial urinary tract infections caused by two O-serotypes of *Providentia stuartii* in one hospital. *J Clin Micro* 6:551–554, 1977.

21. Schaberg DR, Weinstein RA, Stamm WE: Epidemics of nosocomial urinary tract infection caused by multiply resistant gram-negative bacilli: Epidemiology and control. *J Infect Dis* 133:363–366, 1976.

22. Finland M: Nosocomial epidemics seriatim: Multidrug-resistant bacteria and R factors. *Arch Intern Med* 137:585–587, 1977.

23. Schaberg DR, Haley RW, Highsmith AK, et al: Nosocomial bacteriuria: A prospective study of case clustering and antibiotic resistance. *Ann Intern Med* 93:420–424, 1980.

24. Britt MR, Garibaldi RA, Miller WA, et al: Antimicrobial prophylaxis for catheter-associated bacteriuria. *Antimicrob Agents Chemother* 11:240:253, 1977.

25. Clayton CL, Chawla JC, Stickler DJ: Some observations on urinary tract infections in patients undergoing long-term bladder catheterizations. *J Hosp Infect* 3:39–47, 1982.

26. Garibaldi RA, Burke JP, Dickman ML, et al: Factors predisposing to bacteriuria during indwelling urethral catheterization. *N Engl J Med* 291:215–219, 1974.

27. Haldorson AN, Keys TF, Maker MD, et al: Nonvalue of neomycin instillation after intermittent urinary catheterization. *Antimicrob Agents Chemother* 14:368–370, 1978.

28. Warren JW, Platt R, Thomas RJ, et al: Antibiotic irrigation and catheter-associated urinary tract infections. *N Engl J Med* 299:570–573, 1978.

29. Smith PW, Rusnak PG: Aminoglycoside-resistant *Pseudomonas aeruginosa* urinary tract infections: Study of an outbreak. *J Hosp Infect* 2:71–75, 1981.

30. Hirsh DD, Fainstein V, Musher DM: Do condom catheter collecting systems cause urinary tract infections? *JAMA* 242:340–341, 1979.

31. Lapides J, Diokno AC, Gould FR, et al: Further observations on self-catheterization. *J Urol* 116:169–171, 1976.

32. Centers for Disease Control: Guidelines for prevention of catheter-associated urinary tract infections. *Infect Control* 2:119–130, 1981.

33. Burke JP, Garibaldi RA, Britt MR, et al: Prevention of catheter-associated urinary tract infections: Efficacy of daily meatal care regimens. *Am J Med* 70:655–658, 1981.

34. Maizels M, Schaeffer AJ: Decreased incidence of bacteriuria associated with the periodic instillation of hydrogen peroxide into the urethral catheter drainage bag. *J Urol* 123:841–845, 1980.

35. Sarubbi FA, Rutala WA, Samsa G: Hydrogen peroxide instillation into the urinary drainage bag: Should we or shouldn't we? *Infect Control* 10:70–73, 1982.

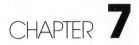

CHAPTER **7**

DECUBITUS ULCERS

Brenda L. W. Hagan

EPIDEMIOLOGY OF DECUBITUS ULCERS

Decubitus ulcer, bedsore, and *pressure sore* are terms that evoke feelings of frustration in the health care team. However, this is an area in which nursing skill can be applied to its fullest measure. Variously referred to as decubitus ulcer (decubitus meaning "lying down") and bedsore (the occurrence being attributed to confinement to bed), the term **pressure sore** more correctly reflects the underlying pathophysiology. Pressure over an area leads to decreased blood flow. Without the nutrients and oxygen supplied by the blood, cells begin to die. When there is a greater cell loss than the immediate healing potential, a pressure sore results.

About 30% of the nursing home population develops a pressure sore (1). Of bedridden patients, 10–15% will develop a pressure sore. The vast majority occur in the lower part of the body (over the sacrum, coccyx, ischial tuberosities, and greater trochanters), and 70–90% are superficial. The healing time ranges from 15 to 55 days and requires very costly medical care. The average cost is several thousand dollars per decubitus ulcer (2).

A pressure sore is not only painful, but it can also lead to serious sequelae. The necrotic debris provides a good growth medium for bacteria, and resultant infections are often caused by multiple bacteria, which complicates the treatment plan. Polymicrobial infections generally include both gram-positive organisms *(Staphylococcus aureus,* enterococcus) and gram-negative bacteria such as *Pseudomonas* spp. and *Enterobacteriaceae.* When there is fecal contamination of the ulcer, anaerobes such as *Clostridium* and *Bacteroides* spp. grow well in deep wounds where oxygen tension is low. Once established, these infections can spread throughout the body by blood and lymphatic systems with resultant septicemia and mortality. When sepsis occurs, the pressure sore should be suspected as a source in the absence of another infection such as a urinary tract infection

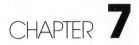

124

or pneumonia (3). Deep ulcers can extend to underlying muscle and bone, causing osteomyelitis (infection of the bone) or joint deformities that compromise weight bearing.

PHYSIOLOGY AND PATHOPHYSIOLOGY

Physiology

The skin is the largest body organ. It warms, cools, exchanges oxygen and carbon dioxide, protects, shapes, excretes toxins, secretes moisturizers, and provides boundaries. This is accomplished by a network of nerves, sweat glands, temperature-sensing mechanisms, pressure sensors, sebaceous glands, hair, and muscles, all beneath a protective outer layer. The skin receives one-third the body's blood supply and is divided into the epidermis and the dermis (see Fig. 7.1). The epidermis ranges in thickness from 0.3 to 1.0 mm. It takes 14 days for the epidermal cell to differentiate and to become a part of the protective horny layer, the stratum corneum. This cell will shed and be replaced in another 14 days.

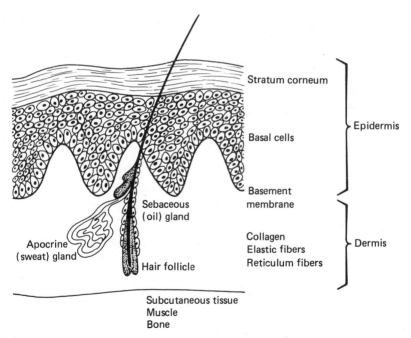

Figure 7.1. Anatomy of normal skin.

The dermis is comprised of connective tissue: Collagen provides strength, elastic fibers provide the mechanical property of elasticity, and reticulin fibers bind these two. The dermis lies above the subcutaneous tissue, muscles, and bone.

The aging process brings with it a decrease in the thickness of the epidermis and dermis (4). The fingerlike projections of the dermis anchor the two together. With aging, these flatten, allowing the layers to slide across one another. The dermis may become avascular, giving the skin a transparent quality. The reduction in subcutaneous tissue also means a loss of resiliency and elasticity. The epidermal turnover rate is reduced by 50%, which leads to a slower repair mechanism and a weak stratum corneum. Decreased production of sebum by the sebaceous glands leads to dry skin. Muscle degeneration, decreased bone calcification, and poor circulation characterize normal aging processes that contribute to the formation of pressure sores.

Pressure is the one factor consistently documented as the cause of pressure sores (5). In addition, there are a myriad of other contributing factors:

Friction (when a patient is dragged across bed sheets) removes the protection of the stratum corneum.

Shearing (when a patient slides down in a bed or Gerichair) provides a horizontal force between the epidermal and the dermal layers, sliding them across in opposite directions, thus disrupting blood supply and skin integrity.

Improper positioning, with weight distributed on bony prominences, compresses the dermal layers, thereby decreasing blood supply.

Incontinence and sweating lead to maceration as moisture lifts the cells of the stratum corneum, thus decreasing its protective property; enzymes in feces digest the skin cells.

Immobility (from sensory loss, weakness, sedation, mechanical restraints, stroke, senile dementia, or fractured bones) interferes with the normal shifting of pressure areas by the patient.

Mechanical abrasives injure skin.

Anemia leads to ischemia due to low hemoglobin for oxygen transport.

Infection, accompanied by exudate, causes irritation and maceration of the surrounding skin, and may also disturb blood flow and nutrition to surrounding skin.

Obesity and emaciation interfere with proper and safe positioning.

Metabolic disorders and dehydration impair the body's resources to cope with assault.

Impaired blood flow leads to cell death and necrosis.

Pressure Points

Pressure sores occur over pressure points, the areas that support body mass: the occipital area, ear rims, shoulder blades, elbows, sacrum, hips (trochanters), inner and outer knees, outer ankles, and heels (6). The localized pressure leads to decreased blood supply and cellular necrosis. Local nerve damage from this impaired blood supply disrupts the normal feedback mechanism that warns if there is too much pressure for too long. Normal individuals will respond to the "pins and needles" sensation with some body movement to relieve pressure.

Initial signs of damaging pressure are erythema, edema, induration, and pinpoint hemorrhages. Ischemic pallor (ischemia meaning "having little blood") is a blanching or pale appearance of the skin due to blood being squeezed from the vessels. Reactive hyperemia (hyperemic meaning "full of extra blood") follows, exhibiting increased reddening of the skin after pressure is released. Hyperemia lasting longer than one hour signals inflammation secondary to cell death that involves one or all layers of the skin. This is the basis for the staging criteria of pressure sores (7):

Stage I—inflammation or reddening (erythema) with no breaks in the skin.

Stage II—inflammation or reddening with ulceration through the epidermis (blister or superficial skin break).

Stage III—inflammation or reddening with ulceration through both layers of the skin (full-thickness skin loss).

Stage IV—ulceration through all skin layers exposing muscle and/or bone.

Stage V—severe ulceration with undermining from one ulcer to another and chronic purulent drainage.

Pressure sores may also be classified as partial- or full-thickness, referring to the extent of epidermal and/or dermal damage.

A crucial consideration in the evaluation of pressure sores is the pressure–cell death–ulcer formation cycle that may be taking place from the inside out. A bony prominence will compress muscle, causing tissue breakdown after which the pressure is transferred to the next layer, subcutaneous tissue, until it deteriorates. The remaining epidermal layer will appear ischemic or hyperemic depending on the extent of the underlying damage. Surrounding tissue will be warm, and the entire area will feel soft or fluctuant on palpation. This process has been likened to an iceberg, in that the greatest mass lies below the surface. Once the epidermal layer breaks, the ulcer should be examined to determine the extent of undermining and the depth of tissue damage.

Figure 1. PRESSURE ULCER ASSESSMENT

Date of Admission: ____________ Date of Onset: ____________
Date and Physician Notified: ____________
Signature of Nurse: ____________

addressograph

Place appropriate score for each category in the space below it and add scores to obtain total. A patient with a score of 11 or below should be considered at risk. Patient should be re-evaluated whenever condition improves or deteriorates.

*RATING SCALE

DATE(S)	MENTAL STATUS 5 Alert 4 Apathetic 3 Confused 2 Stuporous 1 Unconscious	CONTINENCE 4 Fully Controlled 3 Usually Controlled 2 Minimally Controlled 1 Absence of Control	MOBILITY 4 Full 3 Slightly Limited 2 Very Limited 1 Immobile	ACTIVITY 4 Ambulatory 3 Walks with Assistance 2 Chairfast 1 Bedfast	NUTRITION 3 Good 2 Fair 1 Poor	TOTAL SCORE

DESCRIPTION OF ANY PRESSURE ULCERS

	ULCER #1			ULCER #2			ULCER #3			ULCER #4			ULCER #5		
	DATE(S)			DATE(S)			DATE(S)			DATE(S)			DATE(S)		
Location															
Size (in cm)															
Color															
Exudate (describe)															
Odor (+ or ō)															
Inflammation (+ or ō)															
Culture (date done)															
Date Resolved															

*Gosnell DJ: *Nursing Research*, Vol. 22, No.1, 1973
Note: The author wishes to thank Diane Fetherston for her assistance in devising the Pressure Ulcer Assessment Form.

Figure 7.2. Pressure ulcer assessment form. (From Ahmed MC: Preventing and treating pressure ulcers: A nursing challenge. *Nurs Home Infect Control* 1(3): 2, 1982. Reproduced with the permission of Stuart Pharmaceuticals and Healthways Communications, Inc.)

Assessment

Management begins with an assessment of the total patient. Areas that influence the care of an individual at risk to develop pressure sores include the general state of health (i.e., the presence of such predisposing conditions as neuropathies, vascular disease, anemia), mental status, level of activity, mobility, continence, and nutrition/hydration. Tools are available for the assessment of the potential for a pressure sore. These utilize a numerical ranking for each given criterion by which the patient is evaluated to be in good condition or impaired to some degree. The lower the total numerical score, the greater the pressure sore potential (see Fig. 7.2).

A thorough description of the pressure sore is needed in order to devise a care plan and to provide a baseline for future evaluation of the process. Documentation should include stage of development, location, size and depth, color of the wound and surrounding tissue, necrosis, drainage/exudate, and odor. When evaluating a resident with an existing pressure ulcer, previous methods of treatment will provide valuable information for a care plan. A flowchart, checklist, or similar tool is useful to follow the progress of the treatment plan for an evaluation of the intervention being used.

Infection

Normal skin is covered with bacteria. Once the skin is broken, the bacteria will also cover the open area. When bacteria become a part of the wound environment, the wound is colonized. The body may mount an inflammatory response to deal with this assault. Cultures of the pressure sore drainage will tell which organisms are present, but will not indicate if infection has developed. Erythema, edema, pus, malodor, and fever indicate wound infection.

A culture of the pressure sore may be required when a patient is transferred to an extended care facility. The goal should be to treat the wound and not merely the culture report. The natural inflammatory response will deal with contamination. Therapy is aimed at reducing the number of bacteria in the pressure ulcer in order to allow natural responses to proceed. Systemic infection occurs when the bacteria overwhelm the local inflammatory response. Systemic antibiotics are used to eradicate systemic infection, but are not appropriate for the localized pressure sore. The pressure sore has a compromised blood supply, which may result in decreased delivery of systemic antibiotics to the local site.

INTERVENTION

Prevention

Intervention is based on the stage of development of the pressure sore. The key word in pressure sore management is **prevention:** prevention of a pressure sore and prevention of further damage once an ulcer has developed. All care plans should include a reference to turning, positioning, and elimination of pressure. The pressure points to consider in positioning the resident are:

Back-lying (supine) involves the back of the head, scapulae, elbows, sacral area, and heels.

Side-lying involves the ears, greater trochanters (thigh and pelvis), outer aspects of the knees, and ankles.

Lying face down (prone) involves the ears, edges of the sternum and ribs, knees, and top of the feet and toes.

Sitting involves the ischial tuberosities, coccyx, and sacrum.

Pressure is a product of time and force; intervention is geared toward decreasing the amount of time in one position and/or the mass applied over the area of pressure. On an average, the resident should be turned every two hours, day and night. If reactive hyperemia persists after turn-

Pressure Sore Worksheet

Name: John DOE

Date: 10/9/82

Treatment Plan: Ulcer #1 Dial Soap + Water > ① hip
                Skin Prep — layered

                Ulcer #2 Op Site ——> Sacrum

Schedule:

time	treatment	position-prone	supine	right	left	sitting	
8 am	X #1 / #2	X					
9							
10			X				
11							
12				X			
1 pm						lunch	gel pad
2				X			
3							
4	X +1	X					

NOTES: Avoid   Scented   Soap ——> Skin   reaction!

Figure 7.3. Pressure sore worksheet.

ing on this schedule, the individual will need a shorter interval before repositioning. Stryker frames and revolving circular beds can help with turning the body mass from a supine to a prone position, but the resident must be properly positioned once turned to avoid pressure on bony prominences. A position worksheet can be kept at the bedside as a tool to note the time of each previous turn and the positions that have been used most recently. Another approach is for the staff as a team to go through the unit on a scheduled basis and turn all residents (see Fig. 7.3). Even frequent, small shifts of weight on bed or chair may help prevent pressure sores.

Both time and mass need to be addressed. Mass can be manipulated with use of any of several devices that spread the weight over a larger area, thus decreasing pressure at a given point. These include beds (mud-, water-, or air-fluidized), mattresses (air or eggcrate foam), pads (micro-cell flotation, foam, sheepskin, or gel), and products for problem areas (heel and elbow pads). It is necessary to remember that the effectiveness of these devices is inversely related to the thickness of substances between the skin and the device. For instance, Chux pads used on a gel pad will flatten the fluid properties of the gel, negating the value of the gel pad.

Products must be evaluted in terms of the resident's needs. For example, an incontinent resident cannot use a sheepskin pad for long before the natural lanolin will be washed out of it by the hospital laundry, and an obese resident will compress the foam thickness. These products are an additional expense to the resident, since third-party reimbursement may not cover devices that are implemented for the prevention of pressure sores. In some cases, durable products such as special beds will be covered if used in the care of a pressure sore. A physician's order for these products is necessary when submitting requests for reimbursement.

Ambulating the resident, providing passive and active range of motion exercises, and frequent repositioning using rolled towels or pillows will provide relief from pressure, but require personnel time. Draw sheets or turning sheets should be used to lift and position the resident to avoid the friction encountered when the individual is dragged across linen. The draw sheet should not be tucked in, but left hanging loosely, especially when used with pressure-distributing devices. An overhead trapeze is useful if the resident has the ability and the knowledge to use one.

Footboards, with the resident positioned against the board, will prevent slipping/slumping in bed and decrease shear force. Raising the head of the bed more than 30° will allow the individual to slip down and cause a shearing effect on the dermal layers. These effects are not limited to those confined to bed; wheelchair, chair, and Gerichair occupants should be moved or reminded to shift their weight every hour or two. For bedpan use, lift or roll the resident onto the pan. Powder or foam cut to the contour of the bedpan surface serve to reduce friction and pressure.

Finally, it should be remembered that the above pressure-relieving devices do not replace frequent assessments and good nursing care, but are important adjunctive measures.

Interventions by Staging

Stage I and II pressure sores involve partial-thickness skin damage. The supporting dermis is intact, so the process of epithelialization can continue. Healing will take place once the factors contributing to skin breakdown mentioned earlier in this chapter are removed. The treatment consists of first removing the contributing factors, then providing an environment that promotes healing. The skin is washed with water only. Soap leads to drying, although a mild soap can be used for grossly dirty areas. Incontinent stool should be cleaned from the skin immediately to prevent further damage by maceration and enzymatic activity. Avoid vigorous rubbing as this can further damage the skin with the effects of friction. The area should be blotted dry and a skin protector or emollient ointment applied.

Skin protectors come in various forms (see Table 7.1). They prevent friction and provide a barrier to moisture evaporation from the damaged skin. Emollient ointments (e.g., petroleum-based products such as petroleum jelly or A&D ointment that are insoluble in water) protect the skin by preventing skin dehydration. Dry skin leads to cracks, fissures, and flaking of the stratum corneum. Too much moisture (maceration) floats the epithelial cells from the wound. Specific products are reviewed in Table 7.2.

Table 7.1. Nosocomial Skin Care Products—General[a]

Need/Goal	Product	Function
Skin protectors—to permit natural healing	Gelatin pads Polyurethane films "Skin preps" (developed for use in ostomy care) Non–water-soluble ointments	Moisturize (keep skin's secretions from evaporating) Provide protective dressing against environmental factors (friction, excrement, etc.)
Debriding agents—to remove byproducts of healing that retard granulation or epithelialization	Irrigations (normal saline) Enzyme agents (refer to PDR) Wet-to-dry dressing, whirlpool, or scrub	Flush debris with force Selectively debride eschar Provide nonselective debridement
Packing—to fill open space ("dead space") and absorb fluid	Moist, fine mesh gauze High-molecular-weight absorption preparations Sugar, Karaya	Fill open space in order to absorb wound fluids that impede healing and support bacteria

[a]Several manufactures market these products and supply information on their uses. Read all such literature with a critical eye.

Tincture of benzoin and heating lamps were once used to "toughen" the skin, but these approaches actually cause damage by drying the skin. Aluminum paste, also used in pressure sore treatments, traps irritation against the skin and is difficult to remove. Stage II blisters provide a natural dressing for the wound; the fluid cushions the area. They should be ruptured only if the fluid is cloudy (infected).

Stage III and IV pressure sores require the same treatment as described for stages I and II: removal of the contributing factor and promotion of an environment conducive to healing. These ulcers involve full-thickness skin damage, so healing occurs by secondary intention with granulation (i.e., the existing capillary beds give rise to a network of capillaries and supporting cells that later becomes scar tissue) rather than by primary reepithelialization. The goal is healing from the bottom up. Byproducts of wound healing such as serous fluid, dead cells, and bacteria can hinder granulation. If there are healthy wound edges and a good granulation bed, continue to protect the wound using the means previously described, and the wound will often heal. When the debris is overwhelming or interfering with the granulation process, a debriding procedure is needed.

Irrigating the ulcer will remove the wound debris and residue from other treatments used in the ulcer. Always wear gloves when working with an open ulcer. Normal saline flushed forcefully into the wound with a syringe will remove debris. Normal saline is used because it is osmotically similar to the body's own fluids, whereas water would be drawn into the cells by osmosis, causing the cells to burst.

At this point one of several antiseptic solutions may be used to control the overgrowth of bacteria. Use these solutions with discrimination, as they can be irritating and may interfere with topical debriding agents used in ulcer care. Anything that is intended to kill bacteria may also harm other living cells. Normal saline irrigation will mechanically remove bacteria from the wound surface. Povidone–iodine and acetic acid (1% vinegar) are broad-spectrum antiseptics used in ulcer care. Hydrogen peroxide is also used for its effervescence that lifts the necrotic tissue from the ulcer bed and mechanically debrides the crevices. However, it will nonselectively lift newly epithelialized tissue also. Thoroughly rinse any antiseptic solution from the wound afterwards.

In addition to normal wound debris, there may be eschar. Eschar, a thick, leathery crust of dead tissue that often covers an underlying necrotic process, must be removed before healthy tissue can grow. Necrotic tissue is an excellent growth medium for bacteria. Three methods of debridement are available: Sharp or manual debridement is completed with a scalpel by a physician or nurse (if permitted); chemical debride-

Table 7.2. Nosocomial Skin Care Products—Specific Preparations[a]

Product	Description	Stage and Action	Miscellaneous Notes
Skin protectors Op Site (Stuart Pharmaceuticals)	Transparent, polyurethane film sheet permeable to air and moisture vapor; adheres to skin surfaces, conforms to contours	I—Prevents friction II—Holds serous fluid (leukocytes, plasma, and fibrin) intact against the crater surface, allowing it to fight infection, liquefy dead tissue, and cushion exposed nerve endings; moist environment encourages migration of epidermal cells	Dressing can be left in place 3–7 days Not for use with severe infection (gross purulence) or copious exudate (will leak); some accumulated fluid can be aspirated with a syringe
Skin barriers Skin Prep (United Surgical) Bard Protective Barrier Film (Bard) Sween products	Transparent spray or gel	All stages—Provides a barrier against acids, enzymes, water; permeable to O_2, water vapor, and CO_2	Can be layered (spray/dry/spray) for added protection
Sugar paste	Paste composed of 3:1 sugar, povidone–iodine ointment, and antiseptic solution; or sugar and antacid (e.g., Maalox, Mylanta)	III—Nutrients delivered directly to healing tissue	Not for use where infection is present (will encourage bacterial growth)
Topical debriding agents: Travase (Flint) Elase (Parke-Davis) Granulex Spray (Hickman)	Ointment applied to eschar	III and IV (for eschar only)—Contains a proteolytic enzyme that accelerates natural autolysis of devitalized and necrotic tissue (Granulex also acts as a protective covering)	Dressings should be changed frequently (accumulated discharge can inactivate the enzyme) Germicides left in ulcer crater will inactivate enzyme
Bard Absorbable Dressing Debrisan (Johnson & Johnson) Helafoam	Granules placed into wound	III and IV—Absorb exudate, small particles, and contaminants leading to increased granulation tissue	Should be covered with light dressing and changed 1–2 times/ day

Product	Description	Uses	Comments
Pressure barriers Karaya (Hollister)	Vegetable gum that is slightly water-soluble; available in rings and wafers that can be cut to fit wound edges or powder that is applied directly into ulcer	II, III, IV—Cushions area to prevent pressure; nutrients delivered directly to healing tissue	Swells with moisture so drainage seems profuse, messy Ring or wafer applied daily; powder applied every 8 hours
Stomahesive (E.R. Squibb & Sons)	Compound of gelatin, pectin, carboxymethylcellulose, and polyisobutylene formed into a thin, pliable wafer that has adhesive on one side; applied directly to affected area	I—Cushions area to prevent pressure II, III, IV—With a hole cut in the wafer to approximate the wound edges, cushions the area	Unless wrinkled or loose, can be left in place 24–48 hours
Topical antibiotics and antiseptics Neosporin	Solution or ointment	III and IV—Controls bacteria directly to a level that host defenses can cope with	Can cause contact dermatitis and encourage the development of resistant organisms
Systemic antibiotics	All modes of administration	Infection—Questionable control of infection in ulcer itself as there is a reliance on compromised vasculature to deliver antibiotic to the site	Should not be used for colonization of wound, but for actual infection.
Wet-to-dry dressings	Gauze pads soaked in normal saline and loosely packed into wound for 3–4 hours, then removed (must not dry in wound)	III and IV—Mechanically debrides wound	

[a]This table is not intended to be a complete listing of all products available for use in skin care and pressure sore management. It should provide the reader with a basis for the development of a pressure sore program. Companies involved in skin care products will generally honor requests for product information.

ment is accomplished by enzymes; and mechanical debridement is effected with wet-to-dry dressings, whirlpool, or scrubbing.

Enzymatic agents are chemicals that interact with the different substrates of wound tissue (see Table 7.1). These pharmaceuticals require a prescription for use. They will not affect intact healthy skin, epithelialization, or granulation. Their effect builds up over time before the tissue begins to slough. Thick eschar can be scored with a knife to encourage penetration of the enzyme.

Wet-to-dry dressings provide nonspecific debridement. The moist gauze is fluffed, packed into the wound, and removed while still slightly damp. It will pull with it the necrotic tissue, leaving healing granulation tissue behind. The ulcer can also be gently scrubbed with a wet gauze sponge. The scrubbing action will debride sloughed tissue. If there is undermining, all areas must be reached when packing or scrubbing, possibly requiring surgical enlargement of the opening for satisfactory access. If there are signs of infection that require treatment, culture the ulcer properly. This is done after the ulcer is cleansed and irrigated, but before an antiseptic solution is used. The ideal method is by aspiration of material from deep in the wound for culture (see Chapter 1); alternatively one may compress the edges to elicit new drainage, then swab the sides and base of the ulcer. Culture results will help in pinpointing a focus of infection when systemic signs are present. The presence of an organism on culture, especially on a swab culture, does not necessarily mean that the organism is causing infection. Clinical correlation is necessary. Blood cultures should be obtained if sepsis is suspected.

Once there is a clean base, the deep wounds or those with undermining pockets require packing. All dead space must be filled or the body will fill it with serous fluid, leading again to the exudate–debris–bacteria cycle that interferes with normal granulation. Wounds can be packed with fine mesh gauze moistened with normal saline that is changed before it dries. All-gauze dressings should be used rather than cotton gauze. High-molecular-weight preparations are available that absorb fluid and expand to fill the space (see Table 7.1). These require less frequent dressing changes. The packing is continued until the ulcer fills in. When granulation is underway, the wound is healing. From this point on, the ulcer should be protected and kept moist as in stages I and II to promote healing.

Continuous assessment of the ulcer is necessary to define a care plan. Stages I and II require protection and promotion of healthy skin. Stages III and IV require a plan for granulation tissue (e.g., protect and promote healthy conditions), wound debris (e.g., irrigation and/or debridement), and dead space (e.g., packing).

Stage V ulcers require intensive intervention. Systemic antibiotics and surgical treatment are indicated at this stage. Skin grafts or pedicle flaps with or without the excision of protruding underlying bone are used to manage these ulcers. After this has been accomplished, it is mandatory to keep pressure off the compromised tissue.

It should be evident that there are a multitude of treatment plans for pressure sores. When selecting an approach, consider the availability of resources, especially time and finances. Although some items require a high initial investment, they may be ultimately cost-saving in terms of personnel time and supplies.

Reevaluate the pressure sore and intervention periodically. Is the intervention meeting the goal it was selected to meet? For example, debridement with enzymatic agents will take longer than sharp debridement, but the same goal will be reached. A new intervention might be appropriate as the condition improves or if there is no improvement. A major pitfall in pressure sore care is the lack of consistency among personnel. There are so many approaches that staff members must communicate among themselves as to which care plan will be used, when it will be reevaluated, and what changes are needed.

SPECIAL CONSIDERATIONS

Pressure sore therapy is not completed with the rendering of good skin care. Other aspects of the total person affect the outcome of topical care. As mentioned above, poor nutrition is associated with anemia, hypoproteinemia, and vitamin deficiencies that influence the development and progress of a pressure sore. These factors are a significant challenge in the elderly, who may have poor appetite due to waning sensory perception of food.

The most obvious result of poor nutrition is the loss of tissue padding over bony prominences. Protein is essential for growth, repair, and maintenance of body tissue. In response to an injury, the body can mobilize protein from various tissues to maintain homeostasis. This process will continue even with protein starvation. However, the mobilized protein must be replaced as soon as possible in order to prevent hypoproteinemia, which leads to negative nitrogen balance (8). Optimal wound healing will not occur when there is a negative balance. Normally, an elderly person requires 0.5 g of protein per kilogram of body weight per day to maintain this protein balance. This should be supplemented with an adequate caloric intake based on the person's activity level. A safety margin of 1.0–1.5 g per kilogram is alloted to allow for the effects of stress. The average elderly man at 70 kg will need approximately 70 g of protein per day (8).

A balanced diet should include meat, fish, dairy products, and vitamin C for the maintenance of skin integrity. Foods such as liver, dark vegetables, or iron supplements will help maintain the ideal hemoglobin level for healing to take place (12–14 g/dl). Feeding the elderly can be an exercise in creativity. Adequate intake cannot be overstressed, even if tube feedings of inhouse pureed foods or commercial preparations are necessary.

Environmental factors also come into play when considering the care of pressure sores in nursing home residents. Special care must be taken not to spread infection from one resident to another. Handwashing is an integral part of pressure sore care. Equipment, solutions, and dressings should be labeled and maintained for an individual, with no sharing among residents. These are precautions that must become a natural part of nursing home care to prevent outbreaks of infection.

SUMMARY

The key word in pressure sore therapy is **prevention.** Identify susceptible residents and pay attention to pressure points, especially when working with the high-risk population. Shift or have the resident shift the body mass at least every two hours, and spread the weight if possible to decrease pressure in any one spot. Reassess to make sure that even more frequent shifts are not necessary. Take care of the skin from the inside out. Nutrition is a cornerstone in prevention and healing.

Once a pressure sore develops, careful assessment of the stage of development is needed with an eye toward principles of wound healing. The plan of care should be well-defined, personalized, and communicated to all caring for the resident. Finally, there must be a committment to following through with the goals set by such a plan. An organized plan of attack will make the decubitus ulcer a manageable problem.

REFERENCES

1. Fowler E: Pressure Sores: A deadly nuisance. *J Gerontol Nursing* 8:680–685, 1982.
2. Spence WR, Burke RD, and Roe JW Jr.: Gel support for prevention of decubitus ulcers. *Arch Phys Med Rehabil* 48:283–288, 1967.

3. Galpin J, Chow AW, Bayer AS, et al: Sepsis associated with decubitus ulcers. *Am J Med* 61:346–349, 1976.

4. Gilchrest BA: Age-associated changes in the skin. *J Am Geriatr Soc* 30:139–143, 1982.

5. Reuler, JB, Cooney TG: The pressure sore: Pathophysiology and principles of management. *Ann Intern Med* 94:661–666, 1981.

6. Vasconez LO, Schneider WJ, Jurkiewicz MJ: Pressure sores. *Curr Prob Surg* 14:1–62, 1977.

7. Shea JD: Pressure sores: Classification and management. *Clin Orthoped* 112:89–100, 1975.

8. Wohl MG, Goodhart RS: *Modern Nutrition in Health and Disease,* 3rd ed. Philadelphia, Lea & Febiger, 1964. pp 146–150, 173–176.

SECTION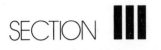

THE INFECTION CONTROL PROGRAM

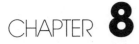

CHAPTER **8**

INFECTION CONTROL PROGRAM ORGANIZATION

Philip W. Smith

REASONS TO HAVE AN INFECTION CONTROL PROGRAM

Protection of Residents and Employees

In Chapter 4, the risk of infection for nursing home residents was delineated. The nosocomial infection rate for nursing homes appears to be at least as high as that for hospitals, with significant morbidity and mortality and considerable financial cost for treatment. Certain nursing home infections pose a threat to the health of employees (see Chapter 15). In view of the frequency of infection and the fact that an important proportion of nosocomial infections may be prevented by an effective infection control program, it is incumbent upon the nursing home to develop such a program for the safety of residents and employees.

Requirements

An infection control program for nursing homes is mandated by the Standards for Certification and Participation in Medicare and Medicaid Programs and the Joint Commission on Accreditation of Hospitals (see Chapter 12). They specifically require an infection control committee responsible for providing all services necessary to maintain a sanitary and comfortable environment and to prevent infection in the nursing home (1,2). The Joint Commission on Accreditation of Hospitals (JCAH) standard addresses such responsibilities as infection surveillance, policies and procedures, employee health program, isolation techniques, housekeeping, laundry, and pest control. Requirements for skilled and intermediate care facilities are different.

Legal Aspects

Several lawsuits have been decided in the area of hospital infections; this has stimulated interest in preventing legal liability by an effective infection control program. The same general principles should be applicable to nursing homes. Malpractice cases are based on the legal theory of negligence. In order to hold the defendant guilty of negligence, the plaintiff must prove that the defendant had a duty to care for the plaintiff, that this duty was breached, that the breach of duty was the proximate cause of the plaintiff's injury, and that the plaintiff suffered damages (3). The health care institution is expected to deliver a standard of care appropriate to the community. Staphylococcal infections transmitted by personnel (4) and roommates (5) have been the basis for successful lawsuits against hospitals.

Lawsuits can be successfully avoided by having rules and regulations that are up-to-date and observed (3). Good record keeping to document compliance with accepted standards is also crucial to effective defense against malpractice in the area of infection control. A strong infection control program demonstrates that the nursing home is interested in providing the resident reasonable protection against the hazards of nursing home–acquired infection.

COMPONENTS OF AN INFECTION CONTROL PROGRAM

There are a number of approaches to infection control in the nursing home setting, depending on the interest and resources of the nursing home. A program needs to assign responsibility for infection control to a person, the infection control practitioner, who is usually a nurse. This person probably will not perform infection control activities on a full-time basis. Ideally this person should receive direction from a multidisciplinary body, the infection control committee.

Infection Control Committee

Most hospitals have an active infection control committee. This committee must have the support of the hospital administration and must also have the written authority to intervene when a dangerous situation (such as an outbreak of *Staphylococcus aureus* infections) arises in the hospital (6). The committee includes representatives from the major medical staff departments, hospital administration, nursing service, and microbiology laboratory, as well as the infection control practitioner. Ideally, the chairman of the committee is a physician with special interest or training in infectious diseases.

The JCAH also mandates an infection control committee in nursing homes; it is their responsibility to provide all services necessary to maintain a sanitary and comfortable environment and to prevent the development and transmission of infection in a nursing home setting (1). The makeup of this committee is similar to that recommended for hospitals, including medical and nursing staffs, administration, and representatives from dietetics, pharmacy, housekeeping, maintenance, and laundry services. The chairman should have knowledge of or special interest or experience in infection control. This committee is responsible for the infection control activities that are discussed in the next section, including review of policies and procedures, employee health, isolation techniques, and environmental control. The infection control committee (ICC) carries out most of these activities through the infection control practitioner and provides medical direction to this person.

Medicare and Medicaid regulations also require skilled nursing facilities to establish an infection control committee with similar responsibilities. The facility must have a program for detecting, preventing, controlling, and reporting infections. The program must address food handling, laundry, waste disposal, employee health, pest control, traffic, visitation, asepsis, quality control, and safety (2).

Through regular meetings the infection control committee brings multidisciplinary skills to bear on the infection control problems of the nursing home.

Infection Control Practitioner

The infection control practitioner (ICP) is the key person who effects the directives of the infection control committee. A background in clinical medicine, usually nursing, is helpful in carrying out the duties of the nurse epidemiologist. Some knowledge of basic microbiology is also beneficial. The ICP is the hub of the infection control program.

In hospitals, one full-time ICP is recommended for every 250 to 300 beds (7). ICPs spend most of their time collecting data on infections in the hospital (surveillance) and on educational activities.

The requirements for an ICP in a nursing home should be similar. The person who performs the duties of infection control should be familiar with the nursing home and familiar with resident care problems; often the director of nursing is chosen. It has been suggested that nursing homes with greater than 150 beds warrant a full-time infection control practitioner (8).

Table 8.1. Elements of an Infection Control Program

Element	Example(s)
Surveillance	Document and record infections
Epidemic control	Investigate clusters of infections
Education	In-service programs
Policy formation	Develop isolation manual
Procedure formation	Catheter care techniques
Employee health	TB screening
Environmental control	Inspect laundry, kitchen
Antibiotic monitoring	Review antibiotic sensitivities
Public health impact	Disease reporting

Source: Adapted from Smith, P.W. et al: Infection control in hospitals, current trends and requirements. *Nebr Med J* 64:62–65, 1979. Used with permission.

The ICP must have well-defined authority and support from the infection control committee. It is also very important that this person be extremely tactful in dealing with nursing home personnel, physicians, and residents. A number of potential problems unique to nursing home ICPs have been identified, including role confusion (because the ICP frequently has many other responsibilities), lack of authority to initiate isolation or to perform cultures, high turnover rate, and lack of visibility of the ICP in the institution (8).

The ICP can play a very exciting and important role in the nursing home. While residents tend to have a number of underlying chronic and degenerative diseases which are not reversible, infectious diseases are frequently preventable, treatable, or reversible. Infections are an important problem in nursing homes (see Chapter 4). Finally, because of decreased physician availability in nursing homes compared to acute care hospitals, the ICP may well have a greater responsibility for the diagnosis and prevention of infection.

ACTIVITIES OF AN INFECTION CONTROL PROGRAM

A number of elements in an infection control program can be defined (see Table 8.1).

Data Collection and Evaluation

One of the most important elements of an infection control program is surveillance. An effective infection control program cannot be conducted without knowledge of the specific and unique problems of each nursing home. Infection rates must be determined and compared to the usual (baseline) infection rate so that epidemics can be detected early.

Infection surveillance information is available from several different sources. Rounds to resident care areas are made to search for clues to the presence of infection, such as fever, abnormal x-rays, indwelling bladder catheters, antibiotic use, and dressing changes. Information is obtained from both the chart and communication with nurses (9). Ward rounds may be supplemented by pharmacy records on antibiotic usage, temperature records, Kardex review, x-ray reports, review of microbiology culture results, and comments by physicians in the medical record. In a small institution, direct observation of residents may be used to supplement the above information. Physician reporting of nosocomial infections tends to grossly underestimate the true incidence even in hospitals (10). In nursing homes, the less extensive medical record makes chart review a very inaccurate way to search for nursing home–associated infections if it is not supplemented with other information.

There are several techniques for data collection, including continuous surveillance and periodic prevalence surveys of the entire nursing home population (see Chapter 9). A number of general points should be remembered in designing a surveillance program:

1. The level of surveillance should be tailored to the personnel and financial needs of the nursing home.
2. In order for consistent information to be collected, standard objective definitions for various types of infection should be used.
3. A basic form should be developed and used for collection of data on infections.
4. Periodic analysis of collected surveillance data is necessary. Ideally, rates should be calculated (see Chapters 1 and 9).
5. Surveillance information should be used in the control activities of the infection control practitioner. For example, an increase in the rate of urinary tract infection may lead to discovery of an epidemic that can be terminated by appropriate measures. Examples of infection control problems in the nursing home may be used in educational programs for personnel.
6. Surveillance by itself may serve to decrease infections in the nursing home by reminding personnel of the importance of adhering to good infection control practices and by demonstrating that the administration of that institution is committed to the infection control program.

Epidemic Investigation

One of the major purposes for having a surveillance program in a nursing home is early detection of epidemics. It is the responsibility of the infection control program to detect, document, evaluate, and hopefully control outbreaks of infections in the nursing home. Chapter 10 provides a detailed discussion of the approach to an epidemic.

Education

Education of the nursing home staff is a major ongoing responsibility of the ICP. Because of high turnover rate in many nursing homes, it is imperative for new employees to be instructed in the problem of infections in the nursing home and the role that personnel play in transmission and prevention of these infections.

In the course of daily routine, employees may become careless about certain infection prevention techniques. The ICP needs to periodically remind personnel about the importance of policies and procedures relating to careful handwashing, aseptic bladder catheter insertion, adherence to isolation procedures, maintenance of good personal hygiene, and the susceptibility of the elderly to infection. This may be accomplished by periodic in-service education on basic infection control practices, including a review of policies and procedures. Educational techniques and resources are discussed in depth in Chapter 13.

Policies and Procedures

The ICP plays a vital role in developing and updating policies and procedures in the nursing home. An example is isolation policies. General guidelines are available for isolation (see Chapter 16), but the ICP can play an important role in adapting these general guidelines to the specific needs of the nursing home and serving as a resource person for answering questions about these procedures.

Many aspects of the nursing home environment that affect resident care will be covered by infection control policies or procedures, including employee health, visitor regulations, isolation, disinfection/sterilization, housekeeping, engineering, food preparation, laundry, waste disposal, handwashing procedures, and policies relating to admission and transfer of residents with infection.

Policies and procedures need to be clearly written, widely distributed throughout the nursing home, and periodically updated, and should contain a provision for monitoring of compliance. Policies and procedures are discussed in more detail in Chapter 12.

Employee Health Program

Employees may serve as a source for spread of infection to nursing home residents or may acquire an infection in the line of duty. An active employee health program will minimize both of these risks.

The majority of employee health problems relate to infectious diseases; hence, the ICP is a logical person to oversee an employee health program in a nursing home. Elements of a nursing home employee health program include screening of new employees for infectious diseases, education of employees about their role in transmission of nosocomial infections, updating employee immunizations, periodic screening for infectious diseases such as tuberculosis, and investigation of employees as potential agents for the spread of infectious diseases during epidemics. Employee health programs are reviewed in Chapter 15.

Environmental Control

The ICP is frequently involved in monitoring the inanimate environment in the nursing home and overseeing the maintenance of an appropriately clean environment. Sanitation, disinfection, or sterilization of various parts of the environment are appropriate; specific procedures and policies for these methods should be delineated and monitored. Almost any part of the nursing home environment that comes in contact with the resident may occasionally serve as a vehicle for spread of infection. As a result, the ICP needs to be somewhat familiar with a number of housekeeping and maintenance areas, including ventilation and air conditioning, water distribution and plumbing, cleaning of environmental surfaces, laundry, waste disposal, kitchen and food operations, insect and rodent control, and safety programs.

Routine microbiologic sampling of the environment is costly and not indicated. Selected environmental cultures do play an important role in epidemic investigations, however. Environmental control is discussed in Chapter 15.

Antibiotic Monitoring

The problems of antibiotic overuse and antibiotic-resistant bacteria are not confined to hospitals but are also of importance in the nursing home (see Chapter 11). The ICP may be able to assist in monitoring antibiotic resistance and usage in the nursing home.

Community Health Impact—Disease Reporting

Infection control programs at individual nursing homes have public health responsibilities and interact with health agencies in several ways.

A number of diseases that may be seen in the nursing home are reportable on national or state levels, including hepatitis A, hepatitis B, tuberculosis, salmonellosis, shigellosis, amebiasis, and Legionnaires' disease. Diseases that are first diagnosed in the nursing home may have been communicable prior to hospitalization; hence, persons in the community would be at risk. The state health department is in a position to take measures to protect public health. In addition, epidemics may involve more than one nursing home or hospital.

Health departments in turn help infection control programs by facilitating various diagnostic tests, coordinating investigations of epidemics, providing literature, serving as liaison with the Centers for Disease Control, and providing information on infectious diseases in the community.

Ideally, nursing home, hospital, and public health officials should work together to solve problems of mutual interest and public health importance. Statewide infection control organizations exist in a number of states. In Nebraska, for instance, the Nebraska Infection Control Network (NICN) is an organization cosponsored by the State Health Department, state nursing home association, state hospital association, and local chapter of infection control practitioners. The network organizes educational seminars and publishes a newsletter.

SPECIAL CONCERNS

Cost Containment—Ideas for Institutions with Limited Resources

In spite of the complex job description of an infection control practitioner and the important role such a person plays in preventing infections in the nursing home, many nursing homes may not have the resources to employ a full-time ICP. A number of shortcuts are available for these institutions.

Perhaps the most time-consuming duty of an infection control practitioner is data collection and evaluation. There is no doubt that surveillance of infections is very important in order to provide accurate data for decisions concerning infection prevention. Surveillance systems vary in complexity and time requirements. Walking rounds with chart review and discussions with nursing personnel on a frequent basis is ideal, but alternatives such as periodic prevalence surveys or screening of high-risk residents (e.g., those with indwelling bladder catheters) may be suitable. Any system that is used must be consistent. A system that removes the ICP from contact with nursing home personnel may dilute the effect of spontaneous teaching and encouragement.

Ideally education should be relevant to the institution's own experience. Prepackaged educational programs, such as self-learning modules or audiovisual instructional programs are available. Time may be saved by borrowing ideas on policies, procedures, and isolation manuals from programs that have already developed them or from other sources (11, 12).

Finally, it may be most practical for the nursing home to combine the role of infection control practitioner with a number of other roles of importance in the nursing home. For instance, the ICP may also be responsible for quality assurance or may oversee the institutional safety program, two functions required by accrediting agencies (1). Guidelines for implementation of a quality assurance program have been published (13). The ICP in a nursing home is frequently also a staff nurse. In view of the predominant concern of employee health issues with infectious diseases, the ICP may also be in charge of the employee health program. Another function is to work with the pharmacists on antibiotic audits, antibiotic appropriateness reviews, or antibiotic resistance surveillance.

How to Start a Program

The development of an effective infection control program usually follows the following sequence:

1. Appoint a responsible individual to be the infection control practitioner (ICP). This person needs to have support from administration and a clearly defined responsibility and time allotment for managing the infection control program. Ideally, this person should have direction from an infection control committee or physician.
2. The ICP will require training and resource materials. Brief introductory courses in infection control are available in many locations, and in-depth courses are offered by the Centers for Disease Control, the University of Iowa, and other institutions. Basic reference materials of great assistance in development of a program are available; several are given in this chapter's Appendix.

3. Generally, the first duty of the new ICP is the development of some sort of surveillance system. Initially, definitions of infection can be obtained from reference sources or other institutions, and a simple recording form may be developed. Knowledge of the infection control problems of the nursing home is essential in order to make intelligent decisions about appropriate control measures. Surveillance also facilitates early detection and prevention of epidemics.

4. Policy and procedure development and review should be the next goal. Every facility should have written policies for isolation/precautions, visitation, disinfection/sterilization, aseptic insertion of bladder catheters, decubitus care, and food sanitation.

5. Educational programs for nursing home personnel should begin quickly, since this is one of the most effective control measures available. Surveillance data should be used in educational programs.

6. As time goes on, the infection control practitioner may well evolve additional roles. The ICP serves as resource person for many employees in the nursing home, including nursing, housekeeping, maintenance, administration, and other personnel.

AN OVERVIEW OF CONTROL MEASURES

The development of nosocomial infection involves (see Chapter 4, Fig. 4.1):

1. A reservoir of the infectious agent;
2. A means of transmission of the infectious agent to the resident; and
3. Actual invasion of the host to produce an infectious disease.

The development of a nursing home–acquired (nosocomial) infection can be blocked at any one of the three stages.

Both animate and inanimate **reservoirs** are important in the nursing home. The control methods address residents, visitors, and employees, all part of the animate reservoir (see Fig. 8.1). Other control measures necessary to maintain an appropriately clean inanimate environment in the nursing home are elaborated in Chapter 15.

The second step that may be interrupted is the **transmission** of agents. The single most important step in preventing transmission of infectious diseases in the nursing home is good handwashing; this measure also acts at the first step by decreasing the cutaneous reservoir. The other methods (see Fig. 8.2) address spread by airborne or direct-contact

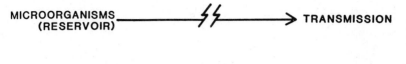

METHODS

Treat established infections   Sterilization

TB screening – new residents   Laundry standards

Bathing residents   Proper food preparation

Visitor checks   Housekeeping

Employee health   Equipment maintenance

Handwashing   Waste disposal

Disinfection of equipment

Figure 8.1. Infection control measures—the reservoir.

methods. Surveillance and education impact transmission by detecting epidemics and reminding personnel of correct infection control practices, respectively. Various aspects of control of transmission of infection are discussed in Chapters 9, 10, and 16.

The final step is the transition from colonization to infection. **Host resistance** may be improved in a number of ways. General resistance may be improved by treating the residents' underlying medical illnesses to the greatest extent possible, providing good nutrition, and minimizing

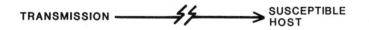

METHODS

Handwashing

Isolation

Closed urinary catheter systems

Air filtration/ventilation

Surveillance

Epidemic investigation

Education

Figure 8.2. Infection control measures—transmission.

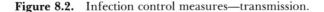

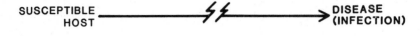

METHODS

Optimal medical care

Minimize invasive devices

Antibiotic control

Nutrition

Immunization against infections

Decubitus care

Respiratory toilet

Figure 8.3. Infection control measures—the host.

antibiotics (see Fig. 8.3). Other options include improving local defenses (e.g., good respiratory toilet) and enhancing specific immunity (e.g., influenza vaccine). Host measures are reviewed in Chapter 14.

Finally, it should be remembered that nosocomial infections cannot be completely eliminated, but they can be minimized by a good infection control program. When nosocomial infections occur in the nursing home and pose a threat to the health of residents, an infection control program must be prepared to detect the problem promptly and apply appropriate control measures. An integrated program will address all major areas that interface with infection control: infection detection (surveillance), epidemic prevention, environment control (e.g., laundry, food preparation, asepsis, waste disposal), policies and procedures (e.g., for isolation or visitation), employee health and safety, antibiotics (usage and resistance), and disease reporting.

The nursing home resources and committment to infection control determine how quickly the above steps take place and how far the infection control program develops. An ICP who is willing to learn and seek advice can overcome deficiencies in training or background.

REFERENCES

1. *Accreditation Manual for Long-Term Care Facilities.* Joint Commission on Accreditation of Hospitals, Chicago, Ill., 1980.

2. U.S. Department of Health and Human Services: Conditions of participation for skilled nursing and intermediate care facilities. *Fed Reg* 45:47368–47382, 1980.

3. Rivkind, RJ: Legal responsibilities in infection control. APIC J 6:23–25, 1978.

4. Nottebart, HC Jr: Hospital acquired staphylococcal infection transmitted by hospital personnel. *Infect Control* 1:190–193, 1980.

5. Nottebart, HC: Staphylococcal infection in hospital roommates. *Infect Control* 1:105–108, 1980.

6. *Accreditation Manual for Hospitals.* Joint Commission on Accreditation of Hospitals, Chicago, Ill., 1983.

7. Mallison GF: A hospital program for control of nosocomial infections. APIC Newslet 2:1–6, 1974.

8. Checko PJ: Infection control in long-term facilities: The state of the art. *Infect Control Urol Care* 5:27–34, 1980.

9. Smith PW, Stoesz PA, Rusnak PG: Infection control in hospitals: Current trends and requirements. *Nebr Med J* 64:62–65, 1979.

10. Hofherr L: Nosocomial infection surveillance techniques: A review. APIC J 7:12–15, 1979.

11. *Infection Prevention and Control for Long-Term Care Facilities,* American Health Care Association, Washington, DC, 1977.

12. *Infection Control in the Extended Care Facility,* American Health Care Association, Washington, DC, 1983.

13. Hoesing, H, Mikolajczak A: *Tools for Effective Management: A Long-Term Care Standard Review.* Joint Commission on Accreditation of Hospitals, Chicago, Ill., 1982.

APPENDIX

Reference Library for the Beginning Infection Control Practitioner

Guidelines for the Prevention and Control of Nosocomial Infections, 1981–1983. U S Department of Health and Human Services, Public Health Service, Centers for Disease Control, Atlanta, GA 30333. Price (1983) = $40.00. Can be ordered by phone (703) 487-4630. (Covers isolation, employee health, environmental control, prevention of urinary tract infections, etc.)

Benenson, AS Ed: *Control of Communicable Diseases in Man,* 13th ed, 1980. American Public Health Association, 1015 Fifteenth Street

NW, Washington, DC 20005. Price (1983) = $7.50. (Lists infectious diseases with signs, symptoms, epidemiology, contagious periods, and treatment.)

Barrett-Connor, E, ed: *Epidemiology for the Infection Control Nurse,* 1978. CV Mosby Co, St Louis, MO. Price (1983) = $19.95. (Discusses basics of epidemiology in health care setting.)

Brachman, PS, ed: *Hospital Infections,* 1979. Little, Brown & Co, Boston, MA. Price (1983) = $23.50. (Discusses basics of nosocomial infections).

Mikat DM, Mikat KW, eds: *A Clinician's Dictionary Guide to Bacteria and Fungi,* 4th ed, 1981. Eli Lilly Co, Indianapolis, IN 46206. Distributed as a service to the medical profession at no charge.

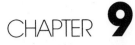

CHAPTER **9**

FINDING AND ANALYZING INFECTIONS IN A NURSING HOME

Nancy J. Haberstich

APPROACH TO SURVEILLANCE

The Importance of Surveillance

As discussed in Chapter 8, surveillance is a critical component of any infection control program. It provides the foundation for the entire program. Surveillance has been defined as the collection, collation, and analysis of data and the dissemination to those who need to know so that an action can result (1). When applied to infection control, **surveillance** identifies the activity that a health care institution employs in order to find, analyze, and control **nosocomial** infections (infections that develop in the nursing home).

Time and energy spent in surveillance activity become an indirect investment in prevention and control of infections. Surveillance data provide a nursing home with valid information for establishing a baseline and determining which control measures are needed. In addition, it provides the nursing home with a system for the early detection of nosocomial epidemics. Infection control policies and procedures may be modified to address problems detected by surveillance. Finally, surveillance activities may even decrease nosocomial infections by reminding personnel of the factors involved in nursing home infections.

In establishing a surveillance program for a nursing home, consideration must be given to the size of the facility, the level of care provided by the facility, and the type and extent of information the program is expected to yield. The availability of resources and personnel to conduct surveillance must also be considered. Committment from the administration of a nursing home to a comprehensive surveillance program is essential; most administrators appreciate the impact of nosocomial infections on residents. Nursing home nosocomial infections occur with a frequency that approximates that of hospital nosocomial infections (see Chapter 4). Requirements by state and other regulatory agencies also stimulate the development of an effective surveillance program.

Who Does Surveillance?

It is essential that one nursing home employee have defined responsibility for surveillance. This person must detect and record nosocomial infections. The person responsible for surveillance in an extended care facility should ideally be a registered nurse with clinical experience. Knowledge of infectious diseases and of their transmission and epidemiology are important qualifications. Background knowledge in microbiology and statistics is helpful.

In hospitals, the amount of time and personnel devoted to surveillance is customarily determined by the number of hospital beds. As a rough rule, at least 20 hours of surveillance per week is necessary for every 250 hospital beds. Most nursing homes can conduct surveillance with more conservative resources. The patient population of a nursing home is generally made up of less critically ill individuals, which eliminates some of the high-risk areas of the hospital setting such as intensive care, surgery, and emergency room. Resources, requirements by regulatory agencies, the number of beds in the facility, occupancy, and the level of care the facility provides will determine the number of personnel-hours dedicated to infection surveillance.

Data collection is the primary surveillance activity and will consume most of the person's time. Since data collection is best performed on a daily basis, the responsibility for surveillance is probably most efficiently accomplished by a nursing supervisor. The infection control committee and administration of the nursing home should make the decision on who performs surveillance within their facility. The designated infection surveillance employee, or infection control practitioner (ICP), is said to be the eyes, ears, and feet of the infection control program.

Establishing Definitions of Infections

In order to find nosocomial infections one must know what to look for, so definitions of nosocomial infections must be established for the institution. The Centers for Disease Control (CDC) in Atlanta, Georgia provide established definitions for nosocomial infection by body site (2). The CDC guidelines published in 1970 are reproduced in this chapter's Appendix. The infection control committee of the nursing home can select the appropriate CDC criteria as they apply to the specific population of the institution. Some of these definitions will not be needed by most nursing homes because of their resident population, services offered, and associated risks. For example, surgical wound infections and intravenous-related infections are much less likely in a nursing home than in a hospital. The definitions are general guidelines that should be adapted to the needs of each institution.

It is important, then, for the infection control committee to review all the sites given by the CDC and decide which could be omitted and which are potential hazards for their nursing home residents. The use of specific criteria for nosocomial infections provides uniformity in determining nosocomial origins and prevents biased individual decisions. The definitions of infection also assist the ICP in deciding if an **infection** is present and in differentiating infection from colonization (see Chapter 1).

DATA COLLECTION

Surveillance activities will vary among nursing homes depending on the extent of the surveillance program developed by the infection control committee. The essential elements of any surveillance program are systematic collection of pertinent data, orderly consolidation and evaluation of data, and prompt dissemination of the results to those who need to know (3).

Sources of Pertinent Data

No single method for data collection has been found to identify all infections or risks in a hospital or nursing home, so a combination of methods is recommended. Committment and participation by the nursing staff are essential for comprehensive and efficient data retrieval. A staff nurse is familiar with the residents assigned to his or her care and can help identify the designated risks, symptoms, and treatment for infection. This important solicitation of the assistance of staff nurses may eliminate daily chart and Kardex review by the ICP, although "walking rounds" with visits to nursing stations is an extremely important part of surveillance (4).

In a nursing home, actual review of all the charts and Kardexes in search of new orders and infectious conditions is far too time-consuming even in a small facility. An alternative method of surveying is usually employed; a resident survey can be done daily by a staff nurse on each nursing area. Some institutions find the night charge nurse on a unit more compliant with the resident survey activity. An individualized **infection surveillance report form** is useful in accumulating the data about residents. Such a report is completed by the staff nurse, signed, and

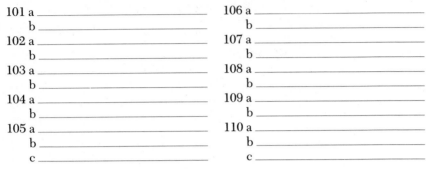

Date _____   Unit _____

DAILY INFECTION SURVEILLANCE REPORT

101 a _____   106 a _____
    b _____   b _____
102 a _____   107 a _____
    b _____   b _____
103 a _____   108 a _____
    b _____   b _____
104 a _____   109 a _____
    b _____   b _____
105 a _____   110 a _____
    b _____   b _____
    c _____   c _____

CODE: A = Pt. on antibiotic
      C = Culture taken today
      I = Isolation or precaution maintained
      U = Urine cloudy or foul; burning with urination
      T = Temperature of 101°F orally or greater
     Dr = Drainage from a wound or lesion
    NVD = Nausea or vomiting or diarrhea
      F = Foley catheter
     FI = Foley catheter put in
     FO = Foley catheter taken out
     IV = Intravenous therapy
     NA = New admission

Nurse Completing Report _____

Figure 9.1.   Infection surveillance report form. (From *Outline for Surveillance and Control of Nosocomial Infections.* Atlanta, Center for Disease Control, 1972.)

given to the ICP at the end of the shift report. The ICP then reviews the reports from all nursing units. An example of an infection surveillance report form is seen in Figure 9.1. Using a code, the significant information is placed next to the designated resident bed.

Communication with nursing staff and infection surveillance report forms are merely devices to help the ICP find clues to infection. Clues that suggest an infection include fever, abnormal x-rays, antibiotic administration, isolation, purulent drainage, and the obtaining of cultures.

If a culture is done, the physician obviously suspects infection; so any resident who has had a culture done will need to be assessed for transmission of the suspected infection. Isolation or precautions may be necessary during the incubation of the culture (see Chapter 16). The mode of transmission of the suspected infection must be determined and the appropriate isolation or precaution immediately instituted. Any resident found to be receiving an antibiotic must be followed for evidence of infection, particularly of nosocomial origin. Symptoms of infection are also identified on the daily infection surveillance report form. Cloudy urine, fever, drainage from a wound, nausea, vomiting, or diarrhea assessed by the staff nurse could be clues to the development of a nosocomial infection or an outbreak within the facility. Obvious risks of infection in geriatric populations include the presence of a Foley catheter, intravenous administration, and decubitus ulcers. These risks are also identified through the use of the form and the code.

Other potential sources of information are laboratory information and radiology reports. It is often useful for the ICP to review all microbiology and radiology reports as they come back to the nursing home from outside facilities.

Forms

After reviewing the resident survey the ICP must then determine where more information is needed. A separate **infection report form** should be initiated for any resident suspected of having a new infection. Some practitioners prefer $8\frac{1}{2} \times 11$ paper for a three-ring looseleaf notebook. Others choose a 5×8 card to be placed in a card file. The looseleaf forms will probably provide for easier storage and filing for small-scale programs. The sheets could be run on a conventional copy machine in quantities as needed without the use of professional services for pre-printing cards. The 5×8 cards, on the other hand, are easier to handle and somewhat more durable.

The infection report form should be initiated by the ICP from the resident survey data. An infection report form like the one seen in Figure 9.2 can be designed to provide a worksheet for the ICP to accumulate data specific to the resident's suspected nosocomial infection. The form should be designed to collect only the data that will be useful in determining nosocomial infections and causes. Liberal use of abbreviations will save the ICP much time in completing the forms.

Most of the information and assessments needed to complete the infection report form will be available from the resident's chart. The form itself is not a part of the resident's medical record; rather, it is a worksheet to help the ICP collect and analyze data. The form is used for any resident experiencing an infection during his stay in the nursing home, any resident confined to isolation or precautions, any resident experiencing a

INFECTION REPORT FORM

Instructions: This form should be inititated for
(1) Any infection that appears during patient's stay
(2) Any isolation or precaution
(3) Any communicable or reportable disease
(4) Any culture ordered

NOTE: This report will NOT be made part of the patient's record.

Date of admission _____ Date of discharge _____ Nsg. unit _____
Patient's name _____ No. _____
Diagnosis _____ Doctor _____
Was infection identified on admission? ____ Yes ____ No
Infectious symptom noted _____ Date noted _____
Culture ordered? ____ Yes ____ No   Type _____ Date _____
Name of patient in same room at onset of infection _____
Predisposing factors _____
Underlying process _____
Culture source _____ Organisms _____
Culture date _____
Antibiotics given & date first used _____
Comments _____

Refer to nosocomial criteria (on back of page) _____
Nosocomial infection? ____ Yes ____No
Apparent cause and recommendation _____
If patient expired, was infection the cause of or related to mortality?
____ Yes ____ No

Signature   Date

Figure 9.2. Infection report form. (From *Outline for Surveillance and Control of Nosocomial Infections.* Atlanta, Center for Disease Control, 1972.)

communicable or reportable disease, and any resident who has a culture ordered.

The form includes the date of admission, a critical factor in determining nosocomial infections. The date of discharge may be important if the resident expires or is transferred to a local hospital. The ICP should record the nursing unit, the resident number, the physician, and the diagnosis. Recognition of the infected resident's roommate is important information in fitting together an outbreak or epidemic within the nursing home. If the resident has a roommate, that name should also be entered on the form.

Identifying the infectious symptoms is also critical, and the date that the infectious symptom was first noted should be placed on the form. Predisposing factors should be listed if they can be identified and will help in the analysis of the infection and prevention of future infections. Examples of predisposing factors are presence of a Foley catheter in a resident with an apparent urinary tract infection or the presence of a decubitus ulcer in a resident with a skin infection. The resident's underlying diseases should be identified; examples of underlying diseases are cerebrovascular accident (stroke), carcinoma, and diabetes.

If a culture is done, the source should be given along with the date that the culture was taken. The organisms isolated from the culture should be obtained and listed on the form. If antibiotic therapy was given, the date it was started should be listed along with any other comments. Results of ancillary tests such as urinalysis, white blood count, and chest x-rays should be recorded if available. Transfer forms should be reviewed by the ICP on newly admitted residents.

Analysis of infection initially involves determining if the resident is truly infected or merely colonized. Information necessary for this decision is based on the symptoms; residents who are merely colonized rarely have symptoms such as fever or wound drainage. The outcome of any cultures that are done is beneficial in identifying true infections. Most nursing homes depend on a commercial laboratory outside the institution. Specimens must be transported outside the building where inoculation of culture media is done. Obtaining accurate results from the culture is dependent upon correct technique in culturing the body site and appropriate transportation of the specimen to the laboratory. Culture techniques are reviewed in Chapter 1.

The nosocomial criteria seen in Figure 9.3 can be printed on the back of the infection report form for easy reference to the ICP. The appropriate criteria should be identified so the determinations can be made whether the case meets the criteria for an infection. If a "yes" is marked in the section for nosocomial determinations, this resident becomes a statistic for the monthly infection report. Apparent cause should be given if ascertainable. If the resident expires, notation should be made as to whether this infection could have been the cause of or related to the resident's mortality. The entire form should be signed and dated. The form can be kept in the ICP's notebook until all information is obtained and the determination is made (see below). Often a report is retained in the surveillance notebook until the resident's clinical condition improves (e.g., temperature drops or drainage subsides).

CRITERIA FOR DETERMINING NOSOCOMIAL INFECTION

A. Urinary tract
   1. Colony count over 10^5 with previous negative culture/UA
   2. New pathogen over 10^5 in repeat culture
   3. Clinical symptoms (dysuria, fever, cloudy urine, frequency, etc.) developed with previous negative culture/UA
B. Respiratory infection—upper: Clinical manifestations of nose, throat, ear infection after admission (interval between admission and onset over incubation period); includes coryzal syndromes, streptococcal pharyngitis, and otitis media
C. Respiratory infection—lower
   1. Signs and symptoms (cough, pleuritic chest pain, fever, purulent sputum) developed after admission
   2. Purulent sputum (with or without pathogen on culture OR suggestive chest x-ray)
   3. Suprainfection with new pathogen AND clincial or x-ray evidence that new organism is associated with deterioration in patient condition
D. Gastroenteritis
   1. Onset of symptoms after admission AND positive culture (interval between admission and onset over incubation period)
   2. Negative stool culture followed by a positive
   3. Viral symptoms AND other cases in-house
E. Other cutaneous infections
   1. Onset of purulent drainage from skin or subcutaneous tissue (after admission)
   2. Change in pathogen if continuing purulent drainage can be attributed to new pathogen
   3. Cellulitis
F. Intravenous site
   1. Purulent drainage
   2. Cellulitis
   3. Inflammation PLUS positive culture of catheter tip OR aspirations of tissue fluid
G. Endometritis: Purulent cervical discharge with either positive culture or systemic manifestations
H. Indicated in chart by physician as nosocomial
 I. An infection on admission directly related to or residual of previous admission

Figure 9.3. Nosocomial infection criteria. (From *Outline for Surveillance and Control of Nosocomial Infections*. Atlanta, Center for Disease Control, 1972.)

Review of the final culture report after 48 hours of incubation is recommended. Preliminary reports are helpful in assessing the need for
control measures, but final reports are more reliable for nosocomial determinations. Culture results assist the ICP in evaluating the infection,
but one must not forget that routine bacterial cultures do not identify
viral or mycoplasma infections. Such diseases are usually identified by
clinical symptoms (see Chapter 1).

Nosocomial Determination

When an infection is found, it must be decided whether or not that infection is nosocomial. Nosocomial determinations can be made by the
ICP once all the data related to the resident's infection are gathered.
However, in complicated cases the ICP may request assistance from the
chairman of the infection control committee or another physician. Such
assistance will often involve differentiating between infection and colonization or determining a feasible incubation period for the resident's
infection. The ICP must keep in mind that a nosocomial infection is one
that was not present or incubating at the time of admission to the nursing
home. It is critical that the date of onset of the resident's signs and symptoms be specifically identified. This date (and sometimes hour) must be
considered along with the known incubation period of the infection. If
the incubation period is unknown and the infection developed more than
48 hours after admission, it is called **nosocomial.** Any infection with obvious signs and symptoms noted upon admission is easily classified as
community-acquired.

Superinfection is a possibility the ICP should be alert for in the already-
infected resident. A resident compromised by infection is vulnerable to
invasion by other microorganisms in that same or another body site.
Similarly, a resident may have more than one simultaneous infection.
An infection report form should be filled out for each nosocomial infection.

DATA ANALYSIS

Recordkeeping

A continuing record of all infections present within the institution must
be kept. The information recorded on the infection report form is then
transferred to a line-listing form. In order to meet the individual needs
of the ICP, a line-listing form can be developed (see the top of Fig. 9.4).

INFECTION CONTROL LINE-LISTING REPORT

Month/Year _____

Patient ID	Room/ Area	Age	Sex	Doctor	Admission Date & Diagnosis	Risk Factors	Site & Type of Infection	Cult. & Date Done	Pathogens	Date of Onset & Symps.	Treatment	Inf. Control Action Taken	Dschg. Date

EMPLOYEE INFECTION LINE-LISTING REPORT

Month/Year _____

Employee ID	Dept/Nsg. Area	Infectious Symptoms	Date of Onset	Days Absent	Treatment	Infection Control Action Taken

Figure 9.4. Infection line listing forms. (From *Outline for Surveillance and Control of Nosocomial Infections*. Atlanta, Center for Disease Control, 1972.)

This form is kept for quick future reference as well as for providing an overview of the infections present within the nursing home for a given month. Sometimes in an outbreak or cluster of infections the index case (first case of an outbreak) may be community-acquired. However, the other cases caused by this infection will be nosocomial. For this reason, all infections occurring within the facility, both nosocomial and community-acquired, should be line-listed.

Liberal use of abbreviations will facilitate the line-listing task. The form can be hand-printed and lined. It can be run on a conventional copying machine using 8½ × 13 paper in order to provide adequate space for data. Once nosocomial determinations have been made from infection report forms, the ICP may wish to lightly shade the resident's infection on the line-listing form with a red pencil. This provides easy reference in locating nosocomial infections on the line-listing form during infection control meetings.

Computing Nosocomial Infection Rates

In Chapter 1, it was pointed out that numbers of infections are not as useful for analysis as infection **rates.** The infection rate takes fluctuation in resident base (denominator) into account. Infection rates are used within an institution to provide a common basis for evaluating surveillance data. In acute care hospitals in the United States, about 5–10% of all patients develop nosocomial infections. Thus, the incidence rate for nosocomial infections is 5–10%. Similar rates have been found in nursing home populations (see Chapter 4). During the first 12 months of a surveillance program, infection rates can be determined in order to develop a data base for future comparisons. Comparison to the nursing home's own prior rates is the most valid standard for evaluating change.

Most acute care hospitals use the number of patient discharges in computing their nosocomial infection rates. Since the number of resident discharges from a nursing home is usually low, the monthly census is a more significant figure for computing infection rates. The number of resident-days may also be used; this would demonstrate the increased risk occurring with increased length of stay within the institution. If monthly census figures or resident-days are used, these figures must be obtained from the administration of the nursing home.

To begin the task of computing a nosocomial infection rate, accumulate infection report sheets and separate out those that have been marked "yes" for meeting the nosocomial criteria. Count these. The total becomes the numerator for the computation. Place this number over the denominator (the monthly census figure) and multiply by 100, as in the example that follows:

Assume a nursing home has an average daily census of 140 for July. The ICP finds 14 nosocomial infections during that month. The nosocomial infection rate for July is

$$\frac{14}{140} \times 100 = 10\% \text{ (infection rate)}$$

or

$$\frac{14}{(140 \times 31)} \times 1000 = 3.2 \text{ (infections per 1000 resident-days)}$$

The same method of calculation is used to compute monthly infection rates by nursing unit or area. Infection report forms termed nosocomial are separated by nursing unit. The number of nosocomial infections from an individual unit is placed over the monthly census for that unit. This product is multiplied by 100, which yields a monthly nosocomial rate for each unit.

An attack rate is a special kind of incidence rate. It is used to document infections from a group within a limited period of risk. Most often it is used in situations where a common source of infection like food poisoning is identified. For example, the attack rate for residents eating spoiled potato salad might be 47%. The most common use of attack rate by a nursing home is in evaluating the risk of urinary tract infection in catheterized residents.

Thus far we have discussed incidence rates, which reflect the number of new infections occurring in the nursing home. A **prevalence** rate may also be used; this is the percentage of persons in a population with a nosocomial infection *at any given time*. For example, if a one-day study reveals 7 residents with active nosocomial infections and the nursing home has 140 residents, then the prevalence rate of nosocomial infection is

$$\frac{7}{140} \times 100 = 5\%$$

Prevalence infection rates may have some value for a nursing home infection control program (4). Prevalence rates may be done at regular intervals in order to test the validity of monthly incidence rates. They may also help to establish priorities for infection control efforts. The prevalence rate identifies the number of infections at a particular point in time. Such a rate is usually determined with data accumulated over a single 24-hour period. All available charts of residents within the facility are systematically reviewed, and any resident with an infection is identified and documented. The criteria for infection used in surveillance can be used in prevalence studies also (see Appendix). Prevalence studies will obviously require more surveillance time and personnel, and they should be carefully undertaken and planned by the infection control committee.

Whatever rate is used in the analysis of infection data, several points should be kept in mind. First, rates should be consistent (i.e., use the same collection methods and denominator data) so that comparisons are valid. Secondly, nosocomial infection rates should be used by the ICP and/or infection control committee to look for deviations from normal that may suggest an outbreak (see Chapter 10) or to solve infection control problems (5).

As surveillance data are accumulated and organized, the ICP should be continually searching for clusters of infection of either the same body site or microorganism. Clusters of residents with similar symptoms are also notable. Surveillance data should be evaluated at the end of each week and especially at the end of the month when infection rates and statistics are made available. The weekly review will be a brief assessment of developing trends. If necessary, these assessments can be made with the assistance of the chairman of the infection control committee or another physician. Monthly evaluation of the infection rate should be done at the infection control committee meeting.

Seasonal trends should be noted. These are annual variations in occurrence of particular diseases that increase when circumstances facilitate the transmission. An example of a seasonal trend is an increase in respiratory infections occurring during the cold winter months when residents are not allowed outside and the closed quarters increase transmission and contact among them.

Care should be taken not to compare statistics such as monthly nosocomial infection rates with other extended care institutions or acute care hospitals. Every facility has its own individualized method of calculating statistics, and to compare rates outside an institution is dangerous and may lead to erroneous conclusions. For this reason, infection rates are usually confidential information of the facility. An exception to this rule might be a situation where a group of nursing homes is managed collectively; comparison among the individual facilities may be requested by administration. This comparison is appropriate only if all facilities use the same method of calculating infection rates and serve comparable resident populations.

Comparison is, however, one of the major reasons for surveillance. The most beneficial and significant comparison is the comparison of the infection rate for one month with that of the same month last year. This analysis deemphasizes seasonal trends. A similar evaluation is the comparison of the rate for one month with that of the previous month. Another potential comparison is the comparison of one nursing unit with another unit, although this is significant only if the units have comparable

NOSOCOMIAL INFECTION MONTHLY REPORT

Month/Year _____

Nsg. Area	UTI	Upper Resp.	Lower Resp.	Cutaneous	Bacteremia	GI	Other	Total	Nosocomial Rate
2 South									
2 North									
3 South									
3 North									
4 South									
4 North									
TOTAL									

Pathogens	UTI	Upper Resp.	Lower Resp.	Cutaneous	Bacteremia	GI	Other	Total
Staph. aureus								
Staph. epidermidis								
Pneumococcus								
Strep. grp A								
Enterococci								
E. coli								
Klebsiella								
Enterobacter								
Pseudomonas								
Proteus								
Serratia								
Bacteroides								
Candida								
Hemophilus								
Other (specify)								
Not Cultured								
TOTAL								

Figure 9.5. Nosocomial infection monthly report form. (From *Outline for Surveillance and Control of Nosocomial Infections*. Atlanta, Center for Disease Control, 1972.)

resident populations and nursing staff. A comparison with other units may emphasize to a nursing unit staff that better compliance with infection control procedure is needed. A desired outcome of surveillance is to generate comparison in order to change the behavior of persons or change environmental factors.

Reporting of Results

A report summarizing the nosocomial infection rate should be prepared for the infection control committee and administration each month. Surveillance data are not useful unless shared with the medical staff, nursing home administration, and employees. The ultimate goal of surveillance is to improve resident care, and infection rates therefore, become a progress report for staff and others concerned with the quality of care. An example of a nosocomial monthly report form is seen in Figure 9.5. Nursing areas can be listed on the vertical axis with common body sites for infection on the horizontal axis. Total numbers of infections and nosocomial rates are tallied on the right. The bottom portion of the report exhibits the statistical summary of pathogens isolated from body sites if cultures were done. After preparing the report, it may be helpful to go over it with another person to insure that it is understandable and clear. Mark the report form with the method used to calculate rates.

The use of visual aids such as graphs may be useful in getting the attention of the infection control committee members and staff. Simple, concise graphs will outline trends that can be visualized and understood by most employees, even those unfamiliar with surveillance methods and computation of statistics. Reporting of nosocomial infection rates can provide positive as well as negative feedback to staff. Infection statistics and reports should not just be filed, because behavior does not change without knowledge of the need for change.

The ICP is usually identified as the liaison with the local health department for disease reporting. Forms or methods specifically outlined by the state in which the nursing home functions must be used. Prompt identification and notification of reportable diseases are most important in assisting the health department in preventing community-related outbreaks and epidemics.

EMPLOYEE SURVEILLANCE

Surveillance within a nursing home should include observation of the employee population as well as the resident population. Comparisons should be made between nosocomial infections occurring in residents and those identified within the employee population. An example of an employee surveillance line-listing form for accumulation of data on employee infections is seen at the bottom of Figure 9.4. The information collected is much the same as the information line-listed for resident infections.

At the end of the month, summaries can be made of the information related to employee infections and reported to the infection control committee. These summaries might include the number of employees absent from work with symptoms of upper respiratory infection, gastrointestinal complaints, and cutaneous infections. Significant comparisons should be noted. Employee health problems are reviewed in Chapter 15.

SUMMARY

The components needed for surveillance are:
1. The infection control practitioner
2. Definitions of infections
3. Surveillance procedures (how to collect data)
4. Data collection forms
5. Data analysis techniques
6. Report forms
7. Communication of surveillance results to appropriate people

A surveillance program must be individually developed for a nursing home. It should be simple and basic at first. After acceptance has been established within the institution, extension of the program can occur. Data collection should be done continually. Weekly and monthly evaluations of data provide the most benefit from the time spent in data collection. Ongoing, prospective surveillance is more beneficial than retrospective methods (e.g., chart reviews) because it permits earlier detection of infection control problems such as epidemics.

Surveillance can be organized through the use of three forms: the daily infection surveillance report, the infection report form, and the infection control line-listing report. A report form should also be developed for bringing surveillance information back to the infection committee meeting monthly. After information is collected it must be analyzed. The relationship among admission date, the onset of symptoms of infection, and any predisposing factors is critical for the determination of nosocomial origin.

Comparison of nosocomial infection rates should be carefully undertaken by the infection control committee. Surveillance of nursing home employees for infections should also be included in the surveillance program. Prevention and control of infection through improved compliance with infection control procedures is the desired outcome of surveillance.

REFERENCES

1. Thacker SB, Keewhan C, Brachman PS: The surveillance of infectious diseases. *JAMA* 249:1181–1185, 1983.
2. *Outline for Surveillance and Control of Nosocomial Infections.* Atlanta, Center for Disease Control, June 1972.
3. Axnick KJ: Surveillance of nosocomial infections, in Barrett-Connor E, Brandt SL, Simon HJ, Dechairo D (eds): *Epidemiology for the Infection Control Nurse.* St Louis, Mosby 1978.
4. Hofherr L: Nosocomial infection surveillance techniques: A review. *APIC J* 7:12–15, 1979.
5. Latham EK, Standfast SJ, Baltch AL, et al: The prevalence survey as an infection surveillance method in an acute- and long-term care institution. *Am J Infect Control* 9:76–81, 1981.

APPENDIX

CDC Guidelines for Determining Presence and Classification of Infection*

URINARY TRACT INFECTIONS

1. Asymptomatic Bacteriuria is applied to those persons having colony counts in urine of greater than 100,000 organisms per ml without previous or current manifestations of infection; such asymptomatic urinary tract infections should be classified as nosocomial if an earlier urine culture was negative at a time when the patient was not receiving antibiotics. If a patient is admitted to the hospital with a urinary tract infection, subsequent culture of a new pathogen in numbers greater than 100,000 organisms per ml should be regarded as a nosocomial infection.

2. Other Urinary Tract Infections—the onset of clinical signs or symptoms of urinary tract infection (fever, dysuria, costovertebral

*source: Center For Disease Control, Atlanta, Ga.

angle tenderness, suprapubic tenderness, etc.) in a hospitalized patient in conjunction with one or both of the following factors developing after admission is sufficient for the diagnosis of nosocomial urinary tract infections.

a. Colony counts of greater than 10,000 pathogens per ml (in midstream urine specimen) or visible organisms on Gram smear of unspun fresh urine.

b. Pyuria of greater than 10 WBC's per high power field in an uncentrifuged specimen, with urinalysis negative for pyuria on admission.

If the patient with a prior negative urinalysis and/or culture develops clinical symptoms of urinary tract infection while hospitalized, and neither urinalysis nor urine culture have been repeated, he should be considered to have a nosocomial urinary tract infection. Also, as described above, the appearance in culture of new organisms in an existing urinary tract infection together with clinical continuation or deterioration constitutes a new nosocomial urinary tract infection.

RESPIRATORY INFECTIONS

1. Upper Respiratory Infections—This category includes clinical manifest infections of the nose, throat or ear (singly or in a combination). The signs and symptoms vary widely and depend on the site or sites involved. Coryzal syndromes, streptococcal pharyngitis, otitis media and mastoiditis are all included in this category; though these diverse entities have been grouped together, the specific diagnosis should be entered on the line listings form to allow separate analysis, if desired. The majority of these infections will be viral or of uncertain etiology. Careful attention must be paid to the incubation period in order to separate community-acquired infections that develop after admission and nosocomial infections.

2. Lower Respiratory Infections—Clinical signs and symptoms of a lower respiratory infection (cough, pleuritic chest pain, fever and particularly purulence) developing after admission are regarded as sufficient evidence to diagnose respiratory infections, whether or not sputum cultures or chest x-rays are obtained. When there is evidence of both upper and lower respiratory infections, concomitantly, entries should be made for both sites on the line listing form.

Other conditions which may result in similar signs or symptoms (congestive heart failure, post-operative atelectasis, pulmonary embolism, etc.) may often be differentiated by the clinical course of the patient. However, even if such entities are suspected to be present, the diagnosis of lower respiratory infection is made in the presence of one or more of the following: purulent sputum (with or without recognized pathogen on sputum culture) or suggestive chest x-ray. Supra-infection of a previously existing respiratory infection may result in a new nosocomial infection when a new pathogen is cultured from sputum and clinical or radiologic evidence indicates that the new organism is associated with deterioration in the patient's condition. Care must be used in distinguishing supra-colonization from supra-infection.

GASTROENTERITIS

Clinically symptomatic gastroenteritis having its onset after admission and associated with a culture which is positive for a known pathogen is regarded as a nosocomial gastroenteritis. If the incubation period for the pathogen is known (i.e., salmonella, shigella, etc.), the interval between admission and the onset of clinical symptoms must be greater than the incubation period. Alternatively, nosocomial gastroenteritis may be diagnosed if a prior stool culture or cultures, obtained on or after admission from a patient with gastroenteritis, were negative for the pathogen in question.

Nosocomial gastroenteritis of viral etiology also occurs—in this instance, the main criteria should rest on epidemiologic data indicating the likelihood of cross-infection.

SKIN AND SUBCUTANEOUS INFECTIONS

1. Burn Infections—Colonization of burn surfaces with bacteria is nearly universal, and the simple isolation of pathogenic organisms is not sufficient, in itself, to allow the diagnosis of infection. Purulent drainage from the burn site and/or clinical evidence of bacteremia in a patient hospitalized for treatment of a burn should lead to a diagnosis of burn infection. Such infections are often caused by organisms carried by the patient on admission; nonetheless, such infections should be regarded as nosocomial if the clinical onset occurs after admission, as nearly all of them do. Supra-infection of burns should be regarded as a separate, new nosocomial infection.

2. Surgical Wound Infections—Any surgical wound which drains purulent material, with or without a positive culture, is considered to be the site of a nosocomial infection. The source of the organisms, whether endogenous or exogenous, is not considered.

3. Other Cutaneous Infections—Any purulent material in skin or subcutaneous tissue first developing after admission is regarded as

indicating a nosocomial infection whether or not a culture is positive, negative, or has not been taken. This category includes nonsurgical wounds, as well as various forms of dermatitis and decubitus ulcers. In patients who are admitted with skin or subcutaneous infections, a change in pathogens cultured from the infected site is regarded as a nosocomial infection if continuing purulent drainage can be attributed to a new pathogen. Cellulitis caused by bacterial agents is usually not accompanied by purulent drainage; in such instances primary reliance must be placed on clinical judgment, which may be confirmed by cultures of tissue fluid aspirates.

OTHER SITES OF INFECTION

1. Any culture-documented bacteremia that develops in a hospitalized patient who was not admitted with evidence of bacteremia is regarded as a nosocomial infection, unless the organism has been judged to be a contaminant. Such nosocomial bacteremias may occur in the absence of recognized underlying infections, or originate from a site of nosocomial infection, or from manipulation of a site which was infected at the time of the patient's admission (i.e., catheters, drains, incision and drainage, etc.).

2. Intravenous Catheters and Needles—Purulent drainage from the site of an intravenous catheter or needle is regarded as nosocomial infection, even if no cultures are obtained. Inflammation of such sites, without purulent material or strong clinical evidence of cellulitis, is not regarded as an infection unless a positive culture is obtained from the catheter tip or from aspirates of tissue fluid.

3. Endometritis—Purulent cervical discharge accompanied by either a positive culture for pathogens or systemic manifestations of infection is regarded as nosocomial endometritis if the onset occurs after admission.

4. Many other possible sites of nosocomial infection must sometimes be considered. Application of the general principles outlined above, however, will generally make classification of these infections possible. It must be re-emphasized that CLINICAL IMPRESSIONS/DIAGNOSIS (if available) always supercede laboratory or radiologic data.

INTRA-ABDOMINAL INFECTIONS

1. Appendicitis, cholecystitis, and diverticulitis should not be coded as infections unless a secondary infectious complication is noted. Abscess formation, peritonitis, and cellulitis are examples of such

complications. The infectious complications will generally be classified as community acquired.

2. If a wound infection develops following surgery for uncomplicated appendicitis, cholecystitis, or diverticulitis, the infection should be classified as nosocomial. Surgical wound infection following surgery involving any infectious complication of the above can be classified as nosocomial only if there is clear anatomical and/or temporal separation of the infectious processes.

CHAPTER 10

EPIDEMIC INVESTIGATION

Philip W. Smith

This chapter is devoted specifically to outbreaks that have been reported in nursing homes and a discussion of the general approach to a nursing home epidemic. As was discussed in Chapter 1, epidemics may be classified broadly into **common-vehicle** outbreaks and outbreaks spread by **cross-contamination.** The latter refers to outbreaks propagated by person-to-person spread, while common-vehicle outbreaks occur when a number of individuals are exposed to the same epidemic source.

Many common vehicles have been responsible for transmission of infections, including food, water, medications, and even air. Cross-contamination may occur by direct contact (person-to-person), indirect contact (with an object such as a bronchoscope transmitting the infection), by airborne spread (e.g., suspension of particles by coughing), or by a vector (e.g., spread of malaria by mosquitoes).

EPIDEMICS IN NURSING HOMES

Most nosocomial infections in the nursing home are endemic, but an important percentage occur in epidemics (1). These are theoretically more easily preventable than endemic nosocomial infections.

One needs to be aware of the great variety of infections that may cause epidemics in a nursing home. Garibaldi (1) noted clustering of cases of upper respiratory tract infections, diarrhea, conjunctivitis, and urinary tract infections, suggesting that outbreaks of these infections frequently occur in the nursing home. Personnel need to consider their potential role in the evolution of epidemics and constantly consider the decreased resistance of the institutionalized elderly resident to infectious diseases.

Airborne Outbreaks

Virtually all airborne outbreaks in nursing homes are spread by cross-infection involving airborne particle spread (see Table 10.1). An occa-

Table 10.1. Airborne Organisms Causing Epidemics in Nursing Homes

Influenza A

Influenza B

Parainfluenza

Respiratory syncytial virus (RSV)

Tuberculosis

Streptococcus, group A

sional common-source airborne outbreak occurs in institutions, such as outbreaks of Legionnaires' disease related to contaminated air-conditioning systems (2).

Reported Outbreaks. **Influenza** spreads rapidly among susceptible persons and causes mortality predominantly among the elderly and the chronically ill (see Table 4.4, Chapter 4). Several outbreaks of influenza A in the nursing home setting have been reported (3–5). In one, 25% of the 120 residents in a nursing home developed an influenzalike illness, nine of the residents died (a case fatality ratio of 30%), and the median duration of illness was nine days (3). Of the 13 residents hospitalized during the outbreak, 12 had clinical pneumonia on physical examination or chest x-ray. An influenza A Bangkok 79 (H_3N_2) virus was isolated from eight residents, most of whom had a fourfold rise in complement fixation antibody titer. In another outbreak, the attack rate was 60% and the case fatality ratio was 8.2% (5).

In the influenza B outbreak described by Hall, the attack rate was 36%, the mean duration of illness was 4.5 days, and temperatures as high as 40.9° C were noted (6). Five residents were hospitalized for treatment of pneumonia, and one resident expired. In searching for epidemiologic clues to their outbreak, it was found that residents requiring only self-care nursing experienced higher attack rates, which may reflect the increased contact among ambulatory residents resulting in a greater opportunity for spread of the influenza virus. Also noted was an increased attack rate with increasing age, an increased attack rate associated with residents on a closed (locked) intermediate care ward, and a temporal association with residents who ate the majority of their meals in a common dining room.

Another influenza B outbreak involved 37% of the residents of a large geriatric facility, and there were 26 outbreak-related deaths (7). Influenza of an unknown type was reported in a Canadian nursing home (8). The attack rate, the complication rate, and the mortality rate were all found to be higher in unvaccinated residents than in those that had received bivalent influenza A/Victoria B/Hong Kong vaccine, an observation also made by others (3,5).

An outbreak at a skilled nursing facility in New York demonstrated the potential for **respiratory syncytial virus** (RSV) to cause respiratory illness in the institutionalized elderly as well as the potential for concurrent epidemics with more than one respiratory virus (4). In outbreaks, residents usually recovered in 3–7 days without major complications (9, 10).

Another virus, **parainfluenza,** has been shown to cause respiratory illness among the elderly in extended care facilities (11,12). Both residents and employees were involved in the outbreaks.

Outbreaks of **bacterial pneumonia** in residential homes are quite unusual, but the potential for spread, particularly of staphylococcal or streptococcal pneumonia, does exist. Two cases of *Streptococcus pyogenes* pneumonia, a rare infection, were encountered in a nursing home and felt to be transmitted by respiratory spread in one case and foodborne spread in another case (13). In both instances, the infections were suspected to be spread from personnel to residents. One of the residents expired.

Tuberculosis is a mycobacterial disease of low to moderate contagiousness that is perhaps the classic example of airborne spread of disease. This disease is more common among the elderly than among any other segment of the population. Stead reported a prevalence of positive TB skin tests of 12% when he tested entering residents in a nursing home in Arkansas (14). Several serious outbreaks of tuberculosis in nursing homes have been reported (15–18), involving both residents and staff. Tuberculosis is discussed further in Chapter 5.

Control Measures.   A number of general control measures for terminating or preventing outbreaks of respiratory infections in nursing homes are suggested from the experience of nursing home respiratory epidemics described above:

1. Maintaining good health among employees is essential. In outbreaks in nursing homes as well as hospitals (19), staff-to-resident transmission of infection has been involved. One needs to keep in mind that a staff member with mild or subclinical infection (e.g., an asymptomatic influenza case) may be the source of severe or even fatal disease in the relatively debilitated and immunocompromised elderly population. Hence, one needs to maintain an effective employee health program with tuberculosis screening and annual influenza vaccination. The nursing home should educate employees

about the hazard of infection transmission to residents and encourage them to report potentially infectious diseases to an employee health nurse and maintain good personal hygiene. Employee health programs are discussed in greater detail in Chapter 15.

2. Simply alerting the staff of the nursing home to the presence of an outbreak and emphasizing standard infection control practices may terminate an outbreak. The staff should be reminded to wash hands before and after contact with every resident, especially during an outbreak.

3. During influenza outbreaks, some have recommended (3) barring the admission of residents from the community with a diagnosis of influenza, restriction of high-risk residents' visitors during community outbreaks, and cohorting residents with influenza (separating residents with influenza from those who are not infected). Residents should receive the influenza vaccine annually (see Chapter 14). In some situations, antiviral prophylaxis with amantadine may be appropriate during an institutional epidemic (20).

4. For outbreaks of influenza or other viral respiratory illnesses, it may be wise to undertake measures that will decrease contact between residents, such as discontinuing social activities, restricting acutely ill residents to one area, serving meals in rooms instead of in a common dining room, and restricting resident-to-resident visitation.

5. When there is an outbreak of tuberculosis in a nursing home, one needs to undertake a rapid and diligent search for an index case or source among residents and personnel.

Outbreaks of Gastrointestinal Disease

As discussed in Chapter 4, epidemic gastrointestinal infections may be classified by the type of reservoir. The reservoir for *Shigella,* amoebae, typhoid fever, *Giardia,* toxin-producing *Escherichia coli,* hepatitis A, hepatitis B, and viral gastroenteritis is people. Spread is generally from person-to-person, and when a foodborne outbreak occurs, it can usually be traced to an infected food handler. The reservoir for *Clostridium perfringens, Staphylococcus aureus, C botulinum,* and non-typhoid *Salmonella* is material used in the preparation of food, such as poultry, meat, or custard products.

Reported Epidemics: Person-to-Person Spread. The most important gastrointestinal infections in nursing homes that are spread from person to person are viral gastroenteritis, hepatitis A, and shigellosis (see Table 10.2).

Table 10.2. Nosocomial Gastroenteritis: Person-to-Person

Viral gastroenteritis
Hepatitis A
Shigellosis
Amebiasis
Giardiasis
Typhoid fever
Hepatitis B

Viral gastroenteritis is usually relatively mild clinically. The leading causes are Norwalk virus (21) and rotavirus (22–24). In a study by the Centers for Disease Control, 11 outbreaks of gastroenteritis due to Norwalk virus were described that resulted in 2 deaths in nursing home residents (21). In the outbreak reported by Marrie, 19 of 34 geriatric residents and 4 of 23 staff assigned to the ward developed gastroenteritis, suggesting staff involvement in transmission of the disease (24).

The **hepatitis A** (infectious hepatitis) virus is excreted in stool, and the risk of spread is significantly increased in the incontinent resident. In a hospital epidemic (25), 10% of susceptible personnel acquired hepatitis A from an incontinent patient. Institutional hepatitis A can occur in large epidemics, especially in mental institutions (26). **Hepatitis B** (serum hepatitis) is rarely involved in nursing home outbreaks. A minor epidemic of hepatitis B at a home for the aged was described in which 6 of 59 residents at a nursing home developed hepatitis B, and the source was felt to be bath brushes that resulted in cross-contamination. One resident died in that outbreak, and the hepatitis virus was demonstrated in a decubitus ulcer (27).

Shigellosis may occur in the nursing home setting. In the United States in 1981, about 70% of *Shigella* isolates were *S. sonnei* (28). Of those isolates, approximately 0.9% were from persons in institutions, where the most common species was *S. flexneri*. *Shigella* gastroenteritis is clinically much more severe than viral gastroenteritis.

Two parasitic diseases have the potential to cause outbreaks of gastrointestinal illness in nursing homes. Outbreaks of **amebiasis** occur in institutions (29), where person-to-person spread is usually involved (30). *Giardia lamblia* is a parasite that causes a milder diarrhea than *Entamoeba histolytica*, the agent of amebiasis. **Giardiasis** has occurred both by person-to-person spread in institutions (31) and in waterborne or foodborne outbreaks (32).

Finally, **typhoid fever,** although relatively uncommon in the United States, accounts for about 2% of human *Salmonella* isolates (33) and can cause nursing home outbreaks. Even a single case of this disease represents an epidemiologic emergency.

Table 10.3.   Nosocomial Gastroenteritis: Common-Source Outbreaks

Nontyphoid *Salmonella*
Clostridium perfringens
Staphylococcus aureus
Shigella

Reported Epidemics: Foodborne Gastroenteritis.   Food poisoning, foodborne gastroenteritis occurring in nursing home epidemics, is most often due to nontyphoid *Salmonella, C. perfringens,* or *Staphylococcus aureus* (see Table 10.3).

Perhaps the most important type of infectious gastroenteritis occurring in the nursing home setting is **salmonellosis.** Between 1963 and 1972, 112 of 395 outbreaks occurring in the United States occurred in institutions (34). Salmonellosis in this study was unusually severe in institutionalized persons, as evidenced by an overall case fatality ratio of 8.7% in nursing homes. There was a total of 48 deaths occurring in the 25 nursing home outbreaks over the 22-year period, and the mean number of residents ill with each outbreak was 22.

Outbreaks of nursing home–associated salmonellosis have been reported with some frequency. In one outbreak (35) a total of 38 residents, 5 staff members and 2 domiciliary contacts of one of the residents were found to be infected. Residents may excrete *Salmonella* in their stool for weeks to months, increasing the chance for secondary person-to-person spread and prolongation of an epidemic. One outbreak (36) demonstrated features of both common-source and person-to-person transmission. Forty-five of 100 residents were found to be harboring *Salmonella St. Paul* in a nursing home outbreak. Thirty-one of the 39 rooms in the nursing home had at least one resident excreting the organism. Residents excreted the organism for a median duration of 35 days. Schroeder reviewed six outbreaks of epidemic salmonellosis in nursing homes (37). The average number ill in each of these epidemics was 18.5, and the case fatality rate was 3.6%. Five of the six nursing home outbreaks were common-vehicle outbreaks. Antibiotics may prolong excretion of the organism in stool. Most cases in the nursing home setting are traced to common vehicles such as poultry, ungraded eggs, red meat, milk, dry coconut, yeast, and even various medical or pharmaceutical products of animal origin (dyes, thyroid extract, liver, vitamins).

Most episodes of food poisoning in the geriatric setting caused by **Clostridium perfringens** were related to preheated meat and poultry dishes that had been cooked one day and inadequately cooled or stored before serving on the following day. Such foods as stews, pies, rolled and minced meats, and chicken dishes were involved in the outbreaks (38). Nursing home outbreaks account for about 3% of all reported epidemics (39). **Staphylococcus aureus** enterotoxin results in nausea and vomiting one to six hours after ingestion; baked goods and custard products are most often implicated. **Shigella** foodborne outbreaks are not common and can usually be traced to a human carrier who inoculates foods during preparation.

Control Measures. The above outbreaks suggest a number of control measures for prevention of gastrointestinal outbreaks in nursing homes:

1. Promptly evaluate clusters of residents with diarrhea, fever, or jaundice. Hepatitis A may be diagnosed serologically, and stools may be examined for parasites or cultured for pathogens such as *Salmonella* or *Shigella.*

2. In special circumstances, reference laboratories may be able to test for a specific viral agent causing gastroenteritis by serologic testing for antibodies (Norwalk agents) or by testing stool for viral particles by immune electron microscopy or radioimmunoassay.

3. Bacterial isolates from stool should be saved by the nursing home or by the reference microbiology lab in the event that future studies of epidemiologic import are required. Leftover foods should be saved for culture.

4. In some instances, it may be appropriate to suspect a human carrier, either a resident or staff member, in an outbreak of viral gastroenteritis, shigellosis, hepatitis A, amebiasis, or typhoid fever. Carriers may be asymptomatic.

5. During outbreaks of hepatitis A, salmonellosis, shigellosis, amebiasis, or viral gastroenteritis, enteric precautions may be appropriate for infected residents (see Chapter 16). Handwashing needs to be emphasized.

6. Ill residents should be treated appropriately. Antibiotics have no place in the treatment of viral gastroenteritis and are rarely helpful in the treatment of nontyphoid *Salmonella* infections, but should be seriously considered for residents with amebiasis, giardiasis, shigellosis, or *Salmonella typhi* infection.

7. Elective admission of residents to a nursing home during an epidemic should be deferred. In addition, all new residents should be questioned with regard to recent diarrhea, and when such a history is positive, stool cultures should be obtained (34).

8. Making the medical staff aware of the potential transmissibility of gastrointestinal agents is important, especially in dietary departments.

9. In a foodborne outbreak, knowledge of the agent involved in the outbreak of gastroenteritis may give a clue as to the type of food to be investigated, such as looking for contaminated custard products in an outbreak of *Staphylococcus aureus* food poisoning or for eggs and poultry products in an outbreak of salmonellosis.

10. Proper food-handling and preparation practices should be specifically outlined and followed (see Chapter 15).

Diseases Spread by Contact

Bacterial Diseases. The reservoir of **gram-negative** bacteria is either residents (e.g., infected bladder or wound) or the environment (e.g., whirlpool tub). Examples of gram-negative bacteria of importance in the nursing home are *E. coli, Klebsiella, Proteus* and *Pseudomonas* (see Chapter 1, Table 1.2). Gram-negative bacteria are the leading cause of nosocomial urinary tract infections in the nursing home and frequently are involved in infections of decubitus ulcers and pneumonias.

The reservoir of **gram-positive** bacteria, on the other hand, is generally people, either those infected with the bacteria or those carrying the organism without apparent harm (colonization). **Staphylococcus aureus** is a cause of skin infections such as cellulitis and abscesses as well as deep infections of decubitus ulcers and wounds. Staphylococci may be spread by the hands of personnel or by individuals who have staphylococcal skin infections. Asymptomatic persons may be nasal carriers of *S. aureus* and may spread the organism. Residents with staphylococcal skin infection frequently require isolation to prevent spread of this organism to others (40).

The group A beta-hemolytic **streptococcus** is a virulent gram-positive bacteria that causes serious skin infections. Like *Staphylococcus aureus,* the reservoir for this organism is persons who are infected or who are carriers of the bacteria.

Cross-infection with any of these bacteria may occur in the nursing home. Both *Staphylococcus aureus* and various gram-negative bacilli may cause infections of decubitus ulcers, urinary tract, or vascular access sites. Cross-contamination between these infected sites has been shown to occur in a number of chronically hospitalized individuals (41). Gram-negative bacteria are more resistant to antibiotics than gram-positive bacteria. A number of gram-negative bacilli, such as *Pseudomonas aeruginosa* and

Klebsiella pneumoniae, may colonize the urethra, perineum, or rectum in the resident who is chronically institutionalized and may be very difficult to remove even by meticulous daily bathing (42). Control measures for residents with bacterial infections involve primarily good handwashing by personnel and physical separation of residents with infected lesions.

Resistant Bacteria.   Outbreaks of infections caused by unusually **resistant bacteria** have occurred in nursing home facilities. The greatest hazard is the spread of multiply antibiotic-resistant gram-negative bacilli, particularly in residents with urinary tract infections who have indwelling bladder catheters, and the spread of methicillin-resistant *Staphylococcus aureus* infections (43, 44). These outbreaks of staphylococcal infection are known to involve both residents and personnel. The spread of resistant bacteria appears to occur primarily via hand carriage by personnel. A number of measures have been used to terminate outbreaks in hospitals and nursing homes (see Chapter 11).

Other Problems.   **Conjunctivitis** due to bacteria or viruses may be quite contagious. Secretion precautions are appropriate (see Chapter 16). Even **scabies** has occurred in nursing home outbreaks (45). Topical treatment is available. A thorough cleaning of the environment is also indicated and should include drapes, floors, walls, and bedding. The standard laundering and drying cycle should be adequate to kill mites in clothing and bedding.

STEPS IN INVESTIGATION OF AN EPIDEMIC

Epidemics in nursing homes affect residents and staff alike. An effective infection surveillance program as described in Chapter 9 permits early detection and control of epidemics. An orderly sequence of steps should be followed when evaluating a possible outbreak (see Table 10.4).

Table 10.4   Steps in Epidemic Investigation

1. Verification of the epidemic
2. Proper communication
3. Case analysis
4. Formation of a tentative hypothesis
5. Institution of control measures
6. Completing the investigation

Verification of the Epidemic

Before one spends time investigating an epidemic, one needs to confirm whether or not there *is* indeed an epidemic. An **epidemic** is defined as the excessive prevalence of a disease in a community. In this case, the community is the nursing home population.

Confirming the Diagnosis.   In some instances, as in an outbreak of staphylococcal infection or *Shigella* gastroenteritis, one may readily confirm the diagnosis by a positive culture. The diagnosis of influenza, encephalitis, or viral gastroenteritis, however, is primarily clinical, and many different etiologies may present with an identical clinical picture. Hence, in order to carry out an objective investigation, one needs a case definition.

Case Definition.   A good case definition will assist in the evaluation of an epidemic. Case definitions may be assigned with differing degrees of stringency, with differing results. For instance, let us assume that there is an outbreak of *Salmonella* gastroenteritis on a nursing home ward. If one defines a case as "a nursing home resident who developed fever and diarrhea on ward A of a nursing home in October," then one has a definition that is specific geographically and temporally, but based on a clinical diagnosis of gastroenteritis. Included in this definition will be the vast majority of the cases of *Salmonella* gastroenteritis that occurred during the epidemic, but, in addition, other cases may be included coincidentally such as residents who have viral gastroenteritis or diarrhea related to medication. A very specific definition may be used such as "a nursing home resident on ward A with a positive stool culture for *Salmonella* during October." In this case, however, one may be excluding from the investigation a number of cases of salmonellosis that were not cultured or were improperly cultured and thus did not fit the microbiological definition of the disease.

One may stratify definitions into definite, probable, and possible cases or classify them according to whether or not they are outbreak-related. It is acceptable to refine a case definition as the investigation goes along. As an example, the initial case definition may encompass "nursing home residents with fever, cough, and a pulmonary infiltrate," but when the involved residents are found to have a positive tuberculosis skin test, the case definition may be refined to include only "residents with fever, cough, pulmonary infiltrate, and a positive purified protein derivative (PPD) test."

Case Finding.   Early in the course of the investigation of a potential epidemic, one needs to search for inapparent cases. A number of resources may be used, including the nursing home nurses or administrators, physicians who care for residents in a nursing home, the reference microbiology laboratory (particularly when a specific organism has been identified), and local or state public health officials who may be aware of outbreaks in other institutions.

The ability to characterize an outbreak depends on complete case finding. An epidemic may be larger than it first appears. A broad search may find cases earlier in time, in other areas of the nursing home, or even in other nursing homes.

Comparison to Normal Frequency.   Knowledge of the baseline frequency of occurrence of an infectious problem is necessary in order to determine whether or not an epidemic exists. The decision as to whether an epidemic is occurring depends on the disease in question and the context. For instance, 20 urinary tract infections in a large nursing home may represent a relatively normal occurrence, whereas a single case of typhoid fever represents an alarming finding. The presence of methicillin-resistant *Staphylococcus aureus* or aminoglycoside-resistant *Pseudomonas aeruginosa* might not be considered unusual in a large hospital intensive care unit, but would be quite disconcerting in a nursing home.

Two additional points need to be made here. First, the comparison to normal frequency is much easier if one deals with **rates** rather than raw numbers. Incidence and prevalence rates (see Chapter 1) facilitate objective decisions.

> *Example 1:*   An observer feels that there are more urinary tract infections (UTIs) at nursing home A than usual. A prevalence survey revealed 15 UTIs compared to 9 during a prevalence survey three months ago. However, the nursing home census was 140 then and is 223 now. The prevalence rates are 15/223 = 6.7% and 9/140 = 6.4%, not significantly different.

It is hazardous to compare rates **between** institutions. A higher UTI rate, for example, may reflect the fact that a nursing home has a more accurate data collection system, performs more urine cultures, or has more residents with urinary catheters, rather than reflecting any deficiency in infection control practices.

As we have seen, the normal incidence and prevalence of disease varies tremendously depending on the disease itself and the setting. As a rough rule, if the incidence or prevalence of a given infectious disease has doubled from the baseline incidence or prevalence, one should suspect an epidemic. A second point to be emphasized is that an epidemic may not become apparent until a more detailed analysis of the data is completed.

> *Example 2:*   Further analysis of the UTIs in Example 1 is done by examining the bacteria causing the infections. Nine of the 15 current UTIs are found by urine culture to be caused by aminoglycoside-resistant *Pseudomonas aeruginosa*, which was not seen in any urine samples in the previous survey. This definitely suggests an outbreak.

The microbiology laboratory can be of great assistance in analysis of organisms to prove whether bacterial isolates in an outbreak are identical or unrelated. Examples of such tests that can be done include antibiotic-sensitivity patterns, phage typing (*S. aureus*), pyocin typing (*Pseudomonas*), serotyping (streptococci), plasmid analysis (resistant bacteria), and restriction enzyme analysis (viruses). These tests are generally available only at reference laboratories (46,47).

Proper Communication

Once it has been decided that there is an epidemic that merits investigation, it is important to communicate to the appropriate individuals early in the course of the investigation. There are several reasons for this. First of all, communication to appropriate physicians, nursing personnel, and nursing home administrators is courteous and avoids misunderstanding and confusion. Misinformation may cause panic about an epidemic. Secondly, this communication may lead to discovery of additional cases that can be included in the epidemic investigation. Finally, communication with public health officials is important because it may lead to recognition of an epidemic that extends beyond the boundaries of the individual nursing home and thereby has public health impact.

Case Analysis

Line Listing of Cases.   An appropriate first step during an epidemic is to perform a line listing of cases that involves listing all cases involved in the epidemic in a column with a few key information bits on each case (see Table 10.5). Examples of baseline information include resident room number, age, name, date of onset of symptoms, and culture results. The line listing permits very rapid assessment of the extent and general nature of the outbreak. Line listings can be expanded to include other relevant

Table 10.5. Sample Line Listing: Outbreak of Diarrhea in Nursing Home, June 1983

Case No.	Patient	Age	Date of Onset	Room
1	JS	84	6/2/83	A-16
2	RB	71	6/2/83	A-16
3	GS	59	6/2/83	A-19
4	AY	92	6/4/83	A-24
5	LL	68	6/10/83	B-3
6	TR	69	6/11/83	B-5

data that may have bearing on the cause of the outbreak. For instance, in a respiratory disease outbreak, one may want to list information on chest x-rays or TB skin test. In an outbreak of gastroenteritis, one may wish to list whether the resident eats in his room or in the common dining room and whether the resident is incontinent. In an outbreak of urinary tract infection, one needs to know whether or not residents have indwelling bladder catheters or are sharing rooms with other residents who have indwelling bladder catheters.

Making an Epidemic Curve.   Often it is easier to characterize an epidemic when results are in graphic form; hence, an epidemic curve is useful in describing an epidemic. The epidemic curve should be plotted with the number of cases on the vertical axis and time on the horizontal axis (see Fig. 10.1). The shape of the curve may facilitate classification of the epidemic in terms of exposure and method of spread. A **person-to-person** epidemic, for instance, is suggested by a bimodal curve with the larger first peak and a smaller secondary wave of disease due to spread from the group of patients who were primarily infected to other susceptibles. This may be seen in influenza outbreaks. Another type of outbreak is a **common-source** outbreak, which may be further divided into single- or continuous-exposure epidemics. A sharply rising and falling curve suggests a **single-point exposure,** as in a staphylococcal food poisoning outbreak. A flat or undulating curve suggests **continuous exposure,** such as an outbreak of Legionnaires' disease related to a contaminated cooling tower.

Demographic Analysis.   A demographic analysis involves the continued search for clues to underlying cause. After the initial line listing and epidemic curve have been done, demographic analysis may involve simply a more complex line listing looking for other common factors. A resident's medical history, geographic location in the nursing home, or con-

EPIDEMIC CURVES

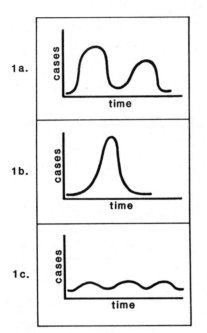

Figure 10.1. Epidemic curves for typical person-to-person (1a), point exposure–common source (1b), and continuous exposure–common source (1c) outbreaks.

tact with other residents or nursing home staff may provide information that gives a clue to the outbreak.

Another aspect of demographic analysis is preparation of frequency distributions and graphs by time, place, and person. Plotting locations of cases geographically may be useful when person-to-person spread is suspected (see Table 10.6). Detailed food histories are necessary when investigating a foodborne outbreak.

Table 10.6. Sample Frequency Listing: Outbreak of Respiratory Disease in Nursing Home, May 1983

Ward Location	No. of Respiratory Disease Cases	No. of Influenza Cases
1E	4	0
1W	8	1
2E	10	2
2W	12	8
3E	7	0
3W	10	2

Statistical Analysis.   A refinement of the data collection process is the calculation of statistical rates. Outbreaks can usually be solved without complex statistics, but some statistical analysis may help the investigation. Basic statistics such as incidence rate, prevalence rate, and attack rate are useful tools (see Chapter 1). More elaborate tests of statistical association are discussed elsewhere (48).

Formation of a Tentative Hypothesis

At this point, one has hopefully characterized the outbreak thoroughly with regard to time, place, person, and possible mode of spread. Estimation of incubation period may be possible by measuring the time from a common-source exposure to the mean date of onset of cases or by measuring the distance between primary and secondary epidemic curves in a person-to-person epidemic.

In order to form a hypothesis, reference sources must be consulted. Background information is gathered from studying the literature or by consulting with others who have experience with the problem. Texts are available that describe diseases in terms of contagiousness, mode of spread, incubation period, period of communicability, symptoms, diagnosis, and control measures (49,50). The literature may also reveal clues to the etiology by describing associations of organisms with certain vehicles, such as *Salmonella* and egg products.

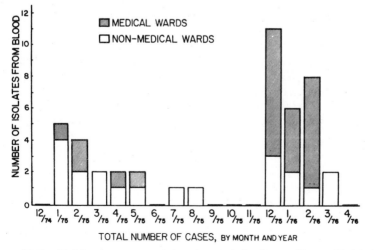

Figure 10.2.   Epidemic curve—*Acinetobacter* infections. (From Smith PW, Massanari RM: Room humidifiers as the source of Acinetobacter infections. *JAMA* 237:795–797, 1977. Copyright 1977, American Medical Association.)

Example 3:   In a published outbreak of *Acinetobacter* infections (51), the epidemic curve displayed peaks in winter months. The institution was located in a cold climate, which led the authors to suspect and investigate room humidifiers as a source of airborne spread (see Fig. 10.2).

Example 4:   The data in Table 10.6 suggest an influenza cluster on ward 2W, probably originating from an infected resident, staff member, or visitor. A listing of respiratory diseases did not provide as much information as a specific listing of influenza cases.

Institution of Control Measures

Testing the Hypothesis.   The hypothesis should be tested either by intervening to see if the epidemic disappears with appropriate control measures or by instituting further steps for data collection. In Example 3 above, the contaminated room humidifiers were removed and the epidemic ceased. More data were gathered by doing laboratory tests on bacterial colonization of room humidifiers as well as the potential of humidifiers to disperse airborne bacteria. It was found that humidifiers in infected patients' rooms were colonized with *Acinetobacter calcoaceticus* and that the contaminated humidifiers could spray the organism at least 10 meters.

Other examples of data collection include culturing equipment or personnel, typing of organisms, and sending out questionnaires to gather more information, as was done in the Legionnaires' disease outbreak in Philadelphia (52). As a general rule, cultures of personnel and environment should not be performed hastily or early in the investigation. They should be performed selectively after a hypothesis has been developed for possible spread of the epidemic organism. Indiscriminate culturing is expensive and may cause panic on the part of personnel or residents. However, collection and saving of specimens for future study may be wise.

Implementing Control Measures.   The goal of an epidemic investigation is, of course, to control or terminate the epidemic. In addition, the best test of the hypothesis frequently is to intervene (e.g., to remove humidifiers, to sterilize respiratory therapy machines, to treat the staphylococcal carrier) and then to see if the epidemic stops. Sometimes epidemics are terminated even if a precise cause is not pinpointed. This may be because the investigation itself reminds personnel of correct procedures (e.g., handwashing or cleaning instruments) about which they may have become lax. A reminder may be enough to improve performance and terminate the epidemic. Alternatively, ancillary control measures (such as isolation for tuberculosis cases) may stop an outbreak. These common-sense measures to protect residents and personnel should be instituted as the epidemic is progressing and not await final investigation results.

Causality.   Because of the occasional random disappearance of epidemics during investigation, one must be cautious about ascribing credit to any particular individual control measure. In addition, it must be remembered that statistical association does not prove causality (48). A nurse who is a staphylococcal nasal carrier may not be responsible for an outbreak of staphylococcal infection among residents, as an example. The nurse may have a different strain of *S. aureus* than the one that caused the epidemic. Secondly, even if the nurse has the epidemic strain, she may have acquired it from a resident with an infected decubitus ulcer rather than the reverse (staff-to-resident transmission). Statistical or microbiological association should not necessarily imply guilt or causality.

Testing Effectiveness of Control Measures.   Control measures, even if they seem logical, may not stop an epidemic. The search for new cases must go on. Failure of control measures requires reconsideration of the hypothesis.

Completing the Investigation

When recommendations to implement certain control measures are made, they should be made specifically and in writing. One may recommend modification of the environment, personnel changes, procedural or policy changes, or implementation of an educational program. Sometimes it is necessary to make interim recommendations until the exact cause of an outbreak has been defined.

During the investigation, one needs to save as much information as possible. All bacterial isolates collected during the investigation should be saved in the event that serotyping, phage typing, or antibiotic sensitivity testing is required. These tests may help to determine whether cultures of organisms found during an epidemic investigation are identical to the epidemic strain. All records, questionnaires, interviews, and line listings should be filed for future reference.

During the course of an investigation, the appropriate persons should be informed of the progress of that investigation. This would include nursing home officials, physicians, and public health officials.

Good records should be kept during the entire epidemic. At the conclusion of an epidemic, a complete and thorough report should be made and sent to all appropriate individuals. This report should include when and how the investigation was initiated, persons involved in the investigation, persons notified during the investigation, all data collected, control measures implemented, and effectiveness of these control measures.

ILLUSTRATIVE EXAMPLE: SALMONELLOSIS IN A NURSING HOME

The following relates the events during an actual epidemic of salmonellosis in a Nebraska nursing home that demonstrates appropriate investigation techniques.*

Background. The nursing home involved is a 72-bed community nursing home. All beds are intermediate care beds. The nursing home employs about 60 employees. A single kitchen prepares food for all residents, and all but the bed feeders consume meals in a central dining room. The home has three wings that share one nursing station adjacent to the lounge and the dining room. The Nebraska State Health Department was requested to intervene in the outbreak. The investigation was carried out by the state epidemiologist, Nebraska State Health Department. He was contacted initially by a physician from the nursing home area when it was noted that during a five-day period, 16 residents and two staff members of the nursing home became ill with diarrhea, fever, and vomiting.

Verification of the Outbreak. The investigating team that visited the nursing home included the state epidemiologist, a representative from the Division of Housing and Environmental Health, and two representatives from the Division of Licensure and Standards, which is responsible for inspection of nursing homes and hospitals in Nebraska.

The records of all suspected cases were reviewed in order to confirm the presence of diarrhea. A case definition was developed. By this time, a number of residents had *Salmonella enteritidis* isolated from their stools. Hence, a case was defined as "a resident having a positive stool culture

*The author wishes to thank Paul A. Stoesz, M.D., Director, Disease Control Division, Nebraska State Health Department, for providing him with this case study.

for *Salmonella* and any two of the following symptoms: abdominal pain, diarrhea, and fever."

Cases were collected by interviews with appropriate nursing home staff, including administrative staff, nurses, and physicians. The records of all suspected cases were reviewed to determine if each met the formulated case definition. It was determined that during a five-day period, 16 residents and two staff members of the nursing home had become ill with diarrhea, and 12 of the 16 cases were found to be stool culture–positive for *Salmonella enteritidis*. Two of the 12 infected residents expired.

No precise baseline statistics had been kept at the nursing home during the previous years. However, all were in agreement that the number of cases of diarrhea in general and *Salmonella* in particular were greatly increased over normal.

Communication.   The investigating team communicated with state public health officials and with all appropriate administrative and medical interests at the nursing home and in the local community.

Analysis of the Cases.   A line listing of cases was compiled (see Table 10.7). The nurses' notes were reviewed to determine the level of nursing care each resident required, type of diet, and other information. An epidemic curve was drawn (see Fig. 10.3). The shape of the curve suggested a common-vehicle outbreak with a single-point source.

An investigation of the food service area was conducted to evaluate the role of sanitation. Food service personnel were interviewed in order to determine the sources of food served and the techniques of handling, storing, preparing, and serving of food to the residents. The menus listing the food served at each meal for 72 hours prior to the first case were also reviewed. Food service personnel were questioned about their own prior gastrointestinal illness history.

At this point, selective stool cultures were performed on all residents suspected of being involved in the epidemic and all food service employees. Some of the food service equipment and several food samples were also cultured. All isolates of *Salmonella* obtained during this outbreak were sent to the Bureau of Laboratories at the Centers for Disease Control for serotyping.

Early in the investigation it was noted that a total of 18 residents were on pureed food and that 15 of the 16 cases fell in this group. Furthermore, none of those who were well had eaten the pureed diet. A review of menus for the 72 hours prior to the first case revealed four foods that were frequently associated with the transmission of *Salmonella*. When each of these foods was served in the pureed state, it was not served to

Table 10.7. Characteristics of Cases of Salmonellosis: Illustrative Example

Case No.	Age	Sex	Onset of Illness	Diarrhea	Fever	Vomiting
1	83	F	8/11/81	+	+	−
2	71	F	8/12/81	+	+	−
3	90	F	8/12/81	+	+	−
4	—	F	8/12/81	+	+	−
5	74	F	8/11/81	+	+	−
6	88	F	8/11/81	+	+	−
7	96	F	8/11/81	+	+	+
8	91	F	8/11/81	+	+	−
9	80	F	8/11/81	+	+	−
10	94	F	8/11/81	+	+	−
11	66	F	8/11/81	+	+	−
12	89	F	8/12/81	+	+	−
13	83	F	8/11/81	+	+	−
14	82	F	8/10/81	+	+	−
15	101	F	8/11/81	+	+	−
16	97	F	8/13/81	+	+	−
17[a]	—	F	8/14/81	+	+	−
18[a]	—	F	8/14/81	+	+	+

[a]Staff members

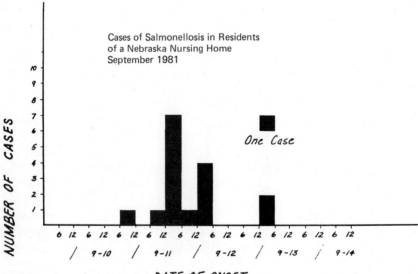

Figure 10.3. Epidemic curve—*Salmonella* cases in a nursing home.

the other residents. All of the food ingredients were from commercial sources, and three were leftovers from previous meals. The suspected foods were pureed in a blender just prior to serving. Roast beef and chicken were contained in the suspected foods. Only one food was available for culturing and was negative for *Salmonella*.

Investigation of the methods used to clean and sanitize food service equipment revealed no written protocol for kitchen help to follow. There was a lack of supervision in the kitchen at all times, lack of monitoring of internal temperatures of foods during cooking and reheating, and lack of knowledge of the proper temperatures. No food service personnel had a history of gastrointestinal illness. All submitted stool cultures, and all were negative for *Salmonella*.

Stool cultures on the 12 cases that were positive for *Salmonella enteritidis* were all confirmed as being serotype *montevideo*.

Formation of a Tentative Hypothesis.   Several facts were evident at this point:

1. There was an outbreak of febrile diarrheal illness due to a certain *Salmonella* strain.
2. *Salmonella* outbreaks are usually foodborne, and deficiencies in food handling and preparation practices were noted.
3. The epidemic curve suggested a single-exposure, common-vehicle outbreak.
4. The only mode of transmission shared by all cases was food, suggesting a foodborne outbreak.
5. The food histories among the residents who had acquired salmonellosis suggested that the food was contaminated during the puree process.
6. It is known that the incubation period of *Salmonella* is 6–72 hours. The median onset of illness was 3:00 p.m., August 11. Hence the range of possible infected meals was 3:00 p.m. on August 8 through 9:00 a.m. on August 11.

Control Measures.   It was impossible to test the impact of control measures on the epidemic curve since the point source exposure period had passed without the occurrence of additional cases. The hypothesis was tested statistically when investigation revealed that 15 of 16 cases had eaten a pureed diet 72 hours prior to the onset of illness compared to none ill who had not eaten the pureed diet. This is highly statistically significant. An effort was made to confirm the theory microbiologically

Table 10.8.   Salmonella Outbreak—Suggested Control Measures

1. Food should be obtained from sources that comply with all laws relating to food inspection and labeling.

2. In food service areas, all food should be protected against contamination during storage, preparation, and serving. Potentially hazardous food requiring cooking should be cooked to heat all parts of the food to a temperature of at least 140°F. However, poultry, poultry stuffings, stuffed meats, and stuffings containing meat shall be cooked to heat all parts of the food to at least 165°F, and pork or any food containing pork shall be cooked to heat all parts of the food to at least 150°.

3. Potentially hazardous foods that have been cooked and then refrigerated or frozen shall be reheated rapidly throughout to 165°F or higher before being served or before being placed in a hot-food-holding unit.

4. A metal stem-type thermometer should be used in order to assure the attainment and maintenance of proper internal cooking, holding, or refrigeration temperatures of all potentially hazardous foods.

5. Potentially hazardous food requiring refrigeration after preparation should be rapidly cooled to an internal temperature of 45°F or below. Potentially hazardous foods of large volume or prepared in large quantities should be rapidly cooled, utilizing such methods as shallow pans, agitation, quick chilling, or water circulation external to the food container so that the cooling period does not exceed four hours.

6. Food service equipment and utensils should be washed, rinsed, and sanitized after each use in order to prevent cross-contamination in the kitchen and to prevent the accumulation of food residue that may decompose or support the development of bacterial pathogens or toxins.

7. Food contact surfaces of equipment and utensils should be easily cleanable, smooth, and free of breaks and open seams that make such a surface impossible to clean and sanitize.

8. All operations of the food service should be supervised at all times. The supervisor should instruct the staff in their responsibilities through in-service training. In order to prevent contamination of food and food contact surfaces, employees must comply with strict standards of cleanliness and personal hygiene. This would include hand-washing, clean clothing, and hair restraints.

9. The development of an infection control committee should be initiated considering the population of the nursing home. The committee could perform surveillance of infections in the facility to assist early epidemic control.

by culturing the blender, but this had been cleaned in the interim, and cultures were negative.

Interim control measures were immediately recommended by the Health Department at the initiation of the investigation. These included cohorting of staff members who treat residents, moving all infected cases into one wing of the nursing home, and recommending that no double rooms be shared by well and ill residents. It was decided that there would be no interchange of staff with resident contact from one wing to another, that no new residents would be allowed into the nursing home until the epidemic was resolved, and that all cases would be placed in enteric precautions. These control measures prevented secondary person-to-person propagation of the epidemic.

Completing the Investigation.   A detailed final report was made that included a number of control measures designed to prevent recurrence of the outbreak (see Table 10.8). Control measures addressed washing, rinsing, and sanitizing of the kitchen equipment as well as proper food handling, holding, reheating, and serving. Cultures of all food service workers were negative. In view of this and the known epidemiology of *Salmonella* infections, it was suspected that the source was not a food service worker, but rather contaminated poultry, eggs, or meat that had been brought into the kitchen and, through inadequate cooking and reheating, had led to infection of those who ate the food. The final report and recommendations were written clearly and specifically, as is ideal.

REFERENCES

1. Garibaldi RA, Brodine S, Matsumiya S: Infections among patients in nursing homes: Policies, prevalence, and problems. *N Engl J Med* 305:731–735, 1981.

2. England AC, Fraser DW: Sporadic and epidemic nosocomial legionellosis in the United States: Epidemiologic features. *Am J Med* 70:707–711, 1981.

3. Goodman RA, Orenstein WA, Munro TF, et al: Impact of influenza A in a nursing home. *JAMA* 247:1451–1453, 1982.

4. Mathur U, Bentley DW, Hall CB: Concurrent respiratory syncytial virus and influenza A infections in the institutionalized elderly and chronically ill. *Ann Intern Med,* 93 (Part 1):49–52, 1980.

5. Centers for Disease Control: Impact of influenza on a nursing home population—New York. *Morbid Mortal Weekly Rep* 32:32–34, 1983.

6. Hall WN, Goodman RA, Noble GR, et al: An outbreak of influenza B in an elderly population. *J Infect Dis* 144:297–302, 1981.

7. Silverstone FA, Libow LS, Duthie E, et al: Outbreak of influenza B in a geriatric long-term care facility, abstracted. *Gerontologist* 20(Part 2):200, 1980.

8. Genesove LJ, Riddiford M: Influenza in a nursing home. *CMA J* 118:1202, 1978.

9. Center for Disease Control: Respiratory syncytial virus—Missouri. *Morbid Mortal Weekly Rep* 26:351, 1977.

10. Garvie DG, Gray J: Outbreak of respiratory syncytial virus infection in the elderly. *Br Med J* 281:1253–1254, 1980.

11. Center for Disease Control: Parainfluenza outbreaks in extended-care facilities—United States. *Morbid Mortal Weekly Rep* 27:475–476, 1978.

12. Parainfluenza 3 spread linked to direct contact. *Hosp Infect Control* 7:16, 1980.

13. Barnham M, Kerby, J: *Streptococcus pyogenes* pneumonia in residential homes: Probable spread of infection from the staff. *J Hosp Infect* 2:255–257, 1981.

14. Stead WW: Infections in nursing homes. *N Engl J Med* 306:302, 1982.

15. Abrahams EW, Edwards FGB, Harris KWH, et al: Minor epidemics of tuberculosis. *Med J Austral* 2:1115–1119, 1967.

16. Center for Disease Control: Tuberculosis—North Dakota. *Morbid Mortal Weekly Rep* 27:523–525, 1979.

17. Center for Disease Control: Tuberculosis in a nuring home—Oklahoma. *Morbid Mortal Weekly Rep* 29:465–467, 1980.

18. Stead WW: Tuberculosis among elderly persons: An outbreak in a nursing home. *Ann Intern Med* 94:606–610, 1981.

19. Van Voris LP, Belshe RB, Shaffer JL: Nosocomial influenza B virus infection in the elderly. *Ann Intern Med* 96:153–158, 1982.

20. Douglas RG, Jr: Amantadine as an antiviral agent in influenza. *N Engl J Med* 307:617–618, 1982.

21. Kaplan JE, Gary GW, Baron RC, et al: Epidemiology of Norwalk gastroenteritis and the role of Norwalk virus in outbreaks of acute nonbacterial gastroenteritis. *Ann Intern Med* 96(Part 1):756–761, 1982.

22. Cubitt WD, Holzel H: An outbreak of rotavirus infection in a long-stay ward of geriatric hospital. *J Clin Path* 33:306–308, 1980.

23. Halvorsrud J, Orstavak I: An epidemic of rotavirus-associated gastroenteritis in a nursing home for the elderly. *Scand J Infect Dis* 12:161–164, 1980.

24. Marrie TJ, Lee SHS, Faulkner RS, et al: Rotavirus infection in a geriatric population. *Arch Intern Med* 142:313–316, 1982.

25. Goodman RA, Carder CC, Allen JR, et al: Nosocomial hepatitis A transmission by an adult patient with diarrhea. *Am J Med* 73:220–226, 1982.

26. Matthew EB, Dietzman DE, Madden DL, et al: A major epidemic of infectious hepatitis at an institution for the mentally retarded. *Am J Epidemiol* 98:199–215, 1973.

27. Braconier JH, Nordenfelt E: Serum hepatitis at home for the aged. *Scand J Infect Dis* 4:79–82, 1972.

28. Centers for Disease Control: Shigellosis—United States, 1981. *Morbid Mortal Weekly Rep* 31:681–682, 1982.

29. Krogstad DJ, Spencer HC Jr, Healy GR, et al: Amebiasis: Epidemiologic studies in the United States, 1971–1974. *Ann Intern Med* 88:89–97, 1978.

30. Sexton DJ: Amebiasis in a mental institution: Serologic and epidemiologic studies. *Am J Epidemiol* 100:414–423, 1974.

31. Thacker SB, Simpson S, Gordon TJ, et al: Parasitic disease control in a residential facility for the mentally retarded . *Am J Pub Health* 69:1279–1281, 1979.

32. Osterholm, MT, Forfang JC, Ristinen TL, et al: An outbreak of foodborne giardiasis. *N Engl Med* 304:24–28, 1981.

33. Centers for Disease Control: Human Salmonella isolates—United States, 1981. *Morbid Mortal Weekly Rep* 31:613–615, 1982.

34. Baine, WB, Gangarosa EJ, Bennett JV, et al: Institutional salmonellosis. *J Infect Dis* 128:357–360, 1973.

35. Anand CM, Finlayson MC, Garson JZ, et al: An institutional outbreak of salmonellosis due to lactose-fermenting *Salmonella newport*. *Am J Clin Pathol* 74:657–660, 1980.

36. Gotoff, SP, Boring JR, Lepper MH: An epidemic of *Salmonella St. Paul* infection in a convalescent home. *Am J Med Sci* 56:16–22, 1966.

37. Schroeder SA, Aserkoff B, Brachman PS: Epidemic salmonellosis in hospitals and institutions: A five year review. *N Engl J Med* 279:674–678, 1968.

38. Sharp JCM, Collier PW: Food poisoning in hospitals in Scotland. *J Hyg Camb* 83:231–236, 1979.

39. Shandera WX, Tacket CO, Blake PA: Food poisoning due to *Clostridium perfringens* in the United States. *J Infect Dis* 147:167–170, 1983.

40. Kunin C: Staphylococcal infection control in a long-term facility. *JAMA* 245:2352, 1981.

41. Vaziri, ND, Cesario T, Mootoo K, et al: Bacterial infections in chronic renal failure occurrence with spinal cord injury. *Arch Intern Med* 142:1273–1277, 1982.

42. Gilmore DS, Jimenez EM, Aeilts GD, et al: Effects of bathing on *Pseudomonas* and *Klebsiella* colonization in patients with spinal cord injuries. *J Clin Micro* 14:404–407, 1981.

43. O'Toole, RD, Drew WL, Dahlgren BJ, et al: An outbreak of methicillin-resistant *Staphylococcus aureus* infection: Observation in hospital and nursing home. *JAMA* 213:257–263, 1970.

44. Aeilts GD, Sapico FL, Canawati HN, et al: Methicillin-resistant *Staphylococcus aureus* colonization and infection in a rehabilitation facility. *J Clin Micro* 16:218–223, 1982.

45. Scabies in Institutions. *J Iowa Med Soc* 71:78–79, 1981.

46. Aber RC, Mackel DC: Epidemiologic typing of nosocomial microorganisms. *Am J Med* 70:899–905, 1981.

47. Goldman DA, Macone AB: A microbiologic approach to the investigation of bacterial nosocomial infection outbreaks. *Infect Control* 1:391–400, 1980.

48. Colton T: *Statistics in Medicine*, 1st ed. Boston Little, Brown, 1974.

49. Benenson AS (ed): *Control of Communicable Diseases in Man*, 13th ed. American Public Health Association, Washington DC, 1980.

50. Wehrle PF, Top FH Sr: *Communicable and Infectious Diseases*, 9th ed. St Louis, Mosby, 1981.

51. Smith, PW, Massanari RM: Room humidifiers as the source of *Acinetobacter* infections. *JAMA* 237:795–797, 1977.

52. Fraser DW, Tsai TR, Orenstein W, et al: Legionnaires' disease: Description of an epidemic of pneumonia. *N Engl J Med* 297:1189–1197, 1977.

CHAPTER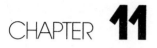

ANTIBIOTICS

Philip W. Smith

OVERVIEW OF ANTIBIOTICS

Mechanisms of Action

The term **antibiotic** includes agents active against microorganisms rang-ing from viruses to parasites. The most commonly used agents are an-tibacterial drugs.

The development of effective antiviral agents has been limited by the difficulty in killing the virus without damaging the human cell in which it lives. As a result, there are a limited number of antiviral agents available. Adenine arabinoside is a moderately effective systemic agent for some serious herpes simplex infections. Acyclovir can be used topically for herpes genitalis. Amantadine hydrochloride has limited application as prophylaxis against influenza A infection during epidemics. These drugs interfere with the penetration of viruses into human cells or with viral nucleic acid replication.

Antibacterial drugs generally act by one of five mechanisms: inter-ference with cell wall synthesis, damaging the bacterial cell membrane, inhibition of DNA synthesis, inhibition of protein synthesis, or interfer-ence with bacterial metabolism.

Penicillins, cephalosporins, and vancomycin are drugs that act by in-terfering with bacterial cell wall synthesis. Penicillin itself is an extremely useful drug against streptococci, *Streptococcus pneumoniae, Neisseria men-ingitidis, Neisseria gonorrhoeae,* syphilis, and anaerobic infections. Because most strains of *Staphylococcus aureus* have become resistant to penicillin, the family of drugs that includes methicillin, oxacillin, nafcillin, cloxacillin, and dicloxacillin have become the drugs of choice for treatment of *S. aureus* infections. Ampicillin and amoxicillin are penicillin derivatives that are very useful against enterococci, *Hemophilus influenzae, Salmonella, Shi-gella, Escherichia coli,* and *Proteus mirabilis* infections. Finally, there are several new broad-spectrum penicillins used parenterally against *Pseu-*

domonas aeruginosa. Included in this group are carbenicillin, ticarcillin, mezlocillin, piperacillin, and azlocillin.

The family of antibiotics known as cephalosporins is of greatest importance in treatment of staphylococcal and other infections in patients who are allergic to penicillin. Newer, broad-spectrum cephalosporins are active against many of the gram-negative bacteria found in hospitals and nursing homes, but they are very expensive and lack consistent activity against *Pseudomonas aeruginosa.*

Bacterial protein metabolism is affected by a number of agents, including the aminoglycosides, tetracyclines, clindamycin, chloramphenicol, and erythromycin. Aminoglycosides are still the most consistently effective antibiotics against the great variety of gram-negative bacteria found in the hospital and nursing home environments. They can be given only parenterally; the most widely used aminoglycosides are gentamicin, tobramycin, and amikacin. Clindamycin and chloramphenicol are appropriate drugs for treating anaerobic infections, and erythromycin may be used for *Mycoplasma* pneumonia and Legionnaires' disease and as an alternative to penicillin for streptococcal infections. Tetracyclines are very broad spectrum oral drugs.

Sulfonamides are examples of antibiotics that act by interfering with bacterial metabolism. Sulfonamides, pyrimethamine, and trimethoprim interfere with folate metabolism in microorganisms. Sulfonamides and trimethoprim are used orally in the treatment of urinary tract infections.

Antifungal agents generally alter the fungal cell membrane. Amphotericin B can be administered only intravenously in the therapy of fungal infections. Two oral drugs of assistance in treatment of fungal infections are flucytosine and ketoconazole. Ketoconazole is indicated for several superficial fungal infections, including severe cutaneous *Candida* infections.

Pharmacokinetics

Patients not requiring hospitalization are usually treated with oral antibiotics. Food, antacids, and malabsorptive disorders often interfere with drug absorption. Intramuscular administration should be avoided in the presence of shock and bleeding disorders. Intravenous administration assures reliable blood levels, but requires the presence of an intravenous cannula.

Antibiotics may also be classified by their route of elimination (see Table 11.1). Drugs excreted by the kidney should be used with extreme caution in the presence of renal disease (1). Drug elimination is measured by the $t_{1/2}$ (half-life), the time it takes a normal person to lower the level

Table 11.1. Antibiotics

Drug	Half-Life	Primary Route of Elimination	Major Side Effects
Penicillins	30–60 min	Renal	Hypersensitivity
Cephalosporins	40–120 min	Renal	Hypersensitivity
Aminoglycosides	2–3 hr	Renal	Nephrotoxicity, ototoxicity
Tetracyclines	6–20 hr	Renal, hepatic	Dental staining, rash, GI intolerance
Erythromycin	1.5 hr	Hepatic	Cholestatic hepatitis, GI intolerance
Clindamycin	4 hr	Hepatic	Diarrhea, colitis
Chloramphenicol	2–3 hr	Hepatic	Bone marrow suppression
Sulfonamides	6–18 hr	Renal, hepatic	Hypersensitivity, crystalluria
Trimethoprim	11 hr	Renal	Anemia, rash
Vancomycin	6 hr	Renal	Nephrotoxicity, phlebitis
Polymyxin	6 hr	Renal	Nephrotoxicity
Metronidazole	7 hr	Renal	GI intolerance

Source: Smith PW: Infectious Diseases, in Kochar MS (ed): *Textbook of General Medicine*, 1st ed. New York, 1983. Used with permission.

of antibiotic in blood by 50%. The longer the $t_{1/2}$, the fewer daily doses of an antibiotic are needed for adequate therapy.

Side Effects

Toxicity.   Toxicity is defined as a dose-related or expected side effect of a drug. This will inevitably occur if a drug is used long enough and at a high enough dosage. Examples of antibiotic toxicity include renal failure and deafness (aminoglycosides), vertigo (streptomycin), optic nerve problems (ethambutol), and aplastic anemia (chloramphenicol). Antibiotic toxic effects may or may not be reversible. Aminoglycoside nephrotoxicity is generally reversible when the drug is discontinued, whereas aminoglycoside ototoxicity is often irreversible. Toxicity can be minimized by a knowledge of drug side effects (see Table 11.1) as well as an awareness of appropriate length of therapy. Adverse reactions to antimicrobial agents have been shown to occur in about 5% of all antibiotic courses and are often severe (2). The elderly appear to be at greater risk of adverse drug reactions (3).

Allergy.   Allergic or hypersensitivity reactions are generally less common, unexpected side effects of antibiotics that do not occur in all persons. Examples of hypersensitivity reactions include rash, serum sickness, anaphylaxis, asthma, and allergic vasculitis. These are most commonly seen with penicillins, cephalosporins, and sulfonamides, but may be seen with almost any antibiotic. Immediate hypersensitivity, which occurs shortly after administration of an antibiotic, can be life-threatening. Urticaria, anaphylaxis, and shock comprise the syndrome. A hypersensitivity reaction to any antibiotic requires discontinuation of the offending drug and avoidance of all related drugs in the future. The medical record should clearly document the presence and nature of a drug allergy; a labeled medical bracelet may be appropriate.

Superinfection. Antibiotics are never completely specific for the intended pathogenic organism but have varying degrees of effect on normal bacterial flora. If the normal flora of the body is disturbed by antibiotic therapy, the host becomes more susceptible to other pathogens. Broad-spectrum antibiotics, such as the broad-spectrum penicillins, third-generation cephalosporins, and the tetracyclines, exert an especially profound influence on normal bacterial flora of the host and are associated with a higher incidence of superinfection. Organisms commonly responsible for superinfections include resistant gram-negative bacteria, yeast (especially *Candida albicans),* and *Clostridium difficile,* the organism responsible for antibiotic-associated colitis.

Resistance Development. Widespread use of antibiotics has resulted in the emergence of many antibiotic-resistant strains of microorganisms (see below).

Cost. In an era of increasing cost awareness, another potential undesirable consequence of antibiotic usage is expense. The cost of new antibiotics, in particular, is great. For instance, a 10-day course of therapy with the third-generation cephalosporin moxalactam, at maximal dosage, would cost several thousand dollars. In view of the marginal therapeutic benefits of many of the new antibiotics, a physician must consider cost when making an antibiotic selection.

Measuring Antibiotic Sensitivities

Antibiotic sensitivity testing for bacteria is most commonly performed by the Bauer–Kirby method. This involves measurement of the zone of inhibition of bacterial growth around an antibiotic-impregnated disk. The size of the zone determines sensitivity or resistance (see Fig. 11.1).

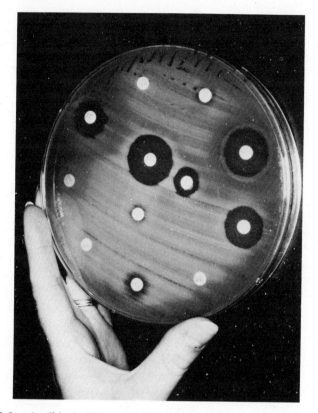

Figure 11.1. Antibiotic disk sensitivity testing. (From Smith PW: Infectious Diseases, in Kochar MS (ed): *Textbook of General Medicine*, 1st ed. New York Wiley, 1983. Used with permission.)

Broth or agar dilution methods enable the laboratory to quantitatively determine the minimum concentration of an antibiotic that is inhibitory (minimum inhibitory concentration, MIC) or bactericidal (minimum bactericidal concentration, MBC) for an organism. Automated MIC measurements are used instead of the disk sensitivity method by a number of laboratories. Comparison to achievable antibiotic levels enables the laboratory to provide a convenient "sensitive" or "resistant" interpretation.

The concentration of an antibiotic in the serum can be measured by a variety of techniques. The microbioassay is the standard method, but more accurate and rapid methods are being developed, such as the radioenzymatic assay for gentamicin.

ANTIBIOTIC RESISTANCE

The Extent of the Problem

Antibiotic resistance is a worldwide problem of great public health import (4). The most serious problem is bacterial resistance, especially hospital strains of gram-negative bacilli resistant to multiple antibiotics and methicillin-resistant *Staphylococcus aureus* (5,6). Other examples of important bacterial resistance include penicillin-resistant gonorrhea, ampicillin-resistant *Hemophilus influenzae,* and chloramphenicol-resistant *Salmonella.*

Resistance problems are not confined to bacteria, however, as demonstrated by dapsone-resistant leprosy, isoniazid-resistant tuberculosis, flucytosine-resistant cryptococcosis, and chloroquin-resistant malaria. Herpes simplex strains resistant to acyclovir lack the thymidine kinase enzyme necessary for drug activity.

Nosocomial antibiotic resistance problems are not confined to hospitals. Reported problems in nursing homes have included antibiotic-resistant gram-negative bacilli, particularly associated with urinary tract infections, and methicillin-resistant *Staphylococcus aureus* (MRSA).

Gram-negative bacilli such as *E. coli, Proteus mirabilis, Klebsiella pneumoniae,* and *Pseudomonas aeruginosa* are leading causes of urinary tract infections (UTIs) in the nursing home resident, especially the catheterized resident. These bacteria are frequently resistant to multiple antibiotics. Gram-negative bacteria causing UTIs in the nursing home are generally more resistant than those found in the community (7,8) and may occur in clusters suggesting epidemic spread (9).

MRSA has the potential for interhospital spread or spread between hospitals and nursing homes (10). O'Toole et al. described an outbreak of MRSA in a hospital that was traced to a nursing home (11). A number of significant points were brought out in their investigation. First, the potential of nursing homes to serve as a source for infection in the hospital setting was confirmed. In addition to the index case, two additional cases of residents who carried the identical strain of MRSA were detected in the nursing home. Secondly, the importance of cutaneous lesions in disseminating bacteria was demonstrated, and temporary hand carriage by personnel was felt to be the most likely mode of spread in the nursing homes. Thirdly, a detailed case analysis suggested that administration of antibiotics encouraged colonization with the methicillin-resistant strain.

Another study of colonization with MRSA involved a rehabilitation facility (12). The authors found 84 episodes of MRSA colonization or infection in 81 residents. The MRSA was capable of causing significant disease, since 28 (34.5%) of the residents developed infection with MRSA.

Many other residents remained colonized for long periods of time; the most common sites of colonization were the anterior nares and wounds. By doing serial cultures, the authors were able to determine that of the 84 cases of MRSA carriage, 65% were nosocomially acquired and 34% were acquired from transferring hospitals.

Mechanisms of Resistance

Some degree of resistance has eventually been seen with virtually every antibiotic developed. Organisms have devised a number of ways to circumvent antibiotics (13). The most common biochemical mechanism is production of an enzyme that inactivates the antibiotic. An example of this is the penicillinase produced by *Staphylococcus aureus, Neisseria gonorrhoeae,* and *Hemophilus influenzae,* which cleaves the penicillin molecule. Aminoglycosides also are enzymatically inactivated. Other mechanisms of resistance include evolution of a target site that is less susceptible to antibiotic action (erythromycin) and decreased uptake and transport of an antibiotic (tetracycline).

Bacteria have several genetic mechanisms for spreading drug resistance. Resistance that is coded for in the bacterial chromosome is passed on to daughter cells. Bacteria, however, have evolved a much more rapid system for transferring drug resistance. A **plasmid** is an extrachromosomal piece of DNA that codes for a number of genetic traits, including drug resistance. Multiple copies of a plasmid may be present per cell, and plasmids may be spread between bacteria of the same or different species. Plasmids greatly increase genetic adaptability of bacteria and enable resistance to be spread from bacterium to bacterium very rapidly.

Another point to be kept in mind is that antibiotic resistance that develops to a given antibiotic is often "linked" to antibiotic resistance to other drugs. In other words, administration of a given antibiotic often encourages development of resistance not just to that antibiotic, but to many other antibiotics as well.

Causes of Resistance

Numerous studies have demonstrated that the extent of resistance can be correlated directly with the extent of antibiotic usage. Antibiotic resistance can appear rapidly; in fact, resistance may appear after a single exposure to an antibiotic. Under the selective pressure of antibiotic administration, resistant bacteria become prominent when antibiotic-sensitive bacteria are eliminated.

Once resistance develops, spread occurs. This is particularly true in the hospital and nursing home environment, where one encounters a population of persons with multiple medical illnesses in close proximity, many of whom are receiving antibiotics. The final common pathway for spread is usually the hands of nursing home or medical personnel. Person-to-person spread of antibiotic-resistant bacteria on the hands of personnel has been implicated in several outbreaks (14–16).

Solutions

Solutions to the problem of antibiotic resistance can be aimed either at preventing development of antibiotic-resistant bacteria or at blocking their spread.

Since antibiotic usage correlates directly with the extent of antibiotic resistance, one potential solution is to decrease the amount of antibiotics used. Several studies have consistently demonstrated a great deal of inappropriate antibiotic usage. In fact, probably only about 50% of antibiotics used both in inpatients and outpatients are appropriate (17–20). Errors in administration of antibiotics include inadequate documentation of indications for antibiotic administration, errors in antibiotic dosing, administration of an antibiotic in spite of documented resistance on sensitivity testing, and even administration of antibiotics when no indication exists, such as in the patient with a viral upper respiratory tract infection.

This very discouraging picture of antibiotic misuse is grounded in several factors. Physicians have a great desire to help the patient and often feel uncomfortable when there is no effective therapy for a disease process. In addition, lack of knowledge of the natural history of various infectious diseases may impel a physician to erroneously prescribe an antibiotic. The physician is often under a great deal of pressure from pharmaceutical companies to prescribe their product and may in fact make antibiotic decisions more on the basis of drug company information than scientific literature (21). Finally, the physician is also frequently under pressure from the patient himself, who desires that "something be done," and from nurses who are concerned about the patient's condition or the presence of a fever.

Education. It is clear that more accurate and conservative administration of antibiotics would result in better medical care, less antibiotic resistance, and considerable cost savings for the patient. One proposed solution is increased education of physicians. While this is a very logical first step, results have been somewhat mixed (22,23). Some have advocated an approach called "counter-detailing" of antibiotics, in which a physician or pharmacist is responsible for presenting an objective review of antibiotics to the practitioner (24).

Antibiotic Control.   When education fails, more drastic measures may be required. Deletion of certain drugs from the hospital formulary is one way to decrease abuse of the substances (25). Some hospitals have required that physicians justify in writing in the hospital record the indication for antibiotic administration (26). Even this simple restraint may substantially decrease the use of antibiotics. Automatic stop orders on antibiotics have been used. Hospitals may also restrict the use of an antibiotic or require infectious disease consultation prior to use of certain widely abused or toxic antibiotics (27,28). In certain extreme cases, all antibiotics have been discontinued when no other measure serves to stop an epidemic of multiply resistant bacterial infections (29).

Isolation.   Other measures may be employed in the nursing home setting to interrupt the spread of antibiotic-resistant bacteria from patient to patient or from environment to patient. Isolation methods have been found to be effective in terminating a number of epidemics. In one outbreak (30), patients who were infected with multiply resistant *Pseudomonas aeruginosa* were admitted to a single room and placed in isolation for resistant bacteria (see Fig. 11.2). Others have found that similar measures have effectively terminated outbreaks (31,32).

Isolation for Resistant Bacteria

1. Private room (physician's order).
2. Wear gloves when having contact with the infected secretion or Foley catheters (urine, sputum, blood, stool, other drainage).
3. Dispose of items contaminated with the resistant bacteria—e.g.:
   a. Urine and feces: Flush directly down toilet, then clean urinal or bedpan with full-strength Lysol solution.
   b. Dressings: Place in paper bag and incinerate.
   c. Oral secretions: Have patient cough into tissue and place tissue in stick bag. Incinerate stick bag.
   Adherence to sterile technique is essential when performing procedures that involve the infected secretion, e.g., suctioning, dressing changes, irrigations, Foley catheter care.
4. Handwashing:
   Patient—following contact with infected secretions.
   Personnel—following any patient contact.

Figure 11.2.   Isolation for resistant bacteria. (From Smith PW, Rusnak P: Aminoglycoside-resistant *Pseudomonas aeruginosa* urinary tract infection: Study of an outbreak. *J Hosp Infect* 2:71–75, 1981. Used with permission.)

ANTIBIOTICS: ASPECTS OF IMPORTANCE IN THE ELDERLY

Drug Usage in the Elderly

Because of age-related diseases, the elderly use more drugs in general and more antibiotics in particular than younger persons. The population over the age of 65 years comprises about 11% of the total population of the United States, and yet they spend approximately 21% of the total national budget for drugs (33). Residents in long-term care facilities are frequently recipients of multiple drugs; in one survey, 73% of nursing home residents received at least three prescription medications daily (34). Two nursing home surveys found that about 10% of residents were receiving antibiotics (9,35), and almost half were receiving sedatives or tranquilizers (9).

Pharmacology

The pharmacokinetics and metabolism of drugs are different in the elderly (36–38). Perhaps the most important change is the decrease in renal function with age, which results in altered elimination of drugs excreted by the kidney. Glomerular filtration rate declines with age, with a mean 35% reduction in the elderly compared with the young. Most commonly used antimicrobial agents are excreted by the kidney; hence, one may expect higher levels and delayed excretion in the elderly.

In the elderly, in general, lean body mass declines and adipose tissue mass increases relative to total body weight, resulting in an altered distribution of drugs. There may be a decrease in serum level of proteins that bind drugs, resulting in a greater level of free antibiotic in the serum. The elderly may also have decreased drug absorption from the intestine or altered hepatic metabolism of drugs.

A number of practical points based on the altered metabolism of drugs in the elderly have been proposed (33), including using smaller doses for the elderly and simplifying the drug regimen. Potentially toxic drugs need to be monitored especially closely. For example, gentamicin pharmacokinetics are quite variable in the elderly, which makes frequent measurement of gentamicin levels prudent (39).

Adverse Drug Reactions

Adverse drug reactions appear to occur more frequently in the elderly. Several studies have found an adverse reaction rate of 10–20% in patients over the age of 60, a figure that is considerably higher than the corresponding rate for patients between the ages of 40 and 50 (3,40).

One reason for the increase in adverse reactions among the elderly may be the altered excretion or metabolism of drugs in this population group. This is felt to explain the increased nephrotoxicity of aminoglycoside antibiotics in the elderly patient (41). Altered hepatic metabolism with age may explain the observation that isoniazid hepatoxicity increases steadily with age (42).

Other factors contributing to the problem of increased adverse drug reactions in extended care facilities include adverse drug interactions, medication errors, and inappropriate therapy (43). Thus, the elderly appear to be more susceptible to adverse drug reactions intrinsically and have an increased risk of such adverse occurrences by virtue of requiring multiple medications.

Drug Interactions

In view of the great number of drugs used by the elderly patient, the risk of the adverse interactions among the drugs is significant. The risk of adverse interaction increases exponentially with increasing numbers of drugs.

The interactions between antibiotics and other drugs have been categorized (44,45):

1. One type of interaction is the displacement of a drug from a protein binding site by an antibiotic that is also protein-bound. An example of this is the displacement of tolbutamide or warfarin from a serum carrier site by sulfonamides, resulting in hypoglycemia or bleeding, respectively, due to increased levels of free (i.e., active) drug.

2. A second type of mechanism is competition for renal tubular secretion. In this instance, probenecid competes with antibiotics such as penicillins and cephalosporins for renal elimination, resulting in elevated antibiotic levels.

3. Antibiotics may affect hepatic enzymes that control elimination of other drugs. As an example, isoniazid inhibits the hepatic enzymes responsible for diphenylhydantoin (dilantin) elimination, resulting in dilantin toxicity.

4. Drugs may interact at tissue sites to potentiate toxicity, as exemplified by the increased nephrotoxicity associated with the use of aminoglycosides with ethacrynic acid or furosemide.

5. Miscellaneous types of interactions that are possible include the effect of one drug on another by alteration of urinary acidity, decreased absorption (e.g., of oral tetracycline by oral antacids and iron), and reactions similar to that with disulfiram (Antabuse) when alcohol is ingested with metronidazole or moxalactam.

Table 11.2. Antibiotic–Drug Interactions

Antibiotic	Drug	Interaction
Penicillin	Probenecid, acetylsalicylic acid	Raised levels
Doxycycline	Phenobarbital, phenytoin	Shortened half-life of doxycycline
Tetracycline	Antacids	Decreased absorption
Aminoglycosides	Cephalosporins	Enhanced renal toxicity
Chloramphenicol	Tolbutamide	Enhanced tolbutamide action
	Oral anticoagulants	Enhanced action
Aminoglycosides	Ethracrynic acid, furosemide	Enhanced nephrotoxicity
Sulfonamides	Tolbutamide, oral anticoagulants, methotrexate	Enhanced drug action

Source: Modified from a table constructed by Ian M. Smith, M.D.

6. Another concern in the administration of antibiotics to patients is the large number of potential physical incompatibilities of antimicrobials in intravenous infusions. Penicillins and aminoglycosides, for instance, are incompatible when mixed together (46).

7. Finally, a special category of potential adverse interactions among antibiotics occurs when multiple antibiotics are used together. Antagonism may result, especially when bactericidal and bacteristatic antibiotics are used in combination.

Table 11.2 lists examples of specific interactions. This problem can be minimized by limiting the number of drugs administered to the elderly and being aware of known drug interactions (47).

Compliance

Noncompliance with prescribed medication is an important problem in the nursing home population. Noncompliance increases with the total number of drugs and the frequency of dosing. Not all noncompliance in the elderly is unintentional and reflective of patient forgetfulness. Intentional prescription nonadherence was found to be more important than unintentional nonadherence in one in-home survey of elderly subjects taking prescription drugs (48). Intentional noncompliance was more likely when the patient used two or more pharmacies or had received prescriptions from two or more physicians. Noncompliance results in potentially hazardous undermedication as well as increased medical costs.

Rational Approach to Antibiotic Usage

Prerequisites of good antibiotic utilization include a knowledge of the underlying infectious disease, an appropriate indication for antibiotic administration, knowledge of the antibiotic properties (mechanisms, pharmacokinetics, side effects, and cost), selection of the least toxic antibiotic, knowledge of patient allergies, use of narrow-spectrum antibiotics, and periodic reassessment of antibiotic efficacy and side effects during treatment. Combination drugs should be avoided if possible, and health care personnel should be aware of marketed antibiotic products that are ineffective and to be avoided (49). Finally, the unique aspects of drug pharmacology and toxicity in the elderly must be kept in mind.

Vestal has suggested some basic principles for prescribing to geriatric patients (33), some of which are particularly relevant to prescription of antibiotics to the nursing home patient: (1) Use smaller doses for the elderly; (2) simplify the therapeutic regimen; (3) explain the treatment plan to both the patient and a friend or relative and give concise, written directions; (4) choose a dosage form that is appropriate to the patient; (5) suggest the use of a diary or calendar to record daily drug administration; (6) label the drug container clearly; (7) encourage the return and destruction of old or unused medications; (8) regularly review drugs in the treatment plan and discontinue those not needed; and (9) keep in mind potential adverse effects and interactions of the antibiotics.

Another option to improve antibiotic utilization and effectiveness in a nursing home setting is involvement of nursing home consultant pharmacists. Consultant pharmacists have been queried most often about antibiotic side effects, generic equivalence, contraindications, and drug interactions (50). In some instances, the use of consultant pharmacists may decrease the average number of drugs used per nursing home resident (51).

Antibiotic Audits

One of the duties of the infection control practitioner or infection control committee is the monitoring of antibiotic utilization and resistance in the nursing home. The latter can be done without much difficulty by inspection of the results of all cultures obtained on residents at the nursing home. A cluster of isolates of the same bacterium (with identical antibiotic sensitivity pattern) suggests an outbreak (see Chapter 10). An increase in antibiotic resistance, particularly methicillin-resistant *Staphylococcus aureus* or aminoglycoside–resistant gram-negative bacilli, poses a real hazard to residents and may be an indication for isolation.

Table 11.3. Sample Criteria: Audit of Urinary Tract Infection Therapy in Nursing Homes

Methods: The nursing home infection control committee will review infection control records for the last three months, analyzing all nosocomial urinary tract infections. All residents in the nursing home during those three months will be included. This audit is a followup audit; a similar audit six months ago revealed an increase in *Pseudomonas* UTIs.

Elements	*Standard*	*Exceptions*	*Instructions for Data Retrieval*
1. Diagnosis of UTI: 100,000 Bacteria/ml urine	100%	—	Review lab sheets (culture)
or			
Fever *and* dysuria or pyuria	—	—	Review clinical notes, lab sheets (urinalysis)
2. Foley catheter present?	Information only	—	Review nurses' notes
3. Antibiotic therapy:			
Organism sensitive	100%	Culture negative	Review lab sheets (cultures)
No less toxic or expensive drug available	100%	Resident allergic to preferred drug	Review lab sheets (antibiotic sensitivities), history
Length of therapy	Information only	—	Review medication orders

An audit of antibiotic utilization may provide useful information for the infection control team about antibiotic use and potential overuse in a nursing home. An area for audit is generally selected on a basis of high antibiotic cost (such as the new cephalosporins), extensive antibiotic usage, well-known potential misuse (such as antibiotic prophylaxis), or antibiotics that have significant toxicity (such as chloramphenicol or aminoglycosides). Examples of potential audits include antibiotic therapy of urinary tract infections in residents with urinary catheters, documentation of infection in medical records, monitoring antibiotic toxicity during therapy, and obtaining proper cultures prior to therapy. Topics of local interest should be selected.

Table 11.4. Sample Results: Audit of Urinary Tract Infection Therapy in Nursing Homes

	Standard	*Result*
1. 200 Residents:		
18 Met criteria for UTI (9%)		
a. Urine culture done	100%	18/18 = 100%
b. Culture positive, sensitivity done	—	16 of 18
2. Foley catheter present	—	15 of 18
3. Antibiotic therapy:		
a. Organism sensitive	100%	16/16 = 100%
b. No less toxic or expensive drug available	100%	13/16 = 81%
c. Length of therapy	—	mean = 9 days

Conclusions: Both the incidence of UTIs (9%) and the percent of infected patients with indwelling Foley catheters (83%) are within the expected range for a large nursing home for this period of time. Appropriate urine cultures were obtained prior to therapy frequently (100%) and were almost always positive. The organisms cultured were:
   Proteus mirabilis—6
   Escherichia coli—5
   Pseudomonas aeruginosa—2
   Enterococci—2
   Klebsiella spp.—1
The increase in *Pseudomonas* isolates noted in the audit six months ago has subsided.

All physicians selected drugs for therapy that were appropriate to sensitivities of the organism, although in three instances (19%) a less toxic or less expensive drug could have been used. In two cases this involved use of an expensive cephalosporin rarely indicated for UTIs.

Plan: Distribute results of audit to all nursing home physicians and nursing personnel. Continue to monitor sensitivity results from urine cultures.

The next step is determination of criteria. Criteria should be objective and nonthreatening. Standard criteria have been developed (52). Although the referenced criteria were developed primarily for hospital antibiotic audits, they are applicable to nursing home audits as well.

Data are then collected (53) and performance at the nursing home is compared to an ideal standard (see Table 11.3). Deficiencies are identified and corrective action is taken, usually in the form of an educational program, newsletter, or further monitoring of antibiotic usage (see Table 11.4). The most valid comparison of performance on audits is internal, such as comparison of results before and after an educational program.

REFERENCES

1. Anderson RJ: Drug prescribing for patients in renal failure. *Hosp Pract* 18:145–160, 1983.
2. Caldwell JR, Cluff LE: Adverse reactions to antimicrobial agents. *JAMA* 230:77–80, 1974.
3. Hurwitz N: Predisposing factors in adverse reactions to drugs. *Br Med J* 1:536–539, 1969.
4. Levy SB: Microbial resistance to antibiotics: An evolving and persistent problem. *Lancet* 2:83–88, 1982.
5. Schaberg DR, Rubens CE, Alford RH, et al: Evolution of antimicrobial resistance and nosocomial infection. *Am J Med* 70:445–448, 1981.
6. Weinstein RA, Nathan C, Gruensfelder R, et al: Endemic aminoglycoside resistance in gram-negative bacilli: Epidemiology and mechanisms. *J Infect Dis* 141:338–345, 1980.
7. Gleckman R, Blagg N, Hibert D, et al: Catheter-related urosepsis in the elderly: A prospective study of community-derived infections. *J Am Geriatr Soc* 30:255–257, 1982.
8. Sherman FT, Tucci V, Libow LS, et al: Nosocomial urinary tract infections in a skilled nursing facility. *J Am Geriatr Soc* 28:456–461, 1980.
9. Garibaldi RA, Brodine S, Matsumiya S: Infections among patients in nursing homes: Policies, prevalence, and problems. *N Engl J Med* 305:731–735, 1981.
10. Haley RW, Hightower AW, Khabbaz RF, et al: The emergence of methicillin-resistant *Staphylococcus aureus* infections in United States hospitals. *Ann Intern Med* 97:297–308, 1982.
11. O'Toole RD, Drew WL, Dahlgren BJ, et al: An outbreak of methicillin-resistant *Staphylococcus aureus* infection: Observations in hospital and nursing home. *JAMA* 213:257–263, 1970.

12. Aeilts GD, Sapico FL, Canawati HN, et al: Methicillin-resistant *Staphylococcus aureus* colonization and infection in a rehabilitation facility. *J Clin Micro* 16:218–223, 1982.

13. Lawrence RN, Hoeprich PD: Microbial development of drug resistance: Mechanisms and clinical significance. *CRC Crit Rev Clin Lab Sci* 5:365–386, 1975.

14. Schaberg DR, Alford RH, Anderson R, et al: An outbreak of nosocomial infection due to multiply resistant *Serratia marcescens:* Evidence of interhospital spread. *J Infect Dis* 134:181–188, 1976.

15. Thomas FE, Jackson RT, Melly MA, et al: Sequential hospitalwide outbreaks of resistant Serratia and Klebsiella infection. *Arch Intern Med* 137:581–584, 1977.

16. Weinstein RA, Kabins SA: Strategies for prevention and control of multiple drug-resistant nosocomial infection. *Am J Med* 70:449–454, 1981.

17. Simmons HE, Stolley PD: This is medical progress? Trends and consequences of antibiotic use in the United States. *JAMA* 227:1023–1028, 1974.

18. Kunin CM: Use of antibiotics: A brief exposition of the problem and some tentative solutions. *Ann Intern Med* 79:555–560, 1973.

19. Robert AW, Visconti JA: The rational and irrational use of systemic antimicrobial drugs. *Am J Hosp Pharm* 29:828–834, 1972.

20. Kunin CM: Antibiotic accountability. *N Engl J Med* 301:380–381, 1979.

21. Avorn J, Chan M, Hartley R: Scientific versus commercial sources of influence on the prescribing behavior of physicians. *Am J Med* 73:4–8, 1982.

22. Jones SR, Burks J, Bratton T, et al: The effect of an educational program upon hospital antibiotic use. *Am J Med Sci* 273:79–85, 1977.

23. Johnson MW, Mitch WE, Heller AH, et al: The impact of an educational program on gentamicin use in a teaching hospital. *Am J Med* 73:9–14, 1982.

24. Hendeles L: Need for "counter-detailing" antibiotics. *Am J Hosp Pharm* 33:918–925, 1976.

25. Martucci HJ, Parry MF: Cephalosporin cost reduction. *Hosp Formulary* 16:396–403, 1981.

26. McGowan JE Jr., Cynamon M: Usage of antibiotics in a general hospital: Effect of requiring justification. *J Infect Dis* 130:165–168, 1974.

27. Recco RA, Gladstone JL, Friedman SA, et al: Antibiotic control in a municipal hospital. *JAMA* 241:2283–2286, 1979.

28. Seligman SJ: Reduction in antibiotic cost by restricting use of an oral cephalosporin. *Am J Med* 71:941–944, 1981.

29. Price DEJ, Sleigh JD: Control of infection due to *Klebsiella aerogenes* in a neurosurgical unit by withdrawal of all antibiotics. *Lancet* 2:1213–1215, 1970.

30. Smith PW, Rusnak PG: Aminoglycoside-resistant *Pseudomonas aeruginosa* urinary tract infections: Study of an outbreak. *J Hosp Infect* 2:71–75, 1981.

31. Gardener P, Bennett JV, Burke JP, et al: Nosocomial management of resistant gram-negative bacilli. *J Infect Dis* 141:415–417, 1980.

32. Weinstein RA, Kabins SA: Strategies for prevention and control of multiple drug resistant nosocomial infections. *Am J Med* 70:449–454, 1981.

33. Vestal RF: Pharmacology and aging. *J Am Geriatr Soc* 30:191–200, 1982.

34. Kalchthaler T, Coccaro E, Lichtiger S: Incidence of polypharmacy in a long-term care facility. *J Am Geriatr Soc* 25:308–313, 1977.

35. Cohen ED, Hierholzer WJ Jr, Schilling CR, et al: Nosocomial infections in skilled nursing facilities: A preliminary survey. *Publ Health Rep* 94:162–165, 1979.

36. Koch-Weser J: Drug distribution in old age. *N Engl J Med* 306:1081–1087, 1982.

37. Crooks J, O'Malley K, Stevenson IH: Pharmacokinetics in the elderly. *Clin Pharmacokin* 1:280–296, 1976.

38. Lamy PP: Comparative pharmacokinetic changes and drug therapy in an older population. *J Am Geriatr Soc* 30:S11–S19, 1982.

39. Zaske, DE: Wide interpatient variations in gentamicin dose requirements for geriatric patients. *JAMA* 248:3122–3126, 1982.

40. Seidl LG, Thornton GF, Smith JW, et al: Studies on epidemiology of adverse drug reactions: Reactions in patients on a general medical service. *Bull Johns Hopkins Hosp* 119:299–315, 1966.

41. Ristuccia AM, Cunha BA: The aminoglycosides. *Med Clin N Am* 66:303–312, 1982.

42. Mitchell JR: Isoniazid liver injury: Clinical spectrum pathology, and probable pathogenesis. *Ann Intern Med* 84:181–192, 1976.

43. Bergman HD: Prescription of drugs in a nursing home. *Drug Intell Clin Pharm* 9:365–368, 1975.

44. Kabins SA: Interactions among antibiotics and other drugs. *JAMA* 219:206–213, 1972.

45. Adverse interactions of drugs. *Med Let* 5:17–28, 1981.

46. Phillips I: Aminoglycosides. *Lancet* 2:311–314, 1982.

47. Block LH: Polymedicine: Known and unknown drug interactions. *J Am Geriatr Soc* 30:S94–S98, 1982.

48. Cooper JK, Love DW, Raffoul PR: Intentional prescription nonadherence (noncompliance) by the elderly. *J Am Geriatr Soc* 30:329–333, 1982.

49. *Prescription Drug Products Currently Classified by the Food and Drug Administration as Lacking Adequate Evidence of Effectiveness.* Rockfield, MD, Department of Health and Human Services, Food and Drug Administration, January 1980.

50. Evens RP, Guernsey BG, Hightower WL: Nursing home consultant pharmacists: Drug information services, opinions, and activity study. *Hosp Formulary* 17:408–420, 1982.

51. Cooper JW Jr., Bagwell CG: Contribution of the consultant pharmacist to rational drug usage in the long-term care facility. *J Am Geriatr Soc* 26:513–520, 1978.

52. Kunin CM, Efron HY: Audits of antimicrobial usage: Guidelines for peer review. *JAMA* 237: March 7–May 2, 1977.

53. Latorraca R, Bartons R: Surveillance of antibiotic use in a community hospital. *JAMA* 242:2585–2587, 1979.

CHAPTER **12**

REGULATIONS, POLICIES, AND PROCEDURES

V. Delight Wreed
Patricia G. Rusnak

REGULATIONS AND STANDARDS

Infection prevention and control have always been important components of health care. Physicians, nurses, sanitarians and other health professionals have established professional standards regarding infection prevention and control as part of their daily practice. The Centers for Disease Control (CDC) Atlanta, Georgia, provides guidelines and influences professional standards. Federal, state, and local regulations have been written for nursing homes based on these professional standards to provide at least minimum protection for residents, visitors, staff, and the community against infections and their spread.

Before 1974, most regulations regarding infection control were either at the local or state level. In January 1974, the Department of Health, Education, and Welfare (HEW), published initial Standards for Certification and Participation in Medicare and Medicaid Programs for both skilled nursing facilities (SNFs) and intermediate care facilities (ICFs). These regulations set, and continue to set through various revisions, minimum standards, (including those specific to infection prevention and control) for those facilities choosing to participate in Medicare and Medicaid. Any nursing home, in order to be licensed in a given state, must meet local, state, and federal sanitation and infection control standards. Those who participate voluntarily in Medicaid and Medicare must meet appropriate federal standards.

The federal standards specific to infection control certification and participation in Medicare and Medicaid are specific for skilled nursing facilities and intermediate care facilities as described.

Skilled Regulatory Standards

Skilled nursing facilities must meet the following Standards for Certification and Participation in Medicare and Medicaid Programs for Skilled Nursing Facilities (1):

405.1135 CONDITION OF PARTICIPATION—INFECTION CONTROL

The skilled nursing facility establishes an infection control committee of representative professional staff with responsibility for overall infection control in the facility. All necessary housekeeping and maintenance services are provided to maintain a sanitary and comfortable environment and to help prevent the development and transmission of infection.

a. Standard: *Infection control committee.* The infection control committee is composed of members of the medical and nursing staff, administration, and the dietetic, pharmacy, housekeeping, maintenance, and other services. The committee establishes policies and procedures for investigating, controlling, and preventing infections in the facility, and monitors staff performance to ensure that the policies and procedures are executed.

b. Standard: *Aseptic and isolation techniques.* Written effective procedures in aseptic and isolation techniques are followed by all personnel. Procedures are reviewed and revised annually for effectiveness and improvement.

c. Standard: *Housekeeping.* The facility employs sufficient housekeeping personnel and provides all necessary equipment to maintain a safe, clean, and orderly interior. A full-time employee is designated responsible for the services and for supervision and training of personnel. Nursing personnel are not assigned housekeeping duties. A facility that has a contract with an outside resource for housekeeping services may be found to be in compliance with this standard provided the facility and/or outside resource meets the requirements of the standard.

d. Standard: *Linen.* The facility has available at all times a quantity of linen essential for proper care and comfort of patients. Linens are handled, stored, processed, and transported in such a manner as to prevent the spread of infection.

e. Standard: *Pest control.* The facility is maintained free from insects and rodents through operation of a pest control program.

Also available to expand on the above standards are some guidelines and survey procedures (2). These are primarily for use by the state survey agency, usually the state department of health, the state Medicaid agency, the providers, SNFs, and any organizations and citizens who are concerned about the care provided the institutionalized elderly in the SNF.

Intermediate Regulatory Standards

Although there is no federal standard specifically entitled "Infection Control" for certification and participation in Medicaid in the general intermediate care facility, included are other standards that make reference to infection control. The following standards reflect infection control aspects, taken from the guidelines and nursing procedures (3):

> *Conformity with Federal, State and Local Laws*—The facility is in conformity with Federal, State, and local laws, codes and regulations pertaining to health and safety, including procurement, dispensing, administration, safeguarding and disposal of medications and controlled substances, building, construction, maintenance and equipment standards; *sanitation; Communicable and reportable diseases;* and post-mortem procedures.
> 45CFR249.12 (a) (7) (vi)
> *Sanitary Conditions*—All food is procured, stored, prepared, distributed, and served under sanitary conditions.
> 45CFR249.12 (a) (b)
> *Environment and Sanitation*—The facility maintains conditions relating to environment and sanitation as set forth below:
> 45CFR249.12 (a) (6) (i)
>> *Favorable Environment for Residents*—Resident living areas are designed and equipped for the comfort and privacy of the resident. Each room is equipped with or conveniently located near adequate toilet and bathing facilities appropriate in number, size, and design to meet the needs of residents. Each room is at or above grade level and each resident room contains a suitable bed, closet space which provides security and privacy for clothing and personal belongings, and other appropriate furniture;
>> 45CFR249.12 (a) (6) (ii)
>> *Linen*—The facility has available at all times a quantity of linen essential for proper care and comfort of residents. Each bed is equipped with clean linen;
>> 45CFR249.12 (a) (6) (v)
>> *Isolation*—Provision is made for isolating residents with infectious diseases.

The ICF is designed to provide a protected environment for persons whose health needs require supervision in an institutional setting to prevent deterioration and disability. Even though there is no one standard specific to infection control, the ICF will need to practice infection prevention and control in order to meet the health needs of those in the institution to prevent deterioration and disability. Good infection control and prevention practices are inseparable from good health care.

State and Local Standards

Depending on the location of the facility, state and local standards governing that individual facility will vary. It is necessary to secure copies of state regulations and standards from the appropriate state agency, most commonly the state department of health. Obtain any local standards for sanitation and infection control from the local health department. These agencies are generally excellent resources, not only for written materials but also for consultation to long-term care (LTC) facilities regarding individual questions pertaining to regulations and standards.

Other Standards and Accrediting Agencies

In addition to federal, state, and local regulatory standards, there are other agencies and organizations that have standards for infection control. Depending on the state and institution, these may be important for licensure or voluntary accreditation. The Joint Commission on Accreditation of Hospitals (JCAH) provides an accreditation program with the following standards for long-term care facilities (4):*

INFECTION/ENVIRONMENTAL CONTROL

Principle

An infection control committee shall be responsible for organizing an *infection control program* within the facility. The facility shall provide all services necessary to maintain a sanitary and comfortable environment and to prevent the development and transmission of infection.

Standard I

The *infection control committee* shall be composed of, but not necessarily limited to, members of the medical and nursing staffs, the administration, and the dietetic, pharmacy, housekeeping, maintenance, and laundry services. The chairman of the committee should be an indi-

*Joint Commission on Accreditation of Hospitals, *Accreditation Manual for Long Term Care Facilities*, 1980, pp. 27–29, Used with permission.

vidual who has knowledge, special interest, or experience in infection control.

The infection control committee shall develop written *policies and procedures* for the prevention and control of infections, and the maintenance of a sanitary environment. The infection control committee shall also develop techniques and systems for identifying infections in the facility, including procedures for reporting the results of infection *surveillance* to appropriate authorities.

The *infection control committee* shall: (*1*) review procedures for handling food, processing laundry, disposing environmental and patient/resident wastes, controlling pests, and controlling traffic; (*2*) review patient/resident care practices, visiting rules for high risk areas, and sources of infection; (*3*) meet not less than quarterly, maintain minutes in sufficient detail to document its proceedings and actions, and submit reports to the administrator; (*4*) monitor the health status of employees; (*5*) monitor staff performance to assure that policies and procedures are being followed.

Standard II

There shall be written procedures for *aseptic and isolation techniques.* These procedures shall be made known to, and followed by, all personnel and shall be reviewed at least annually and revised as necessary.

Standard III

The facility shall employ sufficient housekeeping personnel and provide all necessary equipment to maintain a clean, orderly, and safe *environment.* A full time employee shall be responsible for *housekeeping* services and for supervision and training of housekeeping personnel. If the full-time employee responsible for housekeeping services is assigned other duties, sufficient time shall be alloted to him or her to assure the maintenance of a clean, orderly, and safe environment.

To guide personnel in maintaining a safe environment, procedures shall be developed for: (*1*) the use, cleaning, and care of equipment; (*2*) the selection and proper use of housekeeping and cleaning supplies; (*3*) the maintenance of cleaning schedules; (*4*) the evaluation of cleaning techniques; (*5*) the maintenance of personal hygiene.

There shall be documentation of participation by housekeeping personnel in a relevant continuing education program. If the facility has a contract with an outside resource for housekeeping services, the facility must assure that the requirements of this standard are met.

Standard IV

The facility shall have sufficient linen available at all times for the proper care and comfort of patients/residents. Linen shall be handled, processed, stored, and transported in a manner that prevents the transmission of infection.

To guide personnel in the proper handling of *laundry*, procedures shall be developed for: (*1*) the use, cleaning, and care of laundry equipment; (*2*) the selection and proper use of laundry supplies; (*3*) the maintenance of schedules; (*4*) the proper sorting, handling, processing, and transporting of clean and soiled laundry; (*5*) the evaluation of cleaning techniques; (*6*) the maintenance of personal hygiene.

If the facility uses an outside laundry, it shall assure that the requirements of this standard are met.

Standard V

The facility shall be free of insects and rodents. *Pest control* services shall be provided by maintenance personnel or by contract with a pest control company. Where appropriate, screens shall be provided for windows and doors.

These standards are for facilities that provide in-house patient care with an organized medical staff or medical director and nursing services under the direction of a professional nurse. The JCAH also mandates that a LTC facility provide total preventive, rehabilitative, social, spiritual, and emotional care to patients requiring long-term health care.

The Peer Assistance Program (5), although it may vary from state to state, can assist in providing other sources of standards regarding infection control. Other valuable and often extremely practical resources are neighboring LTC facilities. Although it is not recommended as your only resource, other institutions can be very helpful in preparing standards and explaining the connotations of federal, state, local or other agency standards.

DEVELOPING POLICIES AND PROCEDURES

Areas of Application

There are many policies and procedures related to an infection control program that a facility must establish. These policies and procedures should be based on standards (i.e., federal, state, and local professional) regarding infection control. Policies and procedures are the means to implement the standards. A **Policy** reflects standards and the principles upon which decisions governing the operation of the facility are based; a **Procedure**, also reflecting standards, is the method by which that policy is carried out. Infection control program policies and procedures thus direct the facility as to how they will help prevent the transmission and spread of pathogenic microorganisms within the facility and control them if an outbreak should occur.

The administrator of each facility must decide, as part of its infection control program, whether to have a separate infection control policy and procedure manual or whether all infection control policies and procedures will be integrated into the facility's overall general policy and procedure operations manual. For example, a very small ICF may decide not to have a separate manual, whereas a larger SNF facility may have a separate manual. Whichever format option is taken, the policies and procedures should be based on the same principles of infection prevention and control.

Whether incorporating a separate manual or an integrated manual, many areas should be considered when establishing infection prevention and control policies and procedures, taking into account whether the facility is intermediate care or skilled. These areas might include, but are not limited to, the following:

Role of administration
Role of medical director
Infection control committee
Admission, transfer, discharge
Surveillance and data collection
Internal reporting of infections/diseases
External reporting of infections/diseases
Nursing service—prevention
Housekeeping—prevention
Laundry—prevention
Maintenance—prevention
Initiating isolation precautions
Isolation costs
Isolation/precautions
   Resident care
   Handling contaminated items/trash
Housekeeping
Food service
Managing movement of confused resident
Inservice training/staff development
Visitors

Employee health and personnel practices

Legal matters

The following may be helpful in deciding what kinds of policies and procedures are needed (6):

Role of the Medical Director

1. Policies: What policies should be established and communicated pertaining to the role of the Medical Director, such as relation to the Infection Control Committee, role in surveillance and data interpretation, role in case of diagnosed infection, and relationship to regulatory authorities?

2. Procedures: What formal procedures should be established pertaining to the role of the medical director, such as the medical director's service on and consultation to the Infection Control Committee, periodic review and interpretation of surveillance data, liaison between the Infection Control Committee and other physicians, initiation of emergency and long-term control measures, and evaluation of their effectiveness?

Strict isolation

1. Policy: What policies should be established and communicated pertaining to strict isolation, such as types of communicable diseases requiring strict isolation, space provisions, authority to order and terminate strict isolation, protection of persons in contact with infected resident, reporting, and recordkeeping?

2. Procedures: What formal procedures pertaining to strict isolation should be established, such as for patient care, notification of staff, concurrent and terminal cleaning, movements of instruments and equipment in and out of the isolation room, staff hygiene, disposition of resident's personal belongings and of materials removed from the isolation room, requirements for protective clothing, food and linen service, solid waste disposal, and admission of visitors?

Legal Matters

1. Policies: What policies should be established and communicated pertaining to legal matters related to infection control, such as compliance with all laws, rules, and regulations applicable to infection control from federal, state, and local sources, updating of applicable source material, distribution of pertinent information to the facility personnel, authority for implementation, and review of effectiveness of existing policies?

2. Procedures: What formal procedures should be established pertaining to legal matters related to infection control, such as orientation of residents and staff on legal implications of negligence?

Resource materials are useful aids in addressing policies and procedures. For instance, *Guideline for Isolation Precautions in Hospitals* (7) is an excellent resource for both policies and procedures in the area of isolation.

Writing Policies

In writing policies, begin by looking at the standards that need to be conveyed. Use previous wording as a guideline, and make any necessary changes that address the individual facility's situation. Always keep in mind that a policy reflects standards and is the principle upon which decisions governing the operation of the facility are based.

Another way to explain the definition of a policy, is to think of a policy as defining "Who," "What," "When," and "Where." Usually a policy is written to correct a single repetitive problem, to clarify the limitations on future actions, and to define specific results desired. A few examples of Infection Control Committee policies are listed below.

Committee Composition

The Infection Control Committee of this facility will be composed of members of the medical and nursing staffs, administration, dietary, pharmacy, housekeeping, and maintenance.

Committee Functions
1. The Committee will meet at least quarterly.
2. Minutes will be maintained in sufficient detail to document proceedings.
3. The Committee will develop, approve, and annually review written policies and procedures on aseptic and isolation precautions techniques and maintenance of a sanitary environment.
4. The Committee will develop and monitor a system for identifying infections in the facility (surveillance).
5. The Committee will delegate to the Medical Director the responsibility for reporting all reportable diseases to the appropriate authorities.
6. The Committee will develop a system of monitoring staff performance, assuring that all policies and procedures are carried out.
7. The Committee will monitor the health status of employees, including but not limited to provision of (or referral for) preem-

ployment physicals and periodic health examinations, annual tuberculin screening, treatment of any employee reporting for work with illness or untreated wounds, and providing a mechanism to prevent employees with infectious diseases from working with residents or food.

Housekeeping Department

1. The Housekeeping Department shall be supervised by a full-time employee.
2. The Housekeeping Supervisor shall be responsible for all housekeeping services, including supervision and training of personnel.
3. Written procedures including cleaning and disinfecting schedules and cleaning of equipment will be available to housekeeping personnel to assist them in performing their duties.

The example in Figure 12.1 shows the "Who," "What," "When," and "Where" that needs to be reflected in a policy.

Writing Procedures

After policies are developed, it is necessary to develop the "How" and "Why" the policy will be carried out—in other words, procedures. Procedures should be specific, clearly stated, current, and accessible to the people for whom they are intended. It is difficult for procedures to be carried out unless the responsible individuals know how to effect them and the proper equipment and supplies are available as stated in the procedure. Procedures reflect standards, just as policies do. In general terms, a procedure is a standardized method of performing specified work, usually a single task. Several examples of infection control committee procedures are given below:

Annual Review of the Infection Control Manual

1. Proposed changes to the manual will be submitted by Committee members, in writing, to the Infection Control Committee in August for review and approval.
2. The Chairman will appoint various committee members based on familiarity or expertise, to review selected sections of the manual for completeness, accuracy, understandability.
3. Committee members reviewing the manual will report their recommendations to the Committee, which will be approved by a majority of the members.

Section: INFECTION CONTROL POLICY	**Number** 6
Subject: TERMINAL SURGERY CLEANING	**Effective Date** 1-1-81
Supersedes:	**Page** 1 **of** 1
Approved by: *Mary Lou Deverell*	**Date:** 1-1-81

Proper procedures and frequencies must be observed in cleaning the OR area to control the spread of infection. Everything is to be treated as potentially contaminated.

1. Proper OR gowning technique must be observed.

2. Shoe covers must be worn.

3. Handwashing procedure must be followed.

4. Clean equipment must be used and left in the area.

5. Correct dilution of disinfectant cleaner must be followed.

See: # 4 Product Use and Dilution
      # 1 Handwashing
      #14 Care and Cleaning of Equipment
      #15 Gowning
      #16 Terminal Surgery Cleaning

INFECTION CONTROL COMMIT
FEB 1 1 1981
FEB 1 1 1981

925

Figure 12.1. Example of an infection control policy. (Courtesy of Bishop Clarkson Memorial Hospital, Omaha, Nebraska.)

4. The Infection Control Practitioner will make the appropriate revisions and submit the manual for final approval.
5. The Infection Control Practitioner will provide revised copies of the manual to all departments.

Figure 12.2 depicts the "How" and "Why" needed in writing a procedure. In this particular format, the rationale/amplification area is useful to help explain the "Why."

Forms

The format used for policies and procedures is an institutional decision. Usually a very simple format is chosen because of easier use and understandability. It is important to remember that policies and procedures need to be reviewed consistently, usually on an annual basis, and revised accordingly.

Of particular importance in a LTC facility, when considering infection control policies and procedures, are the questions of what type of residents will be admitted and what information is needed when a resident is to be transferred into or out of the facility.

Admission and Transfer Policies

In the past, admission and transfer policies for LTC facilities often were used only when a bed was available for the resident or when the ambulance could come to provide the transportation for the resident from one facility to another. However, in recent years, due to the emphasis given to infection control by administrators and regulatory agencies, admission and transfer policies in the LTC facility have assumed a new importance.

Stark (8) estimated that over 20% of new admissions to LTCs were from the hospital setting; Egger (9) reported that approximately 50% were from general hospitals. These studies point out the close relationship between hospital and nursing home nosocomial infections.

Nosocomial infections occur in approximately 5% of all patients admitted to acute-care hospitals in the United States (10). With the continuous efforts of hospitals to shorten hospital stays, more of these patients are being transferred back into the community, perhaps still recuperating from a nosocomial infection. Thus, nursing homes need to ensure that they can provide proper care for these patients when they are admitted to LTC facilities.

The first step that LTC facilities have taken is to do preadmission

BISHOP CLARKSON MEMORIAL HOSPITAL
NURSING SERVICE DIVISION

PROCEDURE: (x)TECHNICAL ( )OPERATIONAL

| TITLE: *THERMOMETERS: USAGE AND CLEANING* | NUMBER: *2-8-01* |
| | PAGE: 1 OF: *1* |

| APPROVED BY: | EFFECTIVE DATE: *9-24-80* |
| DATE: *September 24, 1980* | SUPERSEDES: *3-28-79* |

OBJECTIVE: *To cleanse individual patient thermometers and reduce the spread of bacterial contamination.*

EQUIPMENT: *Thermometer*
Thermometer holder
Soap and H₂0 (water)

NURSING ACTION	RATIONALE/AMPLIFICATION
1. *Wash your hands.*	
2. *Place the thermometer, given to each patient at the time of admission, in the thermometer holder found in the Admission Care Kit.*	
3. *Leave the thermometer holder, devoid of any solution, with the thermometer inside, at the patient's bedside.*	*There should not be any type of antiseptic solution for the thermometer holder in the admission kit. If there is, it should be discarded. Any solution that stands for even a short period of time must be considered grossly contaminated.*
4. *Cleanse the thermometer with soap and H₂0 (water) before and after each use.*	
5. *Return the clean, dry thermometer to its holder after each use.*	
6. *Discard the thermometer as patient desires upon her/his dismissal.*	*No thermometers are resterilized or reused in this hospital.*

D998 (BCMH Rev. 2-79)

Figure 12.2. Example of an infection control procedure. (Courtesy of Bishop Clarkson Memorial Hospital, Omaha, Nebraska.)

PATIENT TRANSFER FORM
(INTER-AGENCY REFERRAL)

1. PATIENT'S LAST NAME	FIRST NAME	MI	2. SEX	3. HEALTH INSURANCE CLAIM NUMBER
			☐ M ☐ F	

4. PATIENT'S ADDRESS (Street Number, City, State, Zip Code)	5. DATE OF BIRTH	RELIGION

7. DATE OF THIS TRANSFER	8. FACILITY NAME AND ADDRESS TRANSFERRING TO	10. PHYSICIAN IN CHARGE AT TIME OF TRANSFER
		Will this physician care for patient after admission to new facility? ☐ YES ☐ NO

11. DATES OF STAY AT FACILITY TRANSFERRING FROM		14. PAYMENT SOURCE FOR CHARGES TO PATIENT

ADMISSION	DISCHARGE

A. ☐ SELF OR FAMILY   C. ☐ BLUE CROSS BLUE SHIELD   E. ☐ PUBLIC AGENCY (Give name)

B. ☐ PRIVATE INSURANCE   D. ☐ EMPLOYER OR UNION   F. ☐ OTHER (Explain)

12-A. NAME AND ADDRESS OF FACILITY TRANSFERRING FROM	12-B. NAME AND ADDRESSES OF ALL HOSPITALS AND EXTENDED CARE FACILITIES FROM WHICH PATIENT WAS DISCHARGED IN PAST 60 DAYS.

CLINIC APPOINTMENT	DATE	TIME	ATTACH CLINIC APPOINTMENT CARD	DATE OF LAST PHYSICAL EXAMINATION

RELATIVE OR GUARDIAN:	Name	Address	Phone Number

16. DIAGNOSES AT TIME OF TRANSFER   EMPLOYMENT RELATED   A. ☐ YES   B. ☐ NO

(a) Primary

(b) Secondary

(Check if present)

Disabilities
Amputation
Paralysis
Contracture
Decub. Ulcer

Impairments
Mentality
Speech
Hearing
Vision
Sensation

Incontinence
Bladder
Bowel
Saliva

Activity Tolerance Limitations
None   Moderate   Severe

Patient knows diagnosis?

IMPORTANT MEDICAL INFORMATION
(State allergies if any)

DIET, DRUGS, AND OTHER THERAPY
at Time of Discharge

(Physician, please sign below)

Chest X-ray	date_____	result_____
C.B.C.	date_____	result_____
Serology	date_____	result_____
Urinalysis	date_____	result_____

SUGGESTIONS FOR ACTIVE CARE

BED

Position in good body alignment and

change position every_____hrs.

Avoid_____position

Prone position_____times/day as tolerated.

SIT IN CHAIR

_____hrs._____times/day.

WEIGHT BEARING

Full_____Partial_____None_____

on_____Leg

LOCOMOTION

Walk_____times/day.

EXERCISES

Range of motion_____times/day.

to_____

by patient_____nurse_____family_____
Other as outlined below_____
Stand_____Min._____times/day.

SOCIAL ACTIVITIES

Encourage group_____individual_____

within_____outside_____home.

| Transport. Ambulance_____ | Car_____ |
| Car for handicapped _____ | Bus_____ |

Signature of Physician or Nurse_____Date_____

Form 882   BRIGGS, Des Moines, Iowa 50306   PATIENT TRANSFER FORM

Figure 12.3. Example of a transfer form used by hospitals. (Courtesy of Briggs Corporation, Des Moines, Iowa.)

III. PATIENT INFORMATION

SELF CARE STATUS
(Check level of ability. Write S in space if needs supervision only. Draw line across if inapplicable.)

	Independent	Needs Assistance	Unable To Do	
Bed Activity				Turns
				Sits
Personal Hygiene				Face, Hair, Arms
				Trunk & Perineum
				Lower Extremities
				Bladder Program
				Bowel Program
Dressing				Upper Extremities
				Trunk
				Lower Extremities
				Appliance, Splint
Transfer				Feeding
				Sitting
				Standing
				Tub
				Toilet
Loco-motion				Wheelchair
				Walking
				Stairs

BED Low___ Mattress: Firm___ Reg.___
Other___
Side Rails: Yes___ No___

BEHAVIOR
Alcoholic___ Belligerent___ Noisy___
Senile___ Suspicious___ Withdrawn___

MENTAL STATUS
Alert___ Forgetful___ Confused___

COMMUNICATION ABILITY   Yes   No
Can speak   ___ ___
Can write   ___ ___
Understands speaking   ___ ___
Understands writing   ___ ___
Understands gestures   ___ ___
Understands English   ___ ___
If no, state language spoken:___

DIET
Regular___ Low Salt___ Diabetic___
Bland___ Low Residue___
Other___
Feeds self___ Needs Help___
Part___ All___

PATIENT USES
Appliance___ Catheter___ Colostomy___
Cane___ Crutches___ Prosthesis___
Walker___ Chair___

OTHER EQUIPMENT ___

ADDITIONAL PERTINENT INFORMATION
(Explain necessary details of care, diagnosis, medications, treatments, prognosis, teaching, habits, preferences, etc. Therapists and social workers add signature and title to notes.)

IV. SOCIAL INFORMATION (Adjustment to disability, emotional support from family, motivation for self care, socializing ability, financial plan, family health problem, etc.)

Social Welfare
Agencies Active___ Signature___ Title:___ Date:___

Figure 12.3. (Continued)

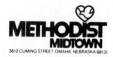

MEDICAL ADMISSION FORM

3612 CUMING STREET, OMAHA, NEBRASKA 68131

PATIENT'S NAME			
	STREET ADDRESS	CITY	STATE

MARITAL STATUS S M W D SEP	DATE OF BIRTH	AGE	CHURCH	TELEPHONE	OCCUPATION

MEDICARE NUMBER	INSURANCE

CLOSEST RELATIVE OR PERSON RESPONSIBLE	RELATIONSHIP	ADDRESS	TELEPHONE

PRESENT LOCATION OF PATIENT	DATE OF ADMISSION

SELF CARE STATUS
(Check Appropriate Space)

		Independent	Needs Assistance	Unable to Do
BED	- Turns			
ACTIVITY	- Sits			
PERSONAL HYGIENE	- Face, Hair, Arms			
	- Trunk, Perineum			
	- Lower Extremities			
DRESSING	- Upper Extremities			
	- Trunk			
	- Lower Extremities			
	- Appliance, Splint			
FEEDING				
TRANSFER	- Sitting			
	- Standing			
	- Tub			
	- Toilet			
LOCOMOTION	- Wheel Chair			
	- Walking			
	- Stairs			

DISABILITIES
(Describe)

AMPUTATION

CONTRACTURE

DECUBITUS ULCER

PARALYSIS

IMPAIRMENTS
(Describe)

HEARING   HEARING AID

SPEECH

VISION   GLASSES

ARTIFICIAL EYE

MENTAL STATUS

ALLERGIES

REV. 12-79

INCONTINENCE   ☐ Bladder   ☐ Bowel   ☐ Saliva

BED   ☐ Siderails   ☐ Bedboards   ☐ Footboards
☐ Overhead Frame   ☐ Restraints

PATIENT USES   ☐ Appliance   ☐ Cane   ☐ Dentures
☐ Walker   ☐ Catheter
☐ Crutches   ☐ Chair
☐ Colostomy   ☐ Prosthesis

MOST RECENT TEST RESULTS
COMPLETE BLOOD COUNT   Date_____

RBC_____/Mil	SEG_____	MONO_____
HGB_____GM%	STAB_____	EOS_____
HT_____%	JUV_____	BASO_____
WBC_____	LYMPH_____	PLATELET_____

URINALYSIS   Date_____

CATHETERIZED_____	PROTEIN_____
APP._____	GLUCOSE_____
COLOR_____	KETONES_____
PH_____	OCCULT BLOOD_____
SP. GR._____	MICRO_____

MS-12   Date_____

NA_____	PROT_____GM%	BILI_____MG%
K_____	ALB_____GM%	BUN_____MG%
CL_____	CA_____MG%	FBS_____MG%
CO2_____	ALK PHOS_____KAU	SGOT_____KU

Other test results that are pertinent: _____

Does patient have any draining areas? _____

Date of last culture _____

Please note: If drainage is present a culture is required within seven days prior to Methodist Midtown transfer.

Other test results that are pertinent:

Signature of person preparing report

Figure 12.4. Example of an admission form used by long term-care facilities. (Courtesy of Methodist Midtown Post-Acute Services, Omaha, Nebraska.)

DIAGNOSIS
(Primary and Secondary)

Date of surgery   Appliance used

☐ History and Physical Attached   ☐ Operative Report Attached (If Applicable)

MEDICATIONS ORDERED	REHABILITATION SERVICES
	☐ Physical Therapy Weight Bearing Status
	☐ Occupational Therapy
	☐ Speech and Hearing
	☐ Therapeutic Recreation
	☐ Social Service
	☐ Psychological Services
DIET ORDERED	☐ Nursing Service
	☐ Bowel & Bladder Program
	☐ Decubitus Care
	Evaluate and follow as indicated
THE PATIENT REQUIRES:	Goals:
☐ Skilled Nursing Service on a daily basis	
☐ Skilled Rehabilitation Services on a daily basis	
☐ Skilled Observation on a daily basis	
☐ Terminal Care	
☐ Chronic Nursing Care	

Estimated Length of Stay_____Days   **Dismissal Plans** ☐ Home ☐ Nursing Home ☐ Other_____

If you wish any other physician to follow this patient at Methodist Midtown, please designate whom _____

Estimated Date of Transfer _____ Mode of Transportation to Methodist Midtown _____

Date   Responsible Physician
Must be member of
Methodist Hosp. Staff

Do not write below this line

Admission   ☐ Approved
              ☐ Disapproved
              ☐ Qualified   Date

SIGNATURE, MEMBER OF ADMISSION COMMITTEE

Comments

Figure 12.4. (Continued)

screeening of hospitalized patients desiring admission to a LTC. This is often done by telephone. In some larger LTC facilities a referral nurse has been hired for the explicit purpose of doing preadmission screening. These nurses actually visit the patients in the hospital, provide a form (see Fig. 12.3) to be filled out by the nurse or attending physician, and check all details with the hospital discharge coordinator before the patient is accepted for transfer to the LTC facility. If the patient, due to a disease or complication, cannot be accepted by the LTC facility, this information needs to be properly communicated. These assessments can be made in a variety of ways, but the importance of written documentation cannot be overemphasized. Most LTC facilities have adopted or developed their own form to suit their needs (see Fig. 12.4).

Admission and transfer policies need to be carefully developed, written, approved, and communicated to all appropriate persons. The policies must be in compliance with the facility's license to practice. Some examples of typical policies might be:

1. Residents with any disease in the communicable stage shall not be admitted to the facility.
2. Residents who develop communicable diseases and who require isolation shall be placed in the appropriate type of isolation immediately.
3. Residents who develop communicable diseases and who require isolation shall be transferred to an appropriate facility as soon as possible.

Disease Reporting

The responsibility for disease reporting in a LTC facility usually rests with the attending physician or medical director. In some areas health departments have provided forms for the facility to fill out and return. Administrators of LTC facilities need to document, in policy form, which diseases need to be reported and who is responsible for reporting.

Few reportable diseases will be encountered in the LTC facility. Nevertheless, the county and state rules and regulations concerning reportable diseases should be known. These are available from state departments of health.

REFERENCES

1. Standards for certification and participation in Medicare and Medicaid program: Skilled nursing facilities. *Fed Reg* 39:2248, 1974.

2. *Interpretive Guidelines and Survey Procedures for the Application of the Standards for Skilled Nursing Facility.* US Department of Health and Human Services, 1974.

3. *Interpretive Guidelines and Survey Procedures for the Application of the Standards in the General Intermediate Care Facility.* US Department of Health and Human Services, 1974.

4. *Accreditation Manual for Long Term Care Facilities.* Chicago, Joint Commission for Accreditation of Hospitals, 1980.

5. *Peer Assistance Program.* American Health Care Association, Washington DC.

6. *Infection Prevention and Control for Long Term Care Facilities,* handbook and instructor's guide. Washington DC, American Health Care Association, 1977.

7. Centers for Disease Control: Guideline for isolation precautions in hospitals. *Infect Control* July–Aug, 1983.

8. Stark AJ, Gutman GM, McCashin B: Acute-care hospitalization and long term care: An examination of transfers. *J Am Geriatr Soc* 30:509–515, 1982.

9. Eggert GM, Bowlyow JE, Nichols CW: Gaining control of the long term care system: First returns from the ACCESS experiment. *Gerontologist* 20:356–363, 1980.

10. Bennett JV, Scheckler WE, Maki DG, et al: Current national patterns—United States, in *Proceedings of the International Conference on Nosocomial Infections,* Center for Disease Control, Atlanta, August 3–6, 1970.

CHAPTER 13

INFECTION CONTROL: EDUCATIONAL ASPECTS

Susan G. Miller

The purpose of this chapter is to help the new infection control practitioner provide an educational program to the personnel of a long-term care facility. The first section is an overview of the principles of learning and education, focusing on the instructor, the learner, and the interaction or communication that takes place between the two. The second section outlines planning, developing, implementing, and evaluating the in-service program itself.

The information presented here should be used to assist the infection control practitioner in developing such a program. The experience and ideas of the presenter are also necessary ingredients—the result being an effective program, one that will be both informative and enjoyable.

EDUCATION

General Considerations

The purpose of education in any health care setting is to change behavior or reinforce a desired behavior so that patient care can be improved. In order to prevent and control infections in the hospital or long-term care facility, education of personnel is vital. For the new practitioner in the field, developing in-service programs on infection control and other related subjects may be viewed as an overwhelming task, especially if educational sessions have never been conducted. These feelings of insecurity and inadequacy are not unusual and will diminish with time and experience. The foremost prerequisite for giving in-services is obviously knowledge of the subjects involved: infection control and the educational process. Finally, it is imperative for the administrators of the nursing home to commit themselves to the education of their employees. They must be willing to confront and solve problems that surface during the educational process.

Infection Control Practitioner/Instructor

The first element in the teaching–learning process is the teacher. The person assigned to organize and implement an infection control program must acquire a working knowledge of the dynamic field of infection control. This individual is called the **infection control practitioner** (ICP).

Historically, the Centers for Disease Control (CDC) have contributed to the growing knowledge in infection control, particularly by the continuous data collected on nosocomial infections and epidemiologic investigations. As this knowledge broadened in scope, the number of practitioners assigned to implement infection control programs also increased. The first formal training course devised primarily for the hospital-based practitioner (Course 1200G) was offered by the CDC in Atlanta, Georgia (1). With the additional influx of nursing home personnel into the field of infection control, the demand on the already established training programs exceeded available spaces.

The Association for Practitioners in Infection Control (APIC), formed in 1972, helped solve this problem by providing and sponsoring educational programs for new ICPs (2). Their curriculum committee (3) identified eight areas in which an ICP must become proficient (see Table 13.1). Although these programs provided opportunities for practitioner education, a need still existed for programs presented geographically close to practitioners. Consequently, state health departments, universities, local APIC chapters, and nonprofit organizations such as the Nebraska Infection Control Network (NICN) began to present their programs on the local level (4). Additionally, regional programs were designed especially for the beginning ICP from the long-term care facility, such as the district programs sponsored by the NICN.

After mastering the basic information required for infection control, the ICP can then develop the role of instructor. Characteristics of the instruction may vary, depending on the information being presented and the method used. Generally, the instructor needs to be the leader in the educational process, deciding the concepts to be taught and the best learning activities suited to the content. The instructor needs to have clear, written objectives that are known to the learner before the in-service begins. The ICP instructor also needs to establish instructor's goals that define the overall objectives for conducting in-services on infection con-

Table 13.1.   Association for Practitioners in Infection Control (APIC) Core Curriculum Subjects

Statistics—Epidemiology—The infection control practitioner (ICP) should have a basic knowledge of epidemiologic principles and statistical methods relevant to infection control.

Microbiology—The ICP should have knowledge of the basic principles of general, clinical, and environmental microbiology in the prevention and control of infection among patients, employees, and visitors within the health care facility.

Patient care practice—The ICP should have a comprehensive knowledge and understanding of therapeutic and diagnostic measures, equipment, and procedures used in patient care as related to infection control.

Sterilization, disinfection, and sanitation—The ICP should have a basic understanding of the principles used in sterilization, disinfection, and sanitation in a health care facility.

Infectious diseases—The ICP should have a basic knowledge of the cause and control of infectious diseases.

Employee health—The ICP should have knowledge of employee health programs as related to infection control.

Education—The ICP should have knowledge of the teaching and learning principles necessary for developing, implementing, and evaluating educational programs related to infection control.

Management and communication skills—The ICP should have knowledge of the management and communication skills necessary for the development, implementation, and coordination of an effective infection control program.

Source: Association for Practitioners in Infection Control: APIC Educational Standards. *Am J Infect Control* 9:42A, 1981. Used with permission.

trol. These are statements identifying what the ICP/instructor believes the personnel of the long-term care facility should learn from each of the in-services (5). Examples of instructor's goals are "to increase understanding of the menace of infection in the long-term health care facility" or "to demonstrate that each employee is personally responsible for infection control."

The materials used for the instruction need to be systematically organized proceeding with small steps. Each educational in-service should cover no more than four or five topics. The learning activity should be approached in a direct, businesslike manner, although the instructor should not be afraid to use humor. Finally, the instructor must be warm and friendly, frequently praising and encouraging the learner.

The Learner

The second element in the teaching–learning process is the learner. In order to facilitate the educational process, it is vital for the ICP/instructor to consider the characteristics of the learners. In the long-term care fa-

Table 13.2. Pedagogy versus Androgogy

Pedagogy	Androgogy
Teacher-directed Learning.	Self-directed Learning.
Nonvoluntary—formal.	Voluntary—informal.
Homogeneous group.	Heterogeneous group—from different backgrounds (ethnic, social, economic, intellectual).
Structured learning process is needed.	Learning process is usually self-directed.
Questions need to be answered unequivocally.	Learners realize questions often have no correct answer.
Correct answers to questions usually mean a higher grade.	Learner's answers to questions may affect others, thus having a more dramatic effect.
Decisions need to be made for the learners.	Learners need only assistance in identifying problems and the various alternative solutions.
Evaluation by instructor.	Evaluation by all involved in the learning process.

cility, the majority of the students will come from various departments, including medical staff (very limited), nursing staff, ancillary resident care, food service, housekeeping, engineering, laundry, maintenance, and administration (6). In the nursing home, employees may have widely differing backgrounds in terms of general knowledge, medical knowledge and interactional skills. Table 13.2 identifies different characteristics in-

Table 13.3. Concepts in Planning Self-Directed Learning Programs

1. There is an acceptance that all human beings can learn.
2. People must be motivated to learn.
3. Learning is an active, not a passive, process.
4. The learner must have guidance.
5. Appropriate materials for sequential learning must be provided.
6. Time must be provided to apply the learning.
7. Learning methods should be varied to avoid boredom.
8. The learner must secure satisfaction from the learning.
9. The learner must get reinforcement from the correct behavior.
10. Standards of performance should be set for the learner.
11. A recognition exists that there are different levels of learning and that these take different times and require different methods.
12. Learners should take something with them from the session.

volved in androgogy (self-directed learning) and pedagogy (teacher-directed learning) (7). The optimal educational approach will generally involve a mixture of these two methods as appropriate to the learners' backgrounds.

In considering the learner, the ICP/instructor will realize that there are employees who are more mature and respond better to learning on a self-directed level, while other employees will respond and learn more from teacher-directed inservice. The ICP/instructor therefore needs to formulate the in-service in such a way as to reach the majority of the learners present. Table 13.3 is a list of general considerations for employees learning by a self-directed method, but the list can and should also be applied to those learning by a teacher-directed method (8,9).

Instructor–Learner Communication

The practice of providing educational programs to the staff of a nursing home has occasionally been limited by several factors: first, a lack of awareness by the administration of the benefits of such a program (e.g., improved resident care); second, a lack of funds for such a program; and third a scarcity of qualified instructors. The ICP needs to assess the educational background of the learners. Learners who have had little education are often uncomfortable with the changes brought about by the educational process. Fear of poor performance on testing, inability to answer questions, and misunderstanding of the needs and purposes of such a program lead to poor retention and application.

There are two major ways the ICP/instructor can interact with learners so that the educational process can take place (10). The "associationists' approach" is frequently used by professional educators and psychologists. It is based on the assumption that learning takes place when the learner experiences repeated associations between a stimulus and the correct response to it. Learning is judged to have taken place if there is a change in either verbal or nonverbal behavior, which occurs as a result of repetition. This educational method uses small steps in presenting new material, and some type of evaluation is scheduled at specific intervals to see if learning has taken place. If not, the material is repeated to the student, perhaps using different audiovisual means. The associationists' approach will work very well with the unsophisticated learner. For example, if the ICP wants to see employees wash their hands more frequently, a brief in-service on handwashing policies and procedures might be presented (see Fig. 13.1). While making rounds, if no increase in the frequency of handwashing is noticed, then the ICP/instructor might put up posters of handwashing. If this does not increase frequency of hand-

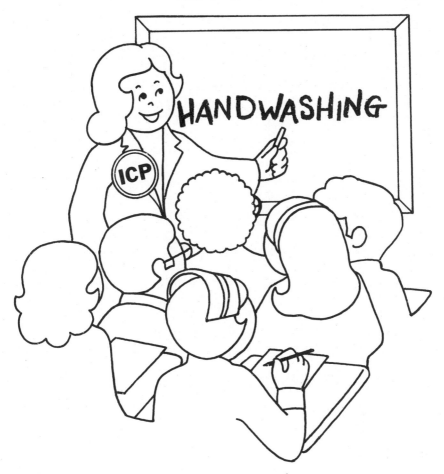

Figure 13.1. Infection control in-service presentation.

washing by the employees, supervisors may be asked to remind their employees to wash their hands. Hopefully, the frequency of handwashing will increase with these repeated reminders.

The "cognitive" or "Gestalt approach" is the second approach used to communicate. It is based on the assumption that learning takes place by people who go beyond the immediate information presented to develop general principles that can then be applied to different situations. It is a purposeful, goal-directed activity involving the gaining of knowledge, skills, or abilities. This approach uses the instructor as a facilitator to assist the learners in examining a problem situation and organizing information and experience into a personal cognitive framework. For example, if the ICP identifies a problem with infrequent handwashing, an opportunity is arranged for the employees (learners) to discuss this problem and develop solutions using round-table discussion so that the frequency of handwashing is increased appropriately.

These are brief summaries of the two major approaches the ICP/instructor can use to communicate or interact with the learner so that learning can take place. Once the instructor has chosen a format for the educational process, the actual in-service preparation can begin.

COMPONENTS OF AN IN-SERVICE

General Considerations

There are four stages or components that must be completed in order to provide a successful education program: planning, developing, implementing, and evaluating. Figure 13.2 depicts the relationship of these

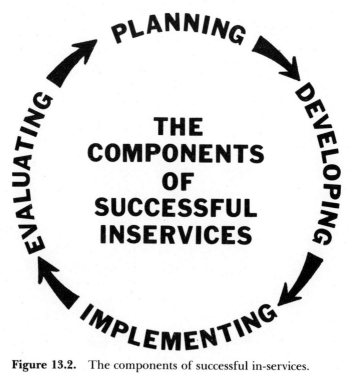

Figure 13.2.   The components of successful in-services.

stages to each other. Note that the educational process does not stop after the evaluating stage, but continues on to directly affect the planning stage of the next in-service.

Planning Stage

During the planning stage, the ICP/instructor must identify the learners' objectives and the material resources needed to help the learners achieve those objectives. Table 13.4 summarizes the steps involved in the planning stage.

First of all, the ICP/instructor must determine the educational needs of the learners (employees, in most cases). There are a variety of ways the instructor can gain this information—for example, evaluations from previous in-services, interviewing each supervisor in the various departments to determine needs, pretests, and infection control deficiencies noted by federal, state, and other accrediting agencies.

However, the most reliable source for determining the educational needs within a long-term care facility is the ICP's personal observation of infection control behaviors within the facility. For example, if the ICP is asked, while making rounds, how to read a culture report, then a need has been established to provide the nursing staff with information regarding culture reports. When doing the needs analysis, the ICP/instructor must keep in mind the amount of time and money budgeted for in-services. This includes considering the instructor's time as well as the learner's time.

After gathering the above data, the ICP/instructor will probably find a large number of subjects that need to be covered in the in-services. Step 2 is to prioritize these needs and select one topic for the in-service.

Step 3 is the developing of objectives. Learner objectives represent what each learner should be able to do after a successful in-service is presented and direct learners' achievement toward meeting the ICP's goals as an instructor. These statements begin with an action word and are followed by a desired behavior or knowledge that the ICP/instructor

Table 13.4. **Steps in the Planning Stage**

1. Determine needs of the audience.
2. Select subject matter.
3. Develop learner objectives.
4. Identify resources.
5. Allocate time.
6. Select instructional methods and materials.

Table 13.5. Examples of Action Words Used to Develop Learner Objectives

After completion of this in-service, the learner will be able to:

1. *Identify* common pathogens in the nursing home environment.
2. *Name* three diseases transmitted by the airborne route.
3. *Use* the double-bagging technique in isolation precautions.
4. *Order* the appropriate isolation precautions for the different types of pneumonias.
5. *Write* a procedure for decubitus care.
6. *Perform* Foley catheter insertion using aseptic technique.
7. *List* the 5 types of isolation precautions.
8. *Compare* the terms *isolation* and *precautions*.

wishes the learner to derive from the in-service (see Table 13.5). Learner objectives can further be defined as minimal competence objectives (which correlate well with the associationists' or repetitive approach) and the problem-solving competence objective (which correlates with the cognitive or Gestalt approach). For example, a learner's minimal competence objective might be "to name the five types of isolation precautions following an in-service on the same subject." A problem-solving competence objective would be "to explain why the door to the isolation rooms must be closed while the door to a precautions' room may be left open." The learner objectives must be known to the learner before the in-service begins.

Step 4 in the planning stage is to identify resources and constraints. For example, is there a classroom available to the ICP/instructor, or will a report room need to be used? Also, the place in which the in-service is to be presented will affect the time and the number of people attending. The ICP/instructor also must adapt the presentation to the audiovisual aids available. A blackboard or flipchart may be used to illustrate points.

In step 5, the ICP/instructor will need to allocate time to prepare for, implement, and evaluate each in-service program. The success of an educational program generally depends on the time committed to it.

The sixth and final step in the planning stage is the selection of instructional methods and materials to be used by the ICP/instructor (see Table 13.6). For example, the ICP/instructor may decide to use a lecture format. Over 70% of all in-service presentations use some variation of this method (11). During a **lecture**, an instructor presents the subject matter to a group of learners, who remain passive during the time the in-service takes place. Generally, a brief orientation to relevant information in past in-services is presented. The lecture is presented in a

Table 13.6. Teaching Methods and Aids

Methods	Aids
Lecture	Tape recorders
Demonstration	Video
Self-programmed instructor	Filmstrips
Slide–sound presentations	Films
Movies	Slides
Audiotapes	Transparencies
Videotapes	Bulletin boards
Learning games	Posters
Case studies	Blackboards
Role playing	Flipcharts

structured manner so the learners can follow. It is important to build in surprise and drama to keep learners from getting bored. The ICP/instructor must limit the lecture to four or five concepts and summarize the important points frequently. The lecture should end with an overview.

Lectures are often used to emphasize and clarify ideas with illustrations and models, introduce a topic, integrate or summarize a problem, cover complex material, share personal experiences, provide enrichment experiences, stimulate the student to further inquiry, show concepts in different perspectives, and extend these solutions to other situations. The ICP/instructor's behavior is most important during a lecture. A conversational tone should be used so that learners do not feel they are being "read to." It is important for the instructor to pace the lecture with the learners' needs for note taking and understanding. The instructor must learn to "read" the audience by looking for facial expressions of boredom, understanding, and interest and then adjusting the lecture as necessary so learning takes place. At the end of a lecture the ICP/instructor must provide time for questions and answers (12).

In addition to lectures, the ICP/instructor can choose from among many other teaching methods and aids. **Television** (videotapes) is a medium that lends itself to learning and creates a feeling in the learner of watching an event as it happens. **Self-study packets** are written materials that allow the learner to study at his or her own pace and ensure standardization of the information transmitted. **Slides/audiotape** is a combined medium that is relatively inexpensive. Slide/audiotape programs are easily modified by changing a slide or the narration. They are easily transported and good for large or small groups. Slides may be used independently for classroom lecture. The audiotape may also be used independently, but is less desirable. Transparencies for use with an **overhead projector** are quickly developed and inexpensive. They are small, portable, and better to use than a blackboard because the ICP/instructor can face the learners as illustrations are made. The planning of an in-service requires the ICP/instructor to decide which of these methods and aids will best help present the particular subject content.

Appropriate selection of these methods, keeping in mind time, money, and learner characteristics, will greatly enhance the educational process for both the learner and instructor. It maximizes the effectiveness of time spent together.

Developing Stage

The developing stage formalizes what the ICP/instructor has done during the planning stage: (*1*) The instructor arranges the in-service schedule, deciding where and when the in-service is to be held (including dates, time of day, and length of the in-service). (*2*) The instructor's goals and the learner objectives are written in final form. (*3*) The content outline of the subject to be presented is developed. (*4*) Handout materials and educational aids are prepared. (*5*) The room and equipment are scheduled. (*6*)The ICP publicizes that an in-service is to take place.

If the ICP is not familiar with the subject being presented, extensive research and preparation are required. The developing stage may be as long as six months or as short as one day. The ICP/instructor must finish each step in this stage before the implementing stage can begin.

Implementing Stage

The implementing stage is thought by some to be the most difficult component for a new ICP/instructor to complete successfully. Anxiety, sleepless nights, and fear of failure often precede the beginning of this stage. The new instructor should remember that almost everyone in the field experiences some insecurity and that with time and experience this will diminish. The new ICP/instructor will feel more confident knowing that the planning and developing stages are completed.

In a health care setting, there is always the possibility that the in-service will be canceled at the last minute due to unforeseen circumstances— for example, insufficient learners on hand, inability of the instructor to be present, weather conditions, or a patient emergency. Soliciting departmental input concerning a "good time and place" during the planning stage can be helpful in anticipating such situations. Other solutions include multiple presentations and scheduling in-services both before and after employees' working shifts.

Before the learners arrive for the session, the instructor should briefly review prepared materials and set up audiovisual aids, checking to make sure they are working properly. Once the students arrive, the instructor should start the in-service on time by introducing her- or himself to the learners and welcoming them. Handout material can then be distributed and the learners' objectives addressed. The instructor should identify the educational format to be used (e.g., lecture) and indicate whether questions may be asked during the session or should be held until the end.

While it is important for the instructor to follow the outline prepared in the developing phase, he or she should also watch for non-verbal clues from learners that indicate whether the material is being understood. Good eye contact with the learners is vital, as is awareness of audience facial expressions. Posturing and head nodding imply that learning is not taking place. The presentation should be adjusted if the instructor senses problems in learning. Then, even while the implementing stage is being completed, the evaluating stage has begun.

Evaluating Stage

The purpose of the evaluating stage is to determine the effectiveness of the previous three stages. The evaluation must not only objectively assess learners to see if learner objectives have been met, but also assess the effectiveness of the teaching process.

There are many ways to determine if learning has taken place, including post-tests, evaluation forms, clinical observations, and verbal feedback. Post-tests must be directly related to the learner objectives stated at the beginning of the in-service. Clinical observation and verbal feedback are most often obtained later, perhaps while the ICP is involved in surveillance activities on the floors.

Evaluation of the instructor is often more difficult. Tape recordings of the presentation can give the instructor feedback. Valuable information may also be gained by asking a colleague to critique the presentation or the audience to evaluate the in-service.

Whatever evaluation method the ICP/instructor uses, the most important item to remember is documentation of the program. The "who," "what," "when," and "where" and the evaluations received are vital to the ICP's infection control educational program and will help identify needed modifications.

PLANNING FUTURE PROGRAMS

This chapter has concentrated on the educational process that takes place between the ICP as instructor and employees of long-term care facilities as learners. After the educational process has been securely established, the ICP may consider the long-range goal of educating residents and their families in the basics of infection control. Establishing such a program requires assessing learner characteristics anew, a task that certainly will challenge the ICP. Residents and families knowledgeable in the basics of infection control practices can only enhance the long-term care facility's infection control program, resulting in a healthier atmosphere for all concerned.

Using the organizational format discussed here, the ICP/instructor can define and resolve new problems through the educational process. In-service programs that are well-organized, practical, and varied will be well received by nursing home staff at any level.

REFERENCES

1. Castle M, Kennicott J: Educating the infection control practitioner, *APIC J* 6:35–37, 1978.
2. *Am J Infect Control* 9:52A, 1981.
3. *Am J Infect Control* 91:42A, 1981.
4. Hospital infection control, *Am Health Consult* 9:27, 1982.
5. *Personnel Education for Infection Control.* Atlanta, Centers for Disease Control.
6. Paulson LG: Education in the nursing home: Practical considerations. *J Am Geriat Soc* 30:600–602, 1982.
7. Robinson RD: *An Introduction to Helping Adults Learn and Change.* Milwaukee, Omni, 1979.
8. Lippitt GL: Conditions of learning affecting training. Unpublished notes, presented in Des Moines, Iowa in 1981.
9. Miller, HL: *Teaching and Learning in Adult Education.* New York, Macmillan, 1964.
10. Knaples HJ: *Approaches to Teaching in the Health Sciences.* Reading, Mass., Addison-Wesley, 1978.
11. Warren MW: *Training for Results.* Reading, Mass., Addison-Wesley, 1969.
12. Stevens BJ: The teaching learning process. *Nurse Educ* 1:9–20, 1976.

SECTION IV

SPECIFIC CONTROL MEASURES

CHAPTER 14

INFECTION CONTROL MEASURES: THE RESIDENT

Philip W. Smith

To prevent infection in the nursing home setting, efforts must be directed at one or more of the three points in the infection sequence (see Chapter 4, Fig 4.1): optimizing the resistance of the resident to infection, controlling the reservoir of infection, and limiting the transmission of infectious agents. This chapter reviews methods of improving the intrinsic resistance of the host to infection (see Chapter 8, Fig 8.3); the other techniques for control of nursing home infections will be discussed in the two subsequent chapters.

A number of areas must be addressed by the nursing home to maximize host resistance in the resident (see Table 14.1).

IMPROVING GENERAL HOST RESISTANCE

Underlying Medical Illnesses

Underlying medical illness often predisposes to nosocomial infection in the nursing home. Treatment of these underlying diseases can be expected to improve the resistance of the host. Cardiac and circulatory disorders are common in the elderly. Congestive heart failure and atherosclerotic vascular disease may impair circulation of extremities, thereby increasing the possibility of skin ulceration and soft tissue infection.

Residents with poorly controlled diabetes mellitus have an increased incidence of certain infections, including nonclostridial gas gangrene, urinary tract infection, respiratory tract infection, and skin infection (1). Infections occur in diabetics for a number of reasons, including peripheral vascular disease (extremity infection), diabetic neuropathy with neurogenic bladder and urine retention (urinary tract infection), and glycosuria (recurrent *Candida* vaginitis). There is also a general correlation

Table 14.1.   Measures to Improve Host Resistance

Control of underlying diseases (e.g., diabetes, heart failure)
Evaluation of medical problems (e.g., incontinence)
Treatment of established infections
Minimization of antibiotic usage
Minimization of other drugs
Nutrition
Local defenses (e.g., avoidance of aspiration, decubiti)
General cleanliness of resident
Identification of specific immune problems
Immunizations

between poor control of blood sugar in diabetes and susceptibility to infection. This may relate to the observation that white blood cells in hyperglycemic diabetics do not ingest and kill bacteria normally (2). A complete discussion of the impact of systemic diseases on immunity to infection can be found in Chapter 2.

Host resistance to pneumonia may be improved by avoidance of cigarette smoke, proper pulmonary toilet in the chronic bronchitis patient, and treatment of pulmonary edema, which impairs lung defenses (3). Many cases of nursing home pneumonia follow aspiration, which is most common in patients with altered states of consciousness, seizure disorders, or dysphagia (4). Feeding a clear liquid diet or elevating the head of the bed after feeding may decrease the chance of aspiration in the high-risk patient.

Finally, it is important to treat established infections in the nursing home resident to prevent secondary infectious complications. For instance, chronic purulent sinusitis may lead to aspiration of the infected sinus drainage with secondary bacterial pneumonia. Recurrent bacterial prostatitis may be the source of relapsing nosocomial urinary tract infection. An infected decubitus ulcer may spread to involve underlying bone. Any uncontrolled local infection carries the risk of a secondary septic complication.

Medication

Antibiotic use has the potential disadvantages of toxic side effects, allergic reactions, disturbance of normal bacterial flora, selection of antibiotic-resistant bacteria, superinfection, and expense. Hence, rational prescription of antibiotics is important to the preservation of health in nursing home residents.

The normal flora is an important defense mechanism in the host. It has been shown that antibiotics may disturb normal flora and facilitate colonization of the pharynx by potentially pathogenic gram-negative bacilli (5). Antibiotics may also lead to overgrowth of organisms such as *Clostridium difficile,* the cause of antibiotic-associated enterocolitis. Antibiotic usage is the primary determinant in the selection of multiply antibiotic-resistant bacteria that can cause epidemics in nursing homes.

Other medications also have potential adverse effects. Anticholinergics may predispose to urinary retention and increase the risk of urinary tract infection. Sedatives and tranquilizers decrease the cough reflex, thereby preventing effective clearance of respiratory tract pathogens. Antacids decrease gastric acid, an important antibacterial defense mechanism. Finally, drugs many interact with antibiotics in a variety of ways. The chance of an adverse effect due to medication is significant in nursing homes where residents tend to be on multiple medications (6).

Nutrition

Malnutrition has an impact on host resistance to infection in a number of areas, including general immunity and wound healing (see Chapter 2). The nutritional requirements of the elderly are different from those of young people (7).

In addition, maintenance of adequate hydration in the elderly patient is very important. Dehydration may diminish urinary flow and mucous production in the respiratory tract, thereby predisposing to infection in these organ systems.

IMPROVING LOCAL DEFENSES

The Skin

Local defenses are the first line of protection against invasive organisms. The skin, for instance, forms an excellent barrier to infection in most individuals. With aging, there is loss of subcutaneous fat and thinning of the skin (8), which along with immobilization predispose to decubitus ulcers (9). Intravenous catheters, when present, also violate the skin barrier.

Control measures designed to maintain this first line of protection, discussed in depth in Chapter 7, include frequent change of position of the immobilized resident and the judicious use of air mattresses or sheepskin to relieve the pressure on bony prominences. Skin lotion is indicated for dry skin. Areas that are already ulcerated should be kept clean and dry. Ambulation and activity should be encouraged within the resident's limits.

Gastric Acid

The elderly resident may have gastric achlorhydria, which negates the potent antibacterial affect of gastric acid, in turn predisposing to a variety of gastrointestinal infections. Antacids accentuate this problem.

Urinary Tract

The most important predisposing factor for nursing home-acquired urinary tract infections is placement of indwelling bladder catheters. Control of urinary tract infections is discussed in Chapter 6. In general, bladder catheters should be minimized. They should be inserted aseptically by trained personnel, and a closed system should be maintained in order to minimize entry of bacteria. Adequate hydration is important, as is treatment of underlying medical diseases predisposing to urinary obstruction (e.g., prostatic hypertrophy).

Respiratory Tract

Local defenses of the upper airway include the cough reflex and the mucociliary system. Factors that interfere with normal upper airway defenses such as cigarette smoking, dehydration, and oversedation are potentially avoidable. Special care of residents receiving gastric tube feedings is recommended to minimize aspiration. This should include elevating the head of the bed during and for one hour after feeding. Good oral hygiene is also vital to local defenses. The prevention of pneumonia is discussed further in Chapter 5.

General Care

General measures of importance include hydration, ambulation, and documentation of skin and catheter care (10). Residents should have their own supplies and equipment and wear fresh clothing daily. Incontinent residents should be diapered. The resident should receive several complete baths per week. During this time, the staff is afforded an opportunity to visualize a number of problems that could lead to nosocomial infections, such as distended bladders, areas of skin erythema that may presage decubitus ulcers, and draining wounds (11).

Good skin care and timely bathing can be expected to delay colonization with resistant gram-negative bacteria. There is some evidence, however, that even meticulous bathing will not eliminate such organisms as *Pseudomonas aeruginosa* from the perineal area once this area has become colonized (12). If the resident's perineum is not kept dry, it may become excoriated.

IMPROVING SPECIFIC IMMUNITY

White Blood Cells

Neutrophils (polymorphonuclear leukocytes) are the first line of defense against bacterial infection. Neutropenia, which is defined as less than 1000 circulating neutrophils per milliliter of blood, is clearly associated with the highest risk of infection. Bacteremia and pneumonia frequently develop, and gram-negative bacilli are the usual cause. Neutropenia is most often caused by cytotoxic chemotherapy, radiation, or bone marrow replacement by tumor. Unfortunately, there are no good preventive measures. White blood cell (granulocyte) transfusions provide short-lived assistance against established bacterial infections in selected neutropenic patients, but are available only in limited circumstances.

A number of medical conditions cause qualitative deficiencies of the white blood cell. Malnutrition, alcoholism, and diabetes are examples of potentially reversible causes of abnormal white blood cell function. Rarely, a well-defined abnormality in white blood cell metabolism or function can be identified in a patient with recurrent infections (13). A great many drugs have also been identified that may adversely effect white blood cell function, either at the level of chemotaxis (directed migration), phagocytosis (ingestion of bacteria), or intracellular killing of ingested bacteria (14).

Antibodies

Antibodies coat (opsonize) bacteria to facilitate their ingestion (phagocytosis) by white blood cells. Other functions include agglutination of organisms, lysis of bacteria, and virus neutralization. IgG is the most important antibody, comprising about 70% of serum immunoglobulin. IgM is the earliest antibody produced in response to infection but is short-lived. IgA is the local antibody of respiratory and gastrointestinal tracts.

IgA deficiency is associated with severe and recurrent respiratory and gastrointestinal tract infections. The severe infections with *Streptococcus pneumoniae* and *Hemophilus influenzae* encountered in IgG deficiency reflect deficient opsonization or coating of bacteria for phagocytosis. Elderly persons who have undergone splenectomy also have an increased susceptibility to pneumococcal and *H. influenzae* infections (15).

A high index of suspicion needs to be maintained in patients with IgA deficiency for possible gastrointestinal or respiratory tract infections. For patients with IgG deficiency, monthly injections of pooled gammaglobulin (antibody harvested from donors) may provide some protection against recurrent infection (16).

Cellular Immunity

Cellular immunity, or delayed hypersensitivity, involves lymphocytes and is the part of the immune system most responsible for fighting tuberculous, fungal and viral infections. Residents with lymphoma or who are receiving corticosteroid therapy have impaired cell-mediated immunity and are at risk for these infections. The dose of corticosteroids should be minimized to decrease the risk of infection.

The nursing staff must be aware that cancer patients have a greatly increased risk of infection; in fact, infection is the leading cause of death in cancer patients (17). The risk of infection relates to the specific immune problems caused by the underlying cancer as well as various treatment modalities.

IMMUNIZATION AND VACCINATION

Passive Immunization

The injection of antibody from an immune donor (see Chapter 2) is passive immunization and provides temporary protection. Passive immunity is useful prophylaxis for those exposed to hepatitis A, hepatitis B, and tetanus and in the treatment of diphtheria and botulism. While passive prophylaxis of nursing home residents on a routine basis against hepatitis A is not recommended, pooled immune globulin may be indicated for residents or personnel who have a significant exposure to hepatitis A or if there is an outbreak of hepatitis A in the institution. The dose is 0.02 ml/kg by the intramuscular route.

Active Immunization

Active immunity is preferable to passive immunity because it is generally long-lasting, involving production of antibody by the host to the vaccine.

The routine immunization schedule that begins in childhood involves administration of the diphtheria–pertussis–tetanus (DPT) vaccine, oral poliomyelitis vaccine (OPV), and measles–mumps–rubella (MMR) vaccine. Adults should receive a standard-dose tetanus, reduced-dose diphtheria (Td) vaccine every 5–10 years throughout adulthood (18). An adult who has never been vaccinated should receive the Td vaccine at times 0, 2 months, and 6 months. Pertussis and polio vaccines are not routinely recommended for adults.

Mumps, measles, rubella, and oral polio vaccines are live viruses that are attenuated (made less pathogenic in the laboratory). Attenuated viruses cause mild disease but induce appropriate immunity. They should not be given to an immunodeficient host. Smallpox vaccine is no longer recommended, since smallpox has been eradicated on a global basis. Rabies, pertussis, and influenza vaccines are inactivated agents. The pneumococcal vaccine consists of a cell wall polysaccharide extract of the organism, and hepatitis B vaccine is composed of surface antigen components of the virus.

Some vaccination preparations (e.g., yellow fever, influenza, and rabies) contain egg products and should therefore be avoided in patients allergic to eggs. Active immunization should be avoided during febrile illness or within three months of passive immunization, when it is less likely to be effective.

Vaccination for the Nursing Home Resident

Several immunizations are of importance to the nursing home resident (see Table 14.2).

Tetanus/Diphtheria.   Tetanus/diphtheria immunization is important because of the increased risk of acquisition of tetanus in the elderly, especially in the setting of vascular insufficiency, skin ulcers of the extremities, or diabetes mellitus (19). The highest risk of tetanus is in persons over 60 years of age (20). Virtually all tetanus cases occur in un-

Table 14.2.   Vaccines of Importance for the Elderly

Vaccine	Recommended Frequency
Tetanus	Every 5–10 years
Diphtheria	Every 5–10 years
Influenza	Yearly
Pneumococcal	Every 5 years (?)

immunized or inadequately immunized persons. Diphtheria still occurs in the United States, and diphtheria vaccination should also be maintained in all elderly persons.

Tetanus and diphtheria vaccines consist of toxoids, substances that resemble the toxins produced by *Clostridium tetani* and *Corynebacterium diphtheriae*, respectively. The resemblance is close enough to induce immunity, and yet the toxoid does not have the detrimental effects of the toxin. Toxoids are produced by formaldehyde treatment of tetanus and diphtheria toxins. Immunization with these toxoids induces an effective antibody response 90% of the time for diphtheria and nearly 100% of the time for tetanus. Adequate antibody levels persist for at least 10 years after effective immunization (21).

Giving tetanus and diphtheria vaccinations more often than every 5 years may be associated with increased incidence and severity of local reactions and has no benefit. The resident who is fully and currently immunized against diphtheria should be safe even during a diphtheria outbreak. The resident who is fully and currently immunized against tetanus is protected from tetanus even after sustaining a dirty wound. Hence, the elderly should receive Td vaccination every 10 years (22).

Influenza.   During influenza epidemics, there is a significant increase in mortality, especially among the elderly and debilitated residents. The development of influenza vaccine is complicated by the fact that antigenic variations of the influenza virus occur frequently. Minor antigenic variations occur every 2 to 4 years and major variations every 10 years, approximately (23). As a result, previous immunity to influenza becomes obsolete. In addition, the short-lived protection induced by the influenza vaccine makes annual revaccination with current strains necessary.

The influenza vaccine strain recommended for 1983–1984 (influenza season is primarily in the winter) was a trivalent vaccine with the three prevalent influenza types. The vaccine contained 15 μg. each of hemagglutinin of influenza A/Brazil/78 (H_1N_1), A/Philippines/82 (H_3N_2), and B/Singapore/79 viruses in a 0.5-ml dose. Adults require only one dose, usually in the late fall. The vaccine is recommended for high-risk groups, including all persons over the age of 65 and persons with underlying disease such as acquired or congenital heart disease, chronic pulmonary disease, chronic renal disease, diabetes mellitus, and immunosuppressive disorders, including malignancies. Side effects are relatively few. About one-third of vaccinees have been reported to have local redness and induration for one to two days at the site of injection. Occasionally, residents will have fever, malaise, myalgia, or other systemic symptoms. Allergic reaction to an egg compound in the vaccine may occur, and very rarely Guillain–Barre syndrome is encountered (24).

It appears that those at greatest risk from influenza, including the elderly, may not respond as well to the influenza vaccine as younger persons (25,26). Others have suggested that vaccine will at least lessen the severity of clinical influenza and decrease morbidity and mortality during an outbreak in an elderly population (25, 27, 28).

In several nursing home outbreaks, clinical attack rates for influenza have averaged 27%. The overall case fatality ratio is 10%. The calculated rates of vaccine efficacy in preventing clinical influenza illness averaged a disappointing 30% (29). The influenza vaccine is somewhat efficacious in preventing clinical influenza in the nursing home setting (29–32), even though the vaccine efficacy in the elderly is somewhat less than the expected 60–80% achieved in the population as a whole. Nevertheless, in view of the extreme susceptibility of the elderly to influenza, the increased morbidity and mortality of influenza in the elderly, and the relative safety of the influenza vaccine, it would seem prudent that nursing home residents over the age of 65 or with serious underlying diseases be vaccinated annually (33).

Occasionally, during an epidemic in a nursing home, the antiviral drug amantadine hydrochloride can play a supplementary role in preventing influenza A. Amantadine protects only against influenza A, not influenza B, and is not a substitute for vaccination. The duration of protection of amantadine lasts only while the individual is receiving the drug. It is thus recommended that amantadine be used only until vaccination can be performed and has taken effect (about 10 to 14 days after vaccination). Amantadine will not interfere with the efficacy of influenza vaccination (24).

Pneumococcal Vaccine. *Streptococcus pneumoniae* is the leading cause of pneumonia in the community. It causes about a half-million to a million cases in the U.S. population per year and is the fifth most common cause of death (34). Pneumococcal pneumonia has an especially high mortality rate in the elderly (28%), even though the organism remains quite sensitive to penicillin. Residents with certain underlying conditions such as antibody deficiency or the postsplenectomy state are at increased risk of contracting this disease.

There are nearly 100 serotypes of the pneumococcus, and immunity is serotype-specific. A vaccine consisting of a polysaccharide extract of the pneumococcal cell wall from each of the 23 leading types in the United States is available. These 23 types represent 90% of bacteremic pneumococcal disease in the United States; the vaccine contains 50 μg of each polysaccharide. It is given as a single dose (0.5 ml) by the intramuscular route. The majority of residents vaccinated develop an antibody response, and antibodies can be detected for three to five years. The vaccine appears to be quite safe. About half of those given pneumococcal vaccine develop side effects such as erythema and mild pain at the site of injection, but severe reactions are extremely rare. The vaccine is currently recommended for persons over the age of two years with splenic dysfunction or anatomic asplenia and for those with chronic diseases that may be associated with an increased risk of pneumococcal disease. These diseases include sickle cell anemia, multiple myeloma, cirrhosis, renal failure, diabetes mellitus, congestive heart failure, chronic lung disease, and immunosuppressive diseases, including malignancies. It is also recommended for mass vaccination of nursing home populations during outbreaks of pneumococcal pneumonia (35).

It should be remembered that the vaccine is far from 100% effective for those serotypes included in the vaccine, and there are many serotypes not included in the vaccine that cause pneumonia. The efficacy of the pneumococcal vaccine in the elderly has been questioned (36–38), although it can be cost-effective if administered to high-risk groups (39,40).

While the efficacy and cost-effectiveness of pneumococcal vaccine in the elderly continue to be studied, at the present time it would seem reasonable to vaccinate all persons over the age of 50 years with underlying chronic diseases and to consider mass vaccination in the nursing home if an outbreak of pneumococcal pneumonia occurs (18,35). The vaccine is quite safe. Simultaneous administration of influenza and pneumococcal vaccines is as safe and effective as giving either vaccine alone (41).

Hepatitis Vaccine.   Hepatitis B vaccine is available for high-risk populations (42). It will have little use in nursing homes, except for frequently transfused residents or in the event of a hepatitis B outbreak. A resident or staff member carrying hepatitis B surface antigen could pose a hazard for those who have contact with that person's blood or secretions.

REFERENCES

1. Rayfield EJ, Ault MJ, Keusch GT, et al: Infection and diabetes: The case for glucose control. *Am J Med* 72:439–449, 1982.

2. Repine JE, Clawson CC, Goetz FC: Bactericidal function of neutrophils from patients with acute bacterial infections and from diabetics. *J Infect Dis* 142:869–875, 1980.

3. LaForce FM, Mullame JF, Boehme RF, et al: The effect of pulmonary edema on antibacterial defenses of the lung. *J Lab Clin Med* 82:634–648, 1973.

4. Bartlett JG, Finegold SM: Anaerobic infections of the lung and pleural space. *Am Rev Resp Dis* 110:56–77, 1974.

5. Mackowiak PA: The normal microbial flora. *N Engl J Med* 307:83–93, 1982.

6. Kalchthaler T, Coccard E, Lightiger S: Incidence of polypharmacy in a long-term care facility. *J Am Geriatr Soc* 25:308–313, 1977.

7. Munro HN: Nutritional requirements in the elderly. *Hosp Pract* 17:143–154, 1982.

8. Gilchrist BA: Age associated changes in the skin. *J Am Geriatr Soc* 30:139–143, 1982.

9. Reuler JB, Cooney TG, et al: The pressure sore: Pathophysiology and principles of management. *Ann Intern Med* 94:661–666, 1981.

10. Magnussen MH, Robb SS: Nosocomial infections in a long-term care facility. *Am J Infect Control* 8:12–17, 1980.

11. Campbell DG: Prevention of infection in extended care facilities. *Nurs Clin N Am* 15:857–868, 1980.

12. Gilmore DS, Jiminez EM, Aeilts GD, et al: Effects of bathing on *Pseudomonas* and *Klebsiella* colonization in patients with spinal cord injuries. *J Clin Micro* 14:404–407, 1981.

13. Graham RC Jr: Disorders of polymorphonuclear leukocytes relevant to infection. *Cleve Clin Q* 42:33–45, 1975.

14. Tauber AI: Current views of neutrophil dysfunction: An integrated clinical perspective. *Am J Med* 70:1237–1245, 1981.

15. Pearson HA: Splenectomy: Its risks and its roles. *Hosp Pract* 15:85–94, 1980.

16. Hermans PE, Diaz-Buxo JA, Stobo JA: Idiopathic late onset immunoglobulin deficiency:·Clinical observations in fifty patients. *Am J Med* 61:221–237, 1967.

17. Bodey GB: Infections in cancer patients. *Cancer Treat Rev* 2:89–128, 1975.

18. Goodman RA, Orenstein WA, Hinman AR: Vaccination and disease prevention for adults. *JAMA* 248:1607–1610, 1982.

19. Irvine P, Crossley K: Tetanus and the institutionalized elderly. *JAMA* 244:2159–2160, 1980.

20. Fraser DW: Preventing tetanus in patients with wounds. *Ann Intern Med* 84:95–96, 1976.

21. Brandling-Bennett AD: Duration of immunity from tetanus and diphtheria toxoid. *JAMA* 225:1400, 1973.

22. Centers for Disease Control: Diphtheria, tetanus and pertussis: Guidelines for vaccine prophylaxis and other preventive measures. *Ann Intern Med* 95:723–728, 1981.

23. Rimland D, McGowan JE Jr, Shulman JA: Immunization for the internist. *Ann Intern Med* 85:622–629, 1976.

24. Centers for Disease Control: Influenza vaccines, 1983–1984. *Morbid Mortal Weekly Rep* 32:333–337, 1983.

25. Howells CHL, Vesselinova-Jenkins CK, Evans AD, et al: Influenza vaccination and mortality from bronchopneumonia in the elderly. *Lancet* 1:381–383, 1975.

26. D'Alessio DJ, Cox PM Jr, Dick EC: Failure of inactivated influenza vaccine to protect an aged population. *JAMA* 210:485–489, 1969.

27. Barker WH, Mullooly JP: Influenza vaccination of elderly persons: Reduction in pneumonia and influenza hospitalizations and deaths. *JAMA* 224:2547–2549, 1980.

28. Ruben FL, Johnston F, Streiff EJ: Influenza in a partially immunized aged population: Effectiveness of killed Hong Kong vaccine against infection with the England strain. *JAMA* 230:863–866, 1974.

29. Centers for Disease Control: Influenza vaccine efficacy in nursing home outbreaks reported during 1981–1982. *Morbid Mortal Weekly Rep* 31:190–195, 1982.

30. Genesove LJ, Riddiford M: Influenza in a nursing home. *CMA J* 118:1202, 1978.

31. Goodman RA, Orenstein WA, Munro TF, et al: Impact of influenza in a nursing home. *JAMA* 247:1451–1453, 1982.

32. Hall WN, Goodman RA, Noble GR, et al: An outbreak of influenza B in an elderly population. *J Infect Dis* 144:297–302, 1981.

33. Ruben FL: Prevention of influenza in the elderly. *J Am Geriatr Soc* 30:577–580, 1982.

34. Rytel MW: Pneumococcal infections and pneumococcal vaccine: An update. *Infect Control* 3:295–298, 1982.

35. Centers for Disease Control: Pneumococcal polysaccharide vaccine. *Morbid Mortal Weekly Rep* 30:410–419, 1981.

36. Bentley DW: Pneumococcal vaccine in the institutionalized elderly: Review of past and recent studies. *Rev Infect Dis* 3(suppl):S61–S70, 1981.

37. Bentley DW, Ha K, Mamot K, et al: Pneumococcal vaccine in the institutionalized elderly: Design of a nonrandomized trial and preliminary results. *Rev Infect Dis* 3(suppl):S71–S81, 1981.

38. Hirschmann JV, Lipsky BA: Pneumococcal vaccine in the United States: A critical analysis. *JAMA* 246:1428–1432, 1981.

39. Willems JS, Sanders CR, Riddiough MA, et al: Cost-effectiveness in vaccination against pneumococcal pneumonia. *N Engl J Med* 303:553–559, 1980.

40. Patrick KM, Woolley FR: A cost-benefit analysis of immunization for pneumococcal pneumonia. *JAMA* 245:473–477, 1981.

41. DeStefano F, Goodman RA, Noble GR, et al: Simultaneous administration of influenza and pneumococcal vaccines. *JAMA* 247:2551–2554, 1982.

42. Centers for Disease Control: Inactivated hepatitis B virus vaccine. *Morbid Mortal Weekly Rep* 31:317–328, 1982.

CHAPTER **15**

INFECTION CONTROL MEASURES: THE ENVIRONMENTAL RESERVOIR

Philip W. Smith

GENERAL MEASURES FOR DECREASING PATHOGENS IN THE ENVIRONMENT

Environmental antimicrobials can be classified on the basis of potency: Sanitation, disinfection, and sterilization refer to increasing levels of antimicrobial activity.

Sanitation

Sanitation may be defined as the act of rendering sanitary by reducing the number of bacterial contaminants to a relatively safe level according to public health requirements (1). This term is commonly used in association with the cleaning of eating and drinking utensils and dairy equipment and has also been applied to a number of cleaning operations. Detergent sanitizers are used in the cleaning of inanimate objects. Application of sanitizing principles to food preparation may prevent food spoilage or foodborne infection. The term *sanitation* has also been used when referring to air purification processes.

Filtration is an effective technique for removing organisms from liquids or gases. Depending on the size of the filter, filtration may be either a sanitizing, disinfecting, or sterilizing process.

Disinfection/Antisepsis

Disinfection can be defined as the process that decreases the number of microorganisms or the microbiological load, including eradication of most pathogens. These agents free a surface from infection by destroying the most potentially harmful organisms, especially the vegetative forms of pathogenic bacteria. A **disinfectant** is a substance that is applied to inanimate surfaces, while an **antiseptic** is a substance that can be applied to the skin. Disinfectants and antiseptics are classified into three groups on the basis of their potency (2). Low-level disinfectants kill bacteria and fungi but not bacterial spores (bacterial spores are the most resistant to disinfection or sterilization), enteroviruses, or mycobacteria. Agents in this category include hexachlorophene, chlorhexidine, mercurial agents, and quaternary ammonium compounds.

Intermediate-level disinfectants and antiseptics are agents that kill bacteria, fungi, mycobacteria, and large viruses such as enteroviruses but do not kill bacterial spores. Chlorine and iodine-containing compounds, phenolics and alcohols are agents that are intermediate-level compounds.

High-level disinfectants, when used under certain conditions, may kill even bacterial spores; hence they can be classified as potential sterilizing agents. Formaldehyde, glutaraldehyde, and stabilized hydrogen peroxide are in this category. These agents are too irritating to be used on the skin as antiseptics.

Disinfectants

A variety of disinfectants may be used in the nursing home and hospital (see Table 15.1).

Formaldehyde is a high-level disinfectant used as an aqueous solution (3–8%) or in 70% alcohol. It has broad activity against organisms and is sporicidal. Disadvantages include noxious fumes and the fact that it is toxic, volatile, corrosive, and irritating to the skin. When diluted to 8%, it is good for emergency spills of infectious materials.

Glutaraldehyde takes 3 to 20 hours to kill bacterial spores but kills other organisms more rapidly. Acid glutaraldehyde is stable longer (i.e., four weeks) but is more corrosive. Alkaline glutaldehyde is more active,

Table 15.1. Commonly Used Disinfectants

Class of Agent	Level of Activity	Examples
Formaldehyde	High	Bard–Parker Germicide
Glutaraldehyde (acid)	High	Sonacide
Glutaraldehyde (alkaline)	High	Cidex, Sporicidin
Phenolic	Intermediate	Lysol, Phenol
Chlorine	Intermediate	Clorox
Alcohol	Intermediate	70% Ethanol
Quaternary ammonium	Low	Benzalkonium chloride (Zephiran)

killing bacteria in two minutes, fungi in five minutes, and spores in three hours. It is stable only for about two weeks, after which time it polymerizes. It is very useful for the cleaning of surfaces, rubber tubing, respiratory therapy and anesthesia equipment, lenses, and bronchoscopes. Either solution may irritate the skin.

Phenolic disinfectants, when used at 0.5–3.0% concentration, kill all organisms except bacterial spores. Their disadvantages are corrosiveness and skin irritation. These agents are widely used for disinfection of smooth surfaces, plastics, rubber, and hinged objects.

Chlorine is a disinfectant that is quite inexpensive, but unstable, corrosive, and inactivated by organic matter. Water is necessary for conversion of chlorine to hypochlorous acid, the active compound. It is used at a concentration of 0.05–0.5% (free chlorine) primarily for cleaning environmental areas such as bathrooms.

Alcohol is a very good antiseptic or disinfectant. Seventy percent alcohol kills better than 95% alcohol; 70% ethanol or 95% isopropanol are the most commonly used substances. Alcohol can be used to clean smooth surfaces and polyethylene tubing.

Quaternary ammonium compounds are relatively weak disinfectants; in addition, these agents can become contaminated with gram-negative bacteria with subsequent outbreaks of infection. They may be inactivated by soaps and organic material, but are appropriate for use on floors, walls, and furniture.

Acetic acid may be used as a 0.25% solution with mild activity against *Pseudomonas* and other gram-negative bacteria. Pasteurization, as applied to milk, refers to the heating of a substance to 60–70°C for 20 to 30 minutes, a process that kills all organisms except bacterial spores.

Antiseptics

Antiseptics are agents that may be used on living tissue (see Table 15.2).

A one- to three-minute wash with 70–90% alcohol will decrease skin bacteria by over 90%. The use of alcohol as an antiseptic has been limited because of its tendency to dry and irritate the skin. Alcohol is also volatile and flammable.

Iodine-containing compounds are effective antibacterial agents; 0.5% iodine in 70% alcohol is called tincture of iodine. It results in fast iodine release but does sting. This substance kills 80–90% of hand bacteria in a two-minute wash. Iodophors (iodine combined with surfactant) permit slow release of iodine to achieve antibacterial activity. Seventy-five to 150 parts per million (ppm) of iodine will decrease skin bacteria 60% in a two-minute scrub. Iodophors do not cause as much skin drying as tincture of iodine but do discolor the skin and may cause iodine allergy.

Table 15.2. Commonly Used Antiseptics

Class of Agent	Level of Activity	Examples
Alcohol	Intermediate	70% Ethanol
Iodine/alcohol	Intermediate	Tincture of iodine
Iodophor	Intermediate	Betadine, Wescodyne
Hexachlorophene	Low	pHisohex
Chlorhexidine	Low	Hibiclens
Mercurials	Low	Mercurochrome

Hexachlorophene is a bisphenolic compound. It is effective especially against gram-positive bacteria when used as a 1–3% solution. The major drawback is its lack of activity against gram-negative bacteria and fungi. In addition, animal toxicity studies indicate that caution must be observed in the use of hexachlorophene in infants and pregnant women. The greatest use of hexachlorophene previously was in prevention of staphylococcal infection in nurseries.

Chlorhexidine is a biguanide compound developed in England. It may be used as an aqueous solution (0.5% in water or alcohol) or as 4% weight per volume of chlorhexidine gluconate emulsion in a detergent. Four percent chlorhexidine gluconate in isopropyl alcohol will eliminate 90% of skin flora in two minutes. The major disadvantage is that weaker solutions may become contaminated with gram-negative bacteria, and mild skin irritation occurs.

Mercurial-containing compounds are weak antiseptics that are inactivated by organic matter. Allergic reactions occasionally occur.

Sterilization

Sterilization is defined as a process that kills all organisms. Since bacterial spores are the most difficult to destroy, they are measured to assure that sterilization has been accomplished. Sterilization may be achieved by a number of techniques. Irradiation (gamma rays, x-rays, or ultraviolet light) are used primarily by industry.

Heat is a very effective way of killing microorganisms. Dry heat, such as 171°C for one hour, 160°C for two hours, or 121°C for six hours kills *Bacillus* spores and is recommended for oils, petroleum products, powders, instruments with cutting edges, needles, greases, and glass syringes. Dry heat sterilizes by denaturing protein in the organisms.

Moist heat kills microorganisms more efficiently than dry heat. Spores are killed by 121°C heat for 15 minutes or 132°C heat for five minutes in the presence of saturated steam at 15–17 lb/in². Steam autoclaving is the preferred method of sterilization in most institutions because of speed and safety.

Ethylene oxide is a gas that sterilizes at lower temperatures; it is preferred for materials that cannot stand high temperatures. It is noncorrosive and penetrates materials well but requires a slow process. Other disadvantages include the fact that ethylene oxide is an explosive gas and long aeration times are required to remove all potentially toxic materials from the sterilized item. If all ethylene oxide metabolites are not removed, they will act as vesicants on skin and mucous membranes. Ethylene oxide kills organisms by alkylating proteins. The process requires ethylene oxide concentration of at least 450–600 mg/liter, moisture (a relative humidity of 30% or greater), appropriate temperature (30–55°C), and appropriate time of exposure (4 to 12 hours). After the sterilization process is finished, aeration at room temperature takes from 24 hours for glass to one week for polyvinyl chloride; the process may be accelerated by forced aeration at higher temperatures.

Chemical sterilization is much less efficient than steam or ethylene oxide sterilization, but has the advantages of being less expensive and more convenient. Most agents classified as high-level disinfectants will sterilize objects if they are used in sufficient concentrations for adequate periods of time. The contact time required for sterilization of an object depends on the chemical agent used and the type of object being sterilized. For example, smooth, hard-surfaced objects, thermometers, and polyethylene tubing/catheters can be sterilized by soaking in 8% formaldehyde (in 70% alcohol) for 18 hours or in 2% alkaline glutaraldehyde for 10 hours (3,4).

Several general concepts should be kept in mind when employing chemical sterilization: (1) Objects must be thoroughly cleaned before any sterilization attempt. (2) All parts of the object must be in contact with the chemical agent. (3) Objects that come into direct contact with residents must be rinsed with sterile distilled water after chemical sterilization. (4) Chemical agents may damage certain types of materials, and manufacturers' recommendations should be checked.

The use of the same agents for shorter periods of time will disinfect (but not sterilize) objects. Most objects can be disinfected by 30 minutes of exposure to 8% formaldehyde (in 70% alcohol), 2% alkaline glutaraldehyde, 2% acid glutaraldehyde, 70–90% alcohol, 3% phenolic solutions, or an iodophor (500 ppm available iodine).

Handwashing

Skin has two types of bacteria: resident and transient flora. **Resident** flora, found on virtually everyone, includes *Staphylococcus epidermidis*, micrococci, and diphtheroids on all skin areas. Anaerobic diphtheroids (e.g., *Propionibacterium acnes*) are found especially on the face because of the sebum there. The numbers of bacteria are greatest on hair, face, axillae, and groin region. Resident bacteria are found on skin surfaces as well as in skin crevices where lipid and cornified epithelium make their removal impossible. Fortunately, resident bacteria are of low virulence in the normal host.

Transient flora includes usual nosocomial pathogens (*S. aureus*, streptococci, *Pseudomonas*) that survive for a short time on open skin. They are readily removed by soap and water or other antiseptics in 30 seconds. *S. aureus* is usually transient flora on the open skin but a resident in the moist areas of the body, especially the nares, axillae, and groin.

Skin cannot be sterilized, but all transient flora and most resident flora can be removed by washing. Soaps and antiseptics facilitate the removal of skin bacteria (see Fig. 15.1).

Soaps are weakly antibacterial agents that are effective at removing transient flora. While bar soap does not appear to transmit bacteria or be responsible for epidemics of infection (5), the bar should be changed frequently and kept on a rack that allows for adequate drainage. Anti-

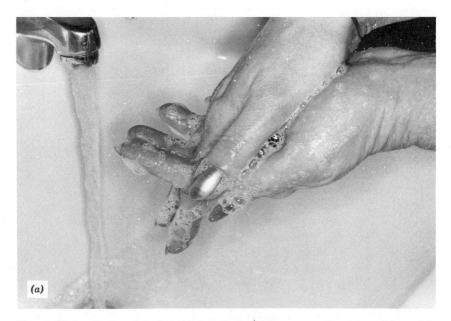

Figure 15.1. Correct handwashing technique, demonstrating (*a*) washing with soap, (*b*) rinsing, and (*c*) turning off faucet with paper towel.

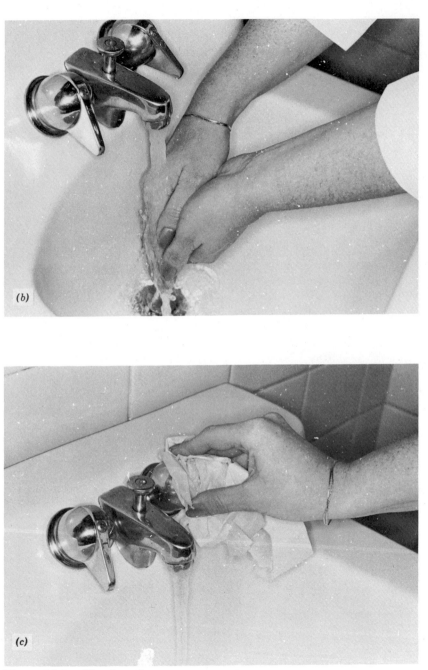

(b)

(c)

Figure 15.1. (Continued)

septics provide additional antibacterial effect when required: Iodophors, chlorhexidine, and hexachlorophene are widely used antiseptics. The antiseptic effect is related to time of contact of the agent with skin (6).

Most epidemics involving hand-to-hand transmission of organisms result from failure to wash hands rather than an incorrect choice of handwashing agent. Medical personnel have been demonstrated in a number of studies to be deficient in handwashing practices, even in intensive care settings in acute care hospitals (7). The hands of personnel may serve not only as a route of transmission for nursing home pathogens but also as a reservoir for gram-negative bacteria (8). Inadequate handwashing has been responsible for many outbreaks of infection in hospitals and nursing homes (see Chapter 10). Finally, the institution of good handwashing practices has interrupted outbreaks in many settings (9).

The correct length of scrub has not yet been determined, but a 5-minute scrub with an antiseptic such as an iodophor is recommended before surgery, while a 15-second scrub with soap and water is adequate between patients (10). Soap leaflets are more expensive but require 10 to 15 seconds to dissolve, thereby insuring lengthy washing. Overuse of antiseptics may lead to dermatitis, which defeats the purpose of handwashing; even antiseptics cannot decrease the flora of dermatitic skin. Virulent organisms such as *S. aureus* may colonize dermatitic skin. Outbreaks of nosocomial infections have also been traced to contaminated hand lotion. Personnel with dermatitis may wish to wear gloves during duty.

Standards for handwashing, including selection of antiseptics, length of washing, and indications for handwashing, have been published by the Centers for Disease Control (11). The most important extrapolation to nursing home personnel includes a recommendation for a 10-second wash with bar soap and water before and after each resident contact. In situations such as performance of minor surgical procedures, insertion of intravenous or urinary catheters, or special dressing changes, use of an antiseptic during handwashing and wearing of sterile gloves may be required.

General Principles

Handwashing/Antiseptics

1. Handwashing is the single most important measure for preventing the spread of nosocomial infections. Studies comparing antiseptics are difficult to interpret because of the variety of techniques used to measure the effectiveness of antiseptics. The type of antiseptic used is much less important than frequent handwashing with cor-

rect technique. In the nursing home setting, handwashing with bar soap is generally adequate, except when invasive procedures such as bladder catheter insertion are undertaken.

2. Virtually any form of soap is appropriate for routine handwashing. Liquid soap dispensers may become contaminated and serve as a source of nosocomial outbreaks (8); hence they should be emptied, cleaned, dried, and filled with a new solution regularly. Disposable cartridge dispensers are available. Hand creams may decrease skin dryness, but they have also served as the source of epidemics when contaminated (8). Personnel with dermatitis involving the hands should probably wear gloves during patient contact.

3. Handwashing with antiseptics and the use of gloves is recommended before urinary tract catheterization, tracheal suctioning, and similar procedures. Iodophors, chlorhexidine, hexachlorophene, and alcohol are all appropriate antiseptics, but quaternary ammonium compounds should not be used (11). Hexachlorophene should not be used by pregnant women.

4. Antiseptic agents, especially if they are not used in the proper concentration, may become contaminated with bacteria and serve as vehicles for outbreaks of infection. Examples include *Pseudomonas* contamination of chlorhexidine (12, 13) and contamination of the usually reliable germicide iodophors (14,15). Bacteria can become resistant to antiseptics just as they can become resistant to antibiotics (16).

Disinfectants

5. Contamination of disinfectants has also occurred, most notably with the quaternary ammonium compounds (17), which is why these agents are no longer recommended as antiseptics.

6. Proper use of a disinfecting agent involves determining the type of agent from the product label, determining the category of effectiveness required for a cleaning function, selecting the proper agent for the job, and using the disinfectant at the directed dilution.

7. In most instances, the process of cleaning (e.g., dishwashing, laundering) is effectively a form of disinfection. The hot laundry cycle at 71°C for 25 minutes will kill all microorganisms except for bacterial spores (18).

8. Semicritical objects in contact with mucous membranes such as endotracheal tubes, thermometers, cystoscopes, and respiratory therapy equipment may be adequately disinfected with an intermediate-level disinfectant.

Sterilization

9. For items that must be sterile such as implantable devices, bladder catheters, intravenous catheters, and surgical instruments, two approaches are available. The safest approach is to use single-use disposable items, but this may not be financially feasible. Patient safety can be guaranteed by adequate sterilization of items between uses.

10. Whether steam or gas is used for sterilization, all equipment must be thoroughly cleaned before the sterilization process, since the presence of gross debris will interfere with sterilization. A number of checks are used to assure that sterilization has taken place, including mechanical checks of time, temperature, and pressure during the sterilization cycle and chemical indicators (19). In addition, biological indicators are employed. Bacterial spores (usually *Bacillus* spp.) are placed inside special containers in the autoclave and tested for growth at the end of the sterilization run. If the spores have been killed, it can be safely assumed that all other microorganisms have been eradicated.

CONTROL MEASURES: ANIMATE ENVIRONMENT

In this and the following sections we discuss the reservoir of infectious agents in the nursing home setting and ways to control that reservoir. The control of nosocomial infections also involves preventing transmission from the nursing home reservoir to the resident (see Chapter 16) and improving host resistance to infection (see Chapter 14). The nursing home reservoir is composed of both animate and inanimate elements.

Residents

Infected residents are an obvious reservoir of pathogenic organisms. In addition, colonization may occur with potentially hazardous bacteria in geriatric facilities (20). Fecal or perineal colonization is most common and may be difficult to eradicate even with meticulous bathing (21). Cross-contamination with staphylococci and gram-negative bacteria may occur between decubitus ulcers, bladder catheters, or vascular access sites (22).

Areas of control to be addressed by the nursing home include (23):

1. Cleanliness of resident's body (bathing two to three times per week, skin care, clipping of nails, oral hygiene, denture care).

2. Supplies and equipment (each resident should have his own bedpan, wash basin, emesis basin, water pitcher, thermometer, medical equipment, and personal care effects).

3. Isolation of infected residents (see Chapter 16).

4. Urinary catheter care (see Chapter 6).

5. Decubitus ulcer care (see Chapter 7).

6. Disposal of body wastes and discharges (especially in residents with infections).

7. Disoriented residents (incontinent residents should wear diapers, and their mattresses should have plastic sheet covers).

8. Resistance of the resident to infection (see Chapters 2 and 14).

9. Treatment of established infections in residents to minimize the reservoir and potential for spread. For instance, antibiotic therapy will usually render a resident with a wound infection or pneumonia noninfectious in several days.

Visitors

Visitors should be taught the basics of infection prevention. Visitors to residents who are in isolation must be instructed in handwashing techniques, the wearing of masks or gowns, and other appropriate infection control practices.

Visitors to a nursing home may introduce infectious diseases from the community, particularly respiratory diseases such as influenza. Common sense dictates that infected persons should not visit residents. Exceptions may be possible on an individual basis, depending upon the contagiousness of the illness and the immune status of the resident who is being visited. A visitor with an infectious disease, however, places not only the resident he is visiting but also other nursing home residents in jeopardy.

Some hospitals and nursing homes have contagion checks in which a member of the nursing home staff queries the visitor about current infectious symptoms. Every nursing home should have a visitation policy that addresses the problems of number of visitors, times of visitation, visitors with infectious diseases, and visits to residents who are in isolation.

Employee Health

Nursing homes are required to provide periodic examinations of employees and ensure the absence of communicable disease (24). Employees and residents are in dynamic equilibrium as far as microorganisms are

Table 15.3.   Nursing Home Employees: Infectious Hazards

Tuberculosis
Hepatitis A
Hepatitis B
Influenza
Herpesviruses
Gastroenteritis
Staphylococcus aureus

concerned. Just as residents may acquire a disease from an employee, an employee may acquire a disease from a resident. Both employees and residents are frequently involved in nursing home outbreaks of influenza, hepatitis, food poisoning, and other contagious diseases (see Chapter 10). Measures to block transmission of infection in the nursing home, such as isolation, are designed to protect both the resident and the employee.

The hospital employee is most concerned about acquisition of hepatitis, tuberculosis, meningococcal meningitis, rubella, and herpesvirus infection (25). There are fewer data on illness in employees of nursing homes, but a number of infections are known to be potential hazards for the nursing home employee (see Table 15.3).

Tuberculosis.   Tuberculosis may spread by the airborne route from a resident with unsuspected tuberculosis to personnel before the institution of appropriate isolation. Since the elderly form the largest reservoir of tuberculosis, nursing home personnel need to be aware of the risk.

Most hospitals in the United States screen for tuberculosis by purified protein derivative (PPD) skin testing or chest x-rays on an annual basis. When an employee's annual skin test for TB converts from negative to positive, it is generally assumed that the person tested has acquired tuberculosis during the past year, and the employee needs a year of isoniazid therapy in order to minimize the chance of developing clinical tuberculosis (see Chapter 5). Once the skin test becomes positive, it usually remains positive for life, and repeat skin tests are not indicated. The employee is a candidate for repeat chest x-ray to rule out pulmonary tuberculosis if new symptoms develop.

Several serious outbreaks of tuberculosis have been reported in nursing homes. On this basis, skin testing of all new residents and employees of nursing homes has been recommended (26). Other aspects of tuberculosis prevention include treating skin test convertors, periodic retesting of employees, and x-rays of employees with positive tuberculin skin tests.

If a nursing home discovers that a resident has active pulmonary tuberculosis, an investigation of possible contacts should be undertaken. The person responsible for infection control or employee health at the nursing home should make a list of all nursing home personnel who had contact with the infected individual and prepare a list of roommates and other residents who may have been exposed before adequate precautions were instituted. Skin testing of exposed individuals should be done six to eight weeks after the last possible exposure, at which time skin tests for TB should be positive if any of the exposed individuals has acquired tuberculosis.

Hepatitis. Hepatitis A is spread by the fecal–oral route. When a nursing home experiences an outbreak of hepatitis A, standard immune serum globulin (ISG) may be administered to residents and staff who have had close contact with infected individuals. This measure may reduce the spread of hepatitis A during an epidemic; ISG is given as a single intramuscular dose of 0.02 ml/kg within two weeks of exposure to hepatitis A. Routine administration in the absence of exposure is not indicated (27).

Hepatitis B is not a major problem in nursing homes but may occasionally be transmitted by accidental percutaneous inoculation. Most needle stick injuries occur during the disposal of used needles, during the administration of parenteral injections or infusion therapy, or while drawing blood, recapping needles after use, or handling linen or trash containing uncapped needles.

A percutaneous (needle stick) or mucous membrane exposure to blood that contains hepatitis B surface antigen is an indication for administration of hepatitis B immuneglobulin (HBIG). HBIG is administered at a dose of 0.06 ml/kg intramuscularly, with a second dose being given one month later. It will prevent or delay hepatitis B when given prophylactically within one week of exposure (27).

Hepatitis B vaccine, consisting of surface antigen of the hepatitis B virus harvested from human carriers of the virus, is available. The vaccine is recommended at three 1.0-ml doses intramuscularly, given at times 0, 1 month, and 6 months. This series stimulates protective antibody production in over 90% of healthy adults. The vaccine is recommended for those at high risk of acquiring hepatitis B, particularly health care workers exposed to blood or blood products (dentists, surgeons, pathologists, operating room staff, phlebotomists, dialysis unit staff), patients who receive frequent transfusions (e.g., those with hemophilia), intravenous illicit drug abusers, homosexual males, and susceptible clients and selected staff of institutions for the mentally retarded (28). The vaccination for hepatitis B is cost-effective in those populations with a high incidence or risk of hepatitis B. Since the incidence of hepatitis B in nursing homes is considerably lower than in hospitals, the vaccine would not appear to be cost-effective in this setting except in the event of an outbreak of hepatitis B.

Influenza.   Influenza poses a serious risk to residents of nursing homes and may occur in epidemics that involve both residents and staff (29). An influenza vaccine is available that annually contains the prevalent strains of influenza virus; it is an inactivated virus vaccine. The vaccine provides moderately effective protection against influenza and is recommended for persons at increased risk of adverse consequences from influenza, including the elderly and those with underlying disease (see Chapter 14). It is also recommended for health care workers, especially in the setting of a community epidemic of influenza (30). Amantadine hydrochloride, an antiviral drug, is active only against influenza A. It may be useful in providing temporary protection until vaccination can be effected during an outbreak of influenza A.

Herpesviruses.   Herpesviruses also pose a potential threat for the nursing home employee. The resident with oral herpes simplex infection excretes herpes simplex virus in oropharyngeal secretions and vesicular fluid. An employee may acquire herpetic whitlow, a painful, vesicular herpetic disease of the finger, from contact with infected secretions. The virus may enter through the skin by traumatic inoculation or through a cut or abrasion.

It has been suggested that in order to prevent acquisition of herpetic whitlow, gloves should be worn if an employee has direct contact with oropharyngeal secretions from a resident with oral herpes simplex lesions. An employee with active herpetic whitlow must also wear a glove on the involved hand to avoid spreading the virus to a resident (31).

The nursing home resident with herpes zoster (shingles) excretes the varicella-zoster virus in secretions from lesions. An employee who has not previously had chickenpox could acquire chickenpox from exposure to a resident with herpes zoster. An employee who has had chickenpox is immune.

Gastroenteritis.   Infectious gastroenteritis, especially that caused by viruses, has been spread between resident and staff in outbreaks (see Chapter 10). Good handwashing is the best preventive measure, since these agents are spread by direct contact.

Staphylococcal Carriers. About 30–50% of the population may be harboring *Staphylococcus aureus* at any one time, frequently without adverse consequences (the **carrier** state). The most common site for carriage of *S. aureus* is the nose. Occasionally, nasal carriers of *S. aureus* will develop clinical manifestations (e.g., boils) or shed the organism into the environment.

Both personnel and residents (32) are not infrequent carriers of *S. aureus* and may disseminate the organism. Personnel with cutaneous infectious lesions caused by *S. aureus* or hemolytic streptococci may also serve as a source for spread of these organisms into the environment. If a staphylococcal or streptococcal outbreak occurs in a nursing home, a member of the staff should be considered a possible source of the epidemic. Since many employees will be innocent carriers of *S. aureus*, one should not implicate an employee as the source of an outbreak until the strain he or she carries has been proven to be identical to the epidemic strain (see Chapter 10).

Personnel with boils or other cutaneous infections should receive appropriate medical care whether or not an outbreak is occurring in the nursing home. Systemic antibiotics do not eradicate the nasal carrier state; rather, nasal carriers should be treated with topical intranasal antibiotic ointment (33). Employees with active staphylococcal infection, however, should be treated with appropriate systemic antibiotics. Infected personnel or carriers who are disseminators of staphylococci into the environment should be removed from resident contact activities during an outbreak until they become noninfectious (34).

Routine microbiologic screening of employees for the staphylococcal carrier state in the absence of an outbreak is not indicated. Recently a few strains of *S. aureus* have become resistant to methicillin and other drugs used in the standard therapy of serious staphylococcal infection (see Chapter 11). These strains are potentially very hazardous and appear predominantly in large hospitals. They may, however, be transferred among hospitals or from hospitals to nursing homes (35). Infected and colonized patients appear to be the major reservoir, and transient carriage on the hands of personnel appears to be the most important mechanism of spread (36).

Employee Health Policies. The majority of hospitals have a formal employee health service, a phenomenon that is much less common in nursing homes. Nevertheless, certain employee health concerns should be addressed by each nursing home (see Table 15.4). New employees in a nursing home should be given a thorough history and physical ex-

Table 15.4. Issues in Employee Health

1. Screening of new employees
2. Health maintenance and hygiene
3. Education in infection control principles
4. Managing employee illness
5. Postemployment screening
6. Employee health policies and procedures
7. Safety

amination with specific attention to past skin diseases, cutaneous infections, recent diarrheal illnesses, and immunization status. They should receive a tuberculin skin test and chest x-ray in addition. New employees should be required to have current immunizations in tetanus, diphtheria, and other childhood diseases, such as measles, rubella, and polio. An individual personnel health record should be kept for every employee. If an employee is working in food services, the nursing home may wish to perform a screening stool culture for enteric pathogens.

Employees should be instructed in how to maintain good health practices and personal hygiene. Specific points include handwashing, body cleanliness, clean clothing, and covering of the nose or mouth when sneezing or coughing. Education in the principles of infection control should ideally cover such topics as the susceptibility of the elderly to infection, how nosocomial infections are spread, and isolation techniques.

Employees should be encouraged to report infectious diseases in residents or in themselves. Infections of greatest concern because of transmissibility to residents or other employees include respiratory viruses, enteric pathogens, *Staphylococcus aureus*, group A streptococcus, herpes simplex virus, tuberculosis, and hepatitis A and B (37). Sick employees should check with the employee health nurse, and employees with infectious diseases should not be penalized financially for missing work. It has been suggested that employees be promptly evaluated for any of the following symptoms that would suggest infection: fever, chills, acute skin eruption, purulent drainage, jaundice, sore throat, productive cough, "flu" syndrome, and diarrhea (38).

Many employees have misconceptions about transmission of infection (39). Decisions about management of sick employees depend on the contagiousness and period of transmissibility of the infection. Employees with upper respiratory tract infection or gastroenteritis are most infectious during the early parts of their illness, for instance, and these infections are much more hazardous than oral herpes simplex lesions (cold sores). Skin infections pose a severe threat, especially if they are staphylococcal or streptococcal in etiology. Guidelines are available for determining the period of communicability of various illnesses (40) and for managing contagious illnesses in hospital employees (38).

Regular health screening of employees ranges in complexity from a periodic TB skin test to an annual checkup. The screening contact is a good time to reinforce infection control principles. Tetanus and diphtheria vaccinations should be maintained (repeated every 10 years), and influenza vaccination may be elected (annually).

A standard approach to employee health problems through appropriate policies and procedures (see Chapter 12) will help ensure the health and safety of personnel and residents.

CONTROL MEASURES: INANIMATE ENVIRONMENT

The inanimate environment includes all elements that surround the resident, such as air, food, water, the room, laundry, and the physical plant of the nursing home. Several general principles should be kept in mind when considering an appropriately clean environment.

First, microbiologic sampling of the inanimate environment on a routine basis is not indicated in nursing homes. Routine cultures of floors, walls, sinks, air, and equipment are expensive and tend to provide information that has little correlation with nosocomial infections (41,42). Routine culturing of personnel is not indicated. In the presence of an outbreak, however, samples of the animate or inanimate environment may be indicated in the course of searching for the source of an outbreak (see Chapter 10). Even then, environmental cultures should be done only after an appropriate epidemiologic investigation has been undertaken, so that culturing can be directed at specific targets.

Second, different levels of cleanliness are appropriate for different parts of the inanimate environment. Sterility is required for such objects as intravenous devices and tracheostomy tubes, whereas low-level disinfection or sanitation is appropriate for noncritical areas of the environment such as walls, floors, and sinks. Guidelines for environmental cleanliness when a resident has a potentially contagious infectious disease (which may contaminate the environment) depend upon the mode of transmission of the disease, the resistance of the infectious agent to disinfection, and the extent of environmental contamination.

Third, it is important to have appropriate policies and procedures for key areas of the nursing home inanimate environment. Periodic inspection of laundry, kitchen, physical therapy, and other areas should be carried out on a regular basis to detect problems and to remind personnel of the importance of maintaining environmental sanitation. In an outbreak of suspected environmental origin, it is important to perform an immediate environmental inspection as part of the epidemic investigation. After any inspection, a written report that contains the date, the area inspected, deviations from existing policies and procedures, potential health hazards, and proposed remedies should be completed and retained.

Design and Construction

Construction or expansion of a nursing home needs to be planned in a fashion appropriate to maintaining good infection control practices in the areas of ventilation systems, waste disposal, equipment, materiel handling, design of surfaces for cleaning, handwashing facilities, and traffic patterns. Basic guidelines are outlined for application to long-term care facilities (43), and others have addressed construction problems related to nursing homes (44). A number of general points of greatest concern to infection control efforts in the nursing home include (see Table 15.5):

1. It is critical to provide adequate handwashing facilities for staff and residents.
2. Clean and dirty utility areas should be separated, and all workrooms should have adequate handwashing facilities.
3. At lease one bathroom should be provided for each four beds, and each resident should have a separate wardrobe locker or closet for clothes. One bathtub or shower including toilet facilities should be provided for each twelve beds. Isolation rooms should have individual bathrooms and sinks.
4. Backflow traps should be installed in plumbing fixtures to prevent backflow of contaminated water.
5. Materials used in construction of the health care facilities should be durable and withstand normal wear, since cracks and crevices will retain microorganisms that are difficult to eradicate. Materials should be easily cleaned and withstand the action of detergents, disinfectants, and other cleaning agents. Floors, especially in food preparation, storage and laboratory areas should be constructed of smooth and easily cleaned materials such as tile or linoleum. Carpeting requires special care since cleaning of carpeting is difficult. Carpeting of closely woven construction that is fairly easy to clean should be selected, and carpeting should not be installed in critical care areas. Carpet cleaning is discussed further on under "Housekeeping and Maintenance."

Table 15.5. Design and Construction: Infection Control Interfaces

Handwashing facilities
Utility areas
Bathrooms/toilets
Plumbing
Surface materials
Waste disposal
Nursing units
Special areas
Engineering service and equipment
Airflow and air conditioning

6. Waste-processing services, including storage, disposal, and incineration, are important.
7. Nursing units impact infection control in the areas of resident care, drug administration, traffic patterns, linen handling, and waste disposal.
8. Special areas such as resident dining areas, recreation areas, physical therapy, dietary facilities, occupational therapy, linen services, central stores, and administration have individual requirements.

Airflow

Excellent technical discussions of airflow problems in health care facilities are available that address such aspects as air quality, particulate matter, types of heating and air-conditioning systems, air cleaning and sterilization, humidity control, air distribution, and ventilation control of toxic agents (45). The requirements for long-term care facilities concerning heating and ventilation systems include specifications for ventilation system design, filter efficiencies, and minimum air exchanges per hour (43). Suggested filter efficiencies for areas relating to resident care, food preparation, and laundry are 80%, while 25% is adequate for administrative, bulk storage, and soiled handling areas. Filters should be changed on a regular basis (see Fig. 15.2).

Soiled work rooms, soiled handling areas, toilet rooms, bathrooms, janitor closets, linen and trash chute rooms, food preparation and storage areas, soiled linen sorting and storage areas, and general laundry are all areas from which all air should be exhausted directly to outdoors. Resident rooms, corridors, physical therapy, occupational therapy, clean workrooms, clean holding areas, and clean linen storage areas may have recirculated air. Clean workrooms, clean holding areas, and clean linen

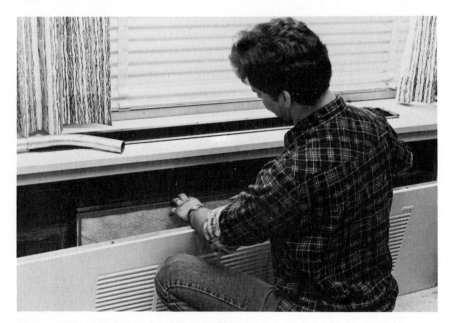

Figure 15.2.   Engineer changing air filter.

storage should be at a positive pressure relative to other parts of the nursing home in order to prevent airborne contamination of the clean materials. Areas such as physical therapy, occupational therapy, soiled workrooms, soiled handling areas, toilet rooms, bathrooms, janitor's closets, linen and trash chute rooms, and soiled linen areas should be at negative pressure to prevent contamination of the general air in the nursing home. If a nursing home has a designated isolation room, this ideally should be exhausted directly to outdoors and be at negative pressure.

The minimal total air exchanges per hour supplied to a given room vary depending on the potential contamination of air in that room. For resident rooms and clean linen storage areas, two exchanges per hour are recommended; for resident corridors and clean workrooms, four are recommended; for examination rooms, physical therapy, and occupational therapy, six are recommended. Ten are suggested for other areas such as soiled workrooms, soiled holding areas, toilet rooms, bathrooms, janitor's closets, linen and trash chute rooms, food preparation centers, general laundry, and soiled linen sorting and storage.

The rationale for the requirements detailed above is the fact that pathogenic microorganisms, such as staphylococci, streptococci, viruses (influenza), and mycobacteria (tuberculosis), tend to spread by the airborne route in a process usually involving attachment to dust, lint, respiratory droplets, or other particles (46). Dilution of contaminated air by fresh outside air and filtration to remove disease-carrying particles are the best means for providing clean and safe air in the nursing home. Exhaustion of contaminated air to the outside is safer than recirculating air, although it is generally more expensive. Filters of varying efficiency are available; high-efficiency filters are suggested in critical areas. There are many examples of an inefficient, poorly designed, or contaminated airflow system causing an epidemic by disseminating infectious particles throughout a health care facility (47,48).

Another potential problem in the nursing home is air-conditioning systems. Both air-conditioning systems and cooling towers may become contaminated and disseminate infectious agents. Contaminated air-conditioning systems, for instance, have served as the source for epidemics of Legionnaires' disease in institutions (49). Proper maintenance of air-conditioning systems is important.

In the event of a possible airborne epidemic, techniques are available for sampling the bacterial and fungal content of air (48). Two commonly used techniques are quantitative colony counts in measured volumes of air and the simpler settle plates, dishes containing nutrient agar that are exposed to the air for a certain period of time. In hospital settings, standard levels of contamination range from fewer than five organisms per cubic foot in operating room areas to 30 to 50 organisms per cubic foot in general patient care areas (50).

Equipment

General guidelines for cleaning, disinfection, and sterilization of hospital equipment have been published by the Centers for Disease Control (51). The recommendations cover critical care objects (e.g., surgical instruments or catheters) that must be sterile, items that require high-level disinfection (e.g., respiratory therapy equipment), and items for which cleaning is sufficient (e.g., bedpans, crutches, water glasses, food utensils, bedside tables, bed rails). Sterilization is required of equipment that has vital contact with the resident, such as surgical instruments, intravenous catheters, and bladder catheters. Non–resident care objects likely to be contaminated with virulent microorganisms should be cleaned with a disinfectant. Objects disinfected with liquid chemicals must be rinsed in sterile water to remove possible toxic or irritating residues. Gloves should be worn when using chemical disinfectants to prevent skin injury.

Respiratory Therapy Equipment. Respiratory therapy equipment may be used in the nursing home, and guidelines are available for the cleaning of such equipment (52). Nasal cannulas for supplying oxygen to the resident should be sterile and preferably disposable. Spirometers and inhalation therapy equipment should be cleansed between uses and sterilized between residents. The potential for respiratory therapy equipment to cause outbreaks of infectious diseases is significant.

Humidifiers are devices that saturate air with water vapor, whereas nebulizers saturate air with water vapor and disperse an aerosol of droplets. Both are intended to provide moist air to residents. Contamination with gram-negative bacteria is relatively common and quite hazardous. Serious outbreaks of respiratory infections may follow contamination of these devices (53–56).

Room humidifiers and nebulizers are difficult to sterilize because of the intricacies of the vaporization devices. Disinfection with normally effective agents has not prevented outbreaks. Nebulizers may become contaminated by the use of distilled water (which can contain bacteria) rather than sterile water. When these machines become contaminated, they have the potential to spread bacteria over long distances by the aerosol route, posing a great hazard (53).

Heating nebulizers above 46°C will decrease contamination by virtue of thermal disinfection. Sterile water should be used in nebulizers, and terminal disinfection of the nebulizer after use is mandatory (56). Widespread use of cold air humidifiers in the nursing home setting is inappropriate, and cold air steam humidifiers have been banned from some hospitals. Central humidification of heated air is preferred.

Thermometers. Any equipment that comes in contact with the resident has the potential for transmission of infection. Even thermometers pose an occasional hazard (57). Recommendations for care of thermometers in the hospital (58) include the following: Personnel should wash their hands before taking a patient's temperature. Each patient should be provided with his or her own thermometer. Between uses on the same patient, the thermometer may be either cleaned with soap and water, and then rinsed and dried, or disinfected with 70–90% alcohol. The thermometer should be stored dry. Terminal cleaning of the thermometer between patients involves either ethylene oxide sterilization or chemical disinfection with at least 30 minutes exposure to 90% ethyl or isopropyl alcohol, glutaraldehyde, 3% phenolic germicidal detergent, or an iodophor germicidal detergent with at least 500 ppm iodine.

Application of the above recommendations to nursing homes is reasonable and should minimize the risk of cross-infection with thermometers.

Food Services

Foodborne outbreaks are fairly common in nursing homes (see Chapter 10). A number of lapses in food handling may be responsible for various types of food poisoning (59). Food poisoning caused by *Clostridium perfringens* is often associated with preheated meat and poultry dishes that have been cooked one day and inadequately cooled or stored before serving on the following day. Salmonellosis is an endemic disease in poultry, and the most common vehicle for transmission to humans is undercooked chicken, turkey, or egg products, especially frozen poultry that is inadequately defrosted, undercooked, or contaminated after cooking. Inadequate cooking facilities, inadequate handwashing facilities, or preparation of food by employees with infectious diarrhea have been implicated in various outbreaks of food poisoning in institutions (60). In other outbreaks, purchase of eggs that were not USDA-approved (e.g., cracked or unwashed eggs) caused food poisoning. Many different organisms and virtually any type of food can serve as a source of a foodborne outbreak of infection.

Control measures fall into two broad categories: measures to address hygiene in food preparers and measures to insure proper preparation of food.

Kitchen Personnel.   Food preparers should use good hygiene and handwashing techniques, wear hair nets, and be in good health. There should be adequate supervision of kitchen personnel. The nursing home needs to provide adequate handwashing and lavatory facilities for kitchen employees.

Ideally, the nursing home should have policies and procedures for maintaining a clean and sanitary work area and hygienic kitchen personnel. It is critical for all employees, especially kitchen personnel, to avoid working when they have infectious diseases such as a diarrheal illness.

Food Handling.   A number of suggestions relative to food storage and preparation can be extracted from the literature (44,46,61):

1. Refrigeration temperatures should be maintained below 40°F. The capacity of the refrigerator equipment should be sufficient so that when large quantities of warm food are placed in the refrigerator, they cool quickly.
2. When foods are heated, they should be maintained at temperatures above 150°F.
3. All ingredients for mixed salads should be prepared from refrigerated ingredients.

4. All foods of questionable quality should be discarded.

5. Equipment should be cleaned betwen uses, and periodically all elements in the kitchen should be cleaned. Cleaning is especially important after equipment is used with raw poultry or meat.

6. All fruits and vegetables should be thoroughly washed before use.

7. Dry food storage should be clean, dry, and above the floor, with temperatures maintained at less than 70°F and relative humidity maintained at less than 40%.

8. Adequate work space should be maintained.

9. Adequate countertop space and ventilation should be provided.

10. The nursing home should purchase eggs from a USDA-approved source, which requires washing of eggs, prohibits the sale of cracked eggs, and requires that egg products be pasteurized.

11. Separation of clean and dirty functions is important, with different clean and dirty dish-handling areas and separation of waste and garbage from food storage areas.

12. Adequate dishwashing facilities should be available. While the exact temperature for appropriate dishwashing is not universally agreed upon, it has been recommended that if dishes are machine-washed, they should be washed at 140°F or higher for 20 seconds and rinsed at 180°F or higher for 10 seconds, and if dishes are manually washed they should be washed with water at 110° to 120°F with an adequate amount of effective soap or detergent (46).

13. Contaminated ice has caused outbreaks of nosocomial infection. Employees who handle ice should wash hands frequently and not handle the ice with their hands. Ice storage compartments should be cleaned on a preset schedule (e.g., weekly). Cleaning should be carried out with a fresh soap or detergent solution, followed by rinsing of all surfaces with water and then a 100 ppm solution of hypochlorite, followed in turn by thorough drying. Mechanical maintenance of ice machines is also important. Periodically, a hypochlorite solution should be circulated through the entire ice-making and storage system for cleaning and sanitizing purposes (62).

Laundry

Soiled laundry is probably the most significant contributor to airborne microbial contamination in the hospital, which underscores the importance of adequate laundry facilities and policies. Bed stripping in nursing homes has been shown to aerosolize significant numbers of bacteria (63).

Employees' uniforms may also carry organisms and should be appropriately clean (64). For the safety of residents and employees, adequate procedures for collection, transportation, processing, and storage of linen are essential. Recommendations for processing of laundry include the following (44,46,65):

1. Laundry may be collected by chute or manual cart collection methods. Laundry must be collected carefully with a minimum of disturbance to decrease airborne contamination. Ideally, soiled linen should be bagged at the location where it is used. Soiled linen should be transported in well-covered and clearly identified carts that have liners that can be cleaned or laundered frequently.

2. Linen should be removed regularly from resident care units, and blankets should be laundered after each resident's use. Mattresses should be enclosed with covers of impervious plastic in order to prevent contamination and to allow for easy cleaning.

3. Soiled linen should be handled and sorted as little as possible. Rooms for handling and sorting soiled linen should be separate from other areas, especially clean functions, and should be at negative pressure and ventilated to the outside with 10 air exchanges per hour.

4. Clean linen should be handled as little as possible and should be covered or wrapped before being stored. Storage in enclosed linen carts is recommended. A separate clean linen storage area should be provided.

5. Good handwashing facilities should be provided.

6. Linen known to be contaminated with infectious microorganisms from isolation areas should be clearly labeled and handled with special care. Ideally, it should be double-bagged in plastic bags that are soluble in hot water and can be placed directly into washing machines; this process minimizes handling.

7. If chutes are used, they should be cleaned on a regular schedule. One method for doing this is the use of a rotating spray head on a hose with high water pressure that can be lowered down the chute (66).

8. Various parts of the washing and drying cycle have antibacterial effects (67): A sudsing cycle of 150–170°F for 30 minutes, a rinsing cycle of 165–170°F for 10–12 minutes, a bleach concentration of 100 ppm chlorine for 10–15 minutes, hot air drying at 160°F for 20–30 minutes, and hot ironing at 330°F for a few seconds have disinfectant effects on many microorganisms. During the washing process, a water temperature above 71°C (160°F) for 25 minutes is recommended and will kill virtually all microorganisms except

spores. Such a temperature is recommended for use with most materials except delicate fabrics, such as woolens and nylon.

Physical Therapy

Physical therapy is frequently an important aspect of chronic and rehabilitative care. Contaminated physical therapy equipment has been responsible for epidemics of infection (68). Physical therapy tank agitators and drains may be colonized by gram-negative bacteria.

Mechanical scrubbing of the Hubbard tank with a detergent disinfectant is an effective way to reduce bacterial contamination (69). Mechanical scrubbing is sufficient to clean the sides of the tank, but an antiseptic is required for cleaning the bottom (see Fig. 15.3). Many patients shed gram-negative bacteria and staphylococci, but these bacteria can be decreased in the bottom of the tank by treatment with a chlorine-containing disinfectant (69). Chlorine 200 ppm is an effective disinfectant for most bacteria contaminating the Hubbard tank, with the exception of spore-forming bacteria (70).

Drying of the whirlpool between uses is also a good sanitizing measure. However, the potential for recontamination is always present, and the

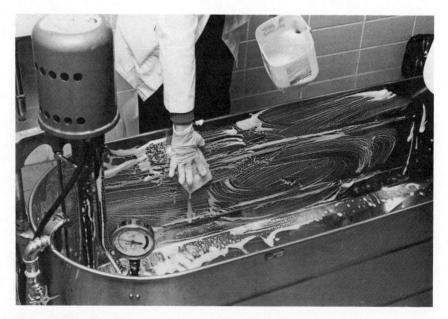

Figure 15.3. Cleaning the physical therapy tank.

most reliable method for controlling potential pathogens is to employ a commercially available disposable plastic liner for the hydrotherapy tank (71), a relatively expensive practice.

Waste Disposal

Nursing homes should provide space and facilities for the sanitary storage and disposal of waste by incineration, mechanical destruction, compaction, or other techniques (41). The incinerator must be placed in a separate room or outdoors and must be adequately ventilated. It is suggested that hazardous wastes from hospitals should be incinerated or autoclaved in the hospital (72). Standards for handling hazardous waste have been developed by the Environmental Protection Agency (73).

For all categories of isolation precautions, it is recommended that urine and feces be flushed directly down the toilet (4). Toilets that are cleaned and have a good flushing system are rarely a source of infection in the hospital or nursing home. If a system for emptying bedpans is employed, it should be designed so that bedpans will be covered and carried a minimum distance.

Housekeeping and Maintenance

The purpose of cleaning the environment is to physically remove microorganisms from various fomites (surfaces, etc.) that might transmit them to patients. Cleaning schedules should be established for walls, floors, windows, window frames and sills, curtains, bedside screens, fixtures, furniture, and waste receptacles throughout the nursing home.

Frequency of Cleaning. In hospitals, it is recommended that all horizontal surfaces in patient areas should be wet-cleaned or damp-cleaned at least daily, and uncarpeted floors should be wet-cleaned daily. Inpatient treatment areas, bathroom fixtures, handwashing facilities, and surface sinks should be thoroughly cleaned at least daily with an appropriate disinfectant. Terminal cleaning of any room that has been occupied by a patient should be thorough. Walls do not need to be cleaned routinely except for spot cleaning of visibly soiled areas.

While the exact frequency of cleaning of environmental surfaces in nursing homes has not yet been determined, some recommendations are available (44). Floors should be cleaned daily with a wet agent, specifically a detergent–germicide. Other objects for which daily cleaning is suggested include bathroom bowls, tops of night stands, chairs, overbed trays, water pitchers, and other objects that come in frequent contact with the residents. Trash should be removed daily, and the carpet vacuumed daily. Weekly disinfection and cleaning is recommended for windows, mirrors, and furniture. On a monthly basis, the ceiling, walls, doors, curtains, drapes, window shades, venetian blinds, and carpet should be cleaned and disinfected. Spot cleaning is necessary when visual soilage has occurred. Terminal cleaning of an isolation room may be more extensive (see Chapter 16).

Cleaning System.   A two-bucket system should be used, with one bucket for the detergent–germicide solution and the other one for warm rinse water (see Fig. 15.4). All housekeeping equipment should be stored

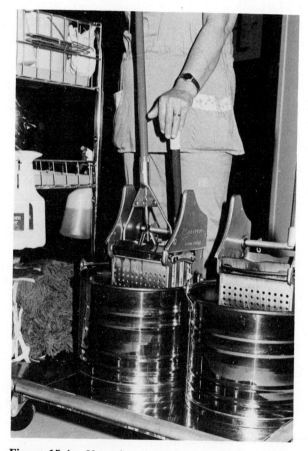

Figure 15.4.   Housekeeping—the two-bucket system.

clean at the end of the day. Clean cloths, sponges, other applicators, and solutions should be supplied frequently during the cleaning process (e.g., every two to three units or four to six beds). Mop heads, cleaning cloths, and cleaning solution should be changed when they become obviously dirty. The nature of the disinfectant–detergent is less important for surface cleaning than physical removal by vigorous scrubbing (74). Antiseptic agents intended for use on the skin should not be used for surface cleaning, and disinfectant fogging should not be done. Gloves should be worn during cleaning procedures.

Floors and Carpets.   Additional cleaning of floors with a detergent–disinfectant should be done when floors have become grossly contaminated or when a patient who has been in isolation has left the room (75).

Carpets consistently have higher microbial contamination than bare floors, and patients in carpeted rooms in institutions may become colonized with bacteria similar to that found in the carpeting (76). It is virtually impossible to adequately disinfect a carpet. Thus, carpeting should ideally not be used in resident care areas, especially in isolation rooms and bathrooms in nursing homes. If carpeting is used, indoor–outdoor carpeting that can be removed for cleaning is suggested. Carpeting should also not be used in areas where wetting or spillage may occur, such as kitchens, lavatories, and utility rooms.

Engineering and Maintenance.   Engineering and maintenance of the nursing home facility are also very important. There should be a regular schedule for checking autoclaves, air filtration systems, air-conditioning units, food service equipment, backflow preventing devices (vacuum breakers), water lines, and environmental surfaces.

Pest Control.   Insects and rodents can transmit infectious diseases to people. Houseflies and cockroaches are the most difficult insects to control in the institutional setting. General measures to decrease pests include elimination of cracks and crevices, checking all paper bags and cartons that enter the facility, proper lighting and ventilation, the use of self-closing screens on doors and windows, the use of tight-fitting, self-closing doors, and proper food storage.

In addition, chemical pesticides are required. Caution must be used in applying pesticides in areas where food is prepared, served, and stored (44). A maintenance contract with a company that provides periodic inspection and pest control is often desirable.

Safety

Health institutions are required by law to insure the safety of both patients and personnel, not only from infections, but also from mechanical, chemical, electrical, radiation, thermal, medicational, or other types of injury. Hospitals have been required to exercise reasonable care with regard to maintenance of buildings and grounds, selection of equipment to insure proper operation, and selection of personnel. The greatest nonmedical hazards are high places, moving machinery, electricity, and transportation.

The nursing home must also address the safety of its staff and residents (24,43). Reasonable initiatives include development of a safety program, a safety checklist (77), and an accident report form (78). Detailed guidelines can be found in the *Life Safety Code* published by the National Fire Protection Association (79) and the standards promulgated by the federal Occupational Safety and Health Administration (OSHA) (80).

REFERENCES

1. Block SS (ed): *Disinfection, Sterilization, and Preservation*, 2nd ed. Philadelphia, Lea & Febiger, 1977.
2. Favero MS: Sterilization, disinfection, and antisepsis in the hospital, in Lennette, EH, et al: *Manual of Clinical Microbiology*, 3rd ed. Washington DC, American Society for Microbiology, 1980.
3. *Infection Control in the Hospital*, 4th ed. Chicago, American Hospital Association, 1979.
4. *Isolation Techniques for Use in Hospitals*, 2nd ed. Atlanta, Center for Disease Control, 1975.
5. Bannan AE, Judge LF: Bacteriological studies relating to handwashing: 1. The inability of soap bars to transmit bacteria. *Am J Pub Health* 55:915–922, 1965.
6. Spaulding EH: Chemical disinfection and antisepsis in the hospital. *J Hosp Res* 9:5–31, 1972.
7. Albert RK, Condie F: Handwashing practices in medical intensive care units. *N Eng J Med* 304:1465–1466, 1981.
8. Knittle MA, Eitzman DV, Baer H: Role of hand contamination of personnel in the epidemiology of gram-negative nosocomial infections. *J Pediatr* 86:433–437, 1975.
9. Black RE, Dykes AC, Anderson KE, et al: Handwashing to prevent diarrhea in day-care centers. *Am J Epidemiol* 113:445–451, 1981.
10. Steere AC, Mallison GF: Handwashing practices for the prevention of nosocomial infections. *Ann Intern Med* 83:683–690, 1975.

11. Centers for Disease Control: Guidelines for hospital environmental control: Antiseptics, handwashing, and handwashing facilties. *Infect Control* 2:131–137, 1981.

12. Sobel JD, Hashman JD, Reinhorz G, et al: Nosocomial *Pseudomonas cepacia* infection associated with chlorhexidine contamination. *Am J Med* 73:183–186. 1982.

13. Wishart MM, Reily TV: Infection with *Pseudomonas maltophilia* hospital outbreak due to contaminated disinfectant. *Med J Aust* 2:710–712, 1976.

14. Craven DE, Moody B, Connoly MG, et al: Pseudobacteremia caused by povidone-iodine solution contaminated with *Pseudomonas cepacia*. *N Engl J Med* 305:621–623, 1981.

15. Centers for Disease Control: *Pseudomonas aeruginosa* peritonitis attributed to a contaminated iodophor solution. *Morbid Mortal Weekly Rep* 31:197–198, 1982.

16. Stickler DJ: Chlorhexidine resistance in *Proteus mirabilis*. *J Clin Path* 27:284–287, 1974.

17. Dixon RE, Kaslow RA, Mackel DC, et al: Aqueous quarternary ammonium antiseptics and disinfectants: Use and misuse. *JAMA* 236:2415–2417, 1976.

18. Reybrouck G: Sterilization. *J Hosp Infect* 2:291–293, 1981.

19. Starkey DH: The use of indicators for quality control of sterilizing processes in hospital practice: A review. *Am J Infect Control* 8:79–84, 1980.

20. Hawkey PM, Penner JL, Potten MR, et al: Prospective survey of fecal, urinary tract and environmental colonization by *Providencia stuartii* in two geriatric wards. *J Clin Micro* 16:422–426, 1982.

21. Gilmore DS, Jiminez EM, Aeilts GD, et al: Effects of bathing on *Pseudomonas* and *Klebsiella* colonization in patients with spinal cord injuries. *J Clin Micro* 14:404–407, 1981.

22. Vaziri ND, Cesario T, Mootoo K, et al: Bacterial infections in patients with chronic renal failure: Occurrence with spinal cord injury. *Arch Intern Med* 142:1273–1276, 1982.

23. Campbell DG: Prevention of infection in extended care facilities. *Nurs Clin N Am* 15:857–868, 1980.

24. US Department of Health and Human Services: Conditions of participation for skilled nursing and intermediate care facilities. *Fed Reg* 45:47368–47382, 1980.

25. Centers for Disease Control: Guideline for Infection Control in Hospital Personnel. *Infect Control* 4:328–349, 1983.

26. American Thoracic Society: Screening for pulmonary tuberculosis in institutions: An official statement. *Am Rev Resp Dis* 115:901–906, 1977.

27. Centers for Disease Control: Immune globulins for protection against viral hepatitis: Recommendation of the Immunization Practices Advisory Committee. *Morbid Mortal Weekly Rep* 30:423–435, 1981.

28. Centers for Disease Control: Inactivated hepatitis B virus vaccine. *Morbid Mortal Weekly Rep* 31:317–328, 1982.

29. VanVoris LP, Belshe RB, Shaffer JL: Nosocomial influenza B virus infection in the elderly. *Ann Intern Med* 96:153–158, 1982.

30. Centers for Disease Control: Influenza vaccines, 1983–1984. *Morbid Mortal Weekly Rep* 32:333–337, 1983.

31. Greaves WL, Kaiser AB, Alford RH, et al: The problem of herpetic whitlow among hospital personnel. *Infect Control* 1:381–385, 1980.

32. Zierdt CH: Long term *Staphylococcus aureus* carrier state in hospital patients. *J Clin Micro* 16:517–520, 1982.

33. Bryan CS, Wilson RS, Meade P, et al: Topical antibiotic ointments for staphylococcal nasal carriers: Survey of current practices and comparison of bacitracin and vancomycin ointments. *Infect Control* 1:153–156, 1980.

34. Franson TR, Hierholzer WJ: Recommendations for management of *Staphylococcus aureus* infections in hospital personnel. *Iowa Dis Bull* September 15, 1981.

35. Haley RW, Hightower AW, Khabbaz RF, et al: The emergence of methicillin-resistant *Staphylococcus aureus* infection in the United States hospitals. *Ann Intern Med* 97:297–308, 1982.

36. Thompson RL, Cabezudo I, Wenzel RP: Epidemiology of nosocomial infections caused by methicillin-resistant *Staphylococcus aureus*. *Ann Intern Med* 97:309–317, 1982.

37. Klein JO: Management of infections in hospital employees. *Am J Med* 70:919–923, 1981.

38. Kaslow RA, Garner JS: Hospital Personnel, in Bennett JV, Brachman PS: *Hospital Infections*, 1st ed. Boston, Little Brown, 1979.

39. Haley RW, Emori TG: The Employee Health Service and infection control in U.S. Hospitals, 1976–1977: II. Managing employee illness. *JAMA* 246:962–966, 1981.

40. Benenson AS: *Control of Communicable Diseases in Man*, 13th ed. American Public Health Association, Washington DC, 1980.

41. Mallison GF, Haley RW: Microbiologic sampling of the inanimate environment in U.S. hospitals, 1976–1977. *Am J Med* 70:941–946, 1981.

42. Maki DG, Alvarado CJ, Hassemer CA, et al: Relation of the inanimate hospital environment to endemic nosocomial infection. *N Engl J Med* 307:1562–1566, 1982.

43. *Minimum Requirements of Construction and Equipment for Hospital and Medical Facilities*, Publication No.76-4000, US Department of Health, Education, and Welfare, 1975.

44. *Infection Prevention and Control for Long-Term Care Facilities*, Handbook and instructors guide. Washington DC, American Health Care Association, 1977.

45. Caplan KJ: Ventilation and air-conditioning, in Bond RG, Michaelsen GS, DeRoos RL: *Environmental Health and Safety in Health-Care Facilities,* 1st ed. New York, Macmillan, 1973.

46. *Infection Control in the Hospital,* 4th ed., Chicago, American Hospital Association, 1979.

47. Walter CW: Prevention and control of airborne infection in hospitals. *Ann NY Acad Sci* 253:312–330, 1980.

48. Ayliffe, GAJ, Lowbury GJL: Airborne infection in hospital. *J Hosp Infect* 3:217–240, 1982.

49. England AC, Fraser DW: Sporadic and epidemic nosocomial legionellosis in the United States: Epidemiologic features. *Am J Med* 70:707–711, 1981.

50. Bartlett RC, Groschel DHM, Mackel DC, et al: Microbiological surveillance, in Lennette EH, Spaulding EH, Truant JP: *Manual of Clinical Microbiology,* 2nd ed. Washington DC, American Society for Microbiology, 1974.

51. Centers for Disease Control: Cleaning, disinfection, and sterilization of hospital equipment. *Infect Control* 2:138–144, 1981.

52. *Methods of Prevention and Control of Nosocomial Infections: Recommendations for the Decontamination and Maintenance of Inhalation Therapy Equipment,* Atlanta, Center for Disease Control, 1975.

53. Smith PW, Massanari RM: Room humidifiers as the source of *Acinetobacter* infections. *JAMA* 237:795–797, 1977.

54. Grieble HG, Colton FR, Bird TJ, et al: Fine-particle humidifiers: Source of *Pseudomonas aeruginosa* infections in respiratory disease unit. *N Engl J Med* 282:531–535, 1970.

55. Kelsen SG, McGuckin M, Kelsen DP, et al: Airborne contamination of fine-particle nebulizers. *JAMA* 237:2311–2314, 1977.

56. Spaepen MS, Bodman HA, Kundsin RB, et al: Microorganisms in heated nebulizers. *Health Sci* 12:316–320, 1975.

57. Im SWK, Chow K, Chau PY: Rectal thermometer mediated cross-infection with *Salmonella wandsworth* in a pediatric ward. *J Hosp Infect* 2:171–174, 1981.

58. *Aseptic Handling of Thermometers and Other Equipment for Measuring Patient Temperatures.* Atlanta, Center for Disease Control, 1978.

59. Sharp JCM, Collier PW: Food poisoning in hospitals in Scotland. *J Hyg Camb* 83:231–236, 1979.

60. Baine WB, Gangarosa EJ, Bennett JV, et al: Institutional salmonellosis. *J Infect Dis* 128:357–360, 1973.

61. Jopke WH: Food Hygiene, in Bond RG, Michaelson GS, De Roos RL: *Environmental Health and Safety in Health-Care Facilities.* 1st ed. New York, Macmillan, 1973.

62. *Sanitary Care and Maintenance of Ice Chests and Ice Machines.* Atlanta, Center for Disease Control, 1975.

63. Litsky BY, Litsky W: Bacterial shedding during bed-stripping of reusable and disposable linens as detected by the high volume air sampler. *HLS* 8:29–34, 1971.

64. Speers R Jr: Contamination of nurses' uniforms with *Staphylococcus aureus*. *Lancet* 2:233–235, 1969.

65. *Guidelines: Nosocomial Infections—Laundry Services,* Atlanta, Centers for Disease Control, 1981.

66. Hoeh KW: Laundry chute cleaning recommendations. *Infect Control* 3:360, 1982.

67. Vesley D: Selected topics in environmental health—laundries, in Bond RG, Michaelsen GS, DeRoos RL: *Environmental Health and Safety in Health-Care Facilities,* 1st ed. New York, Macmillan, 1973.

68. McGuckin MB, Chung S, Humphrey N, et al: Infection control practices in physical therapy. *APIC J* 9:18–19, 1981.

69. Turner AG, Higgins MM, Craddock JG: Disinfection of immersion tanks (Hubbard) in a hospital burn unit. *Arch Env Health* 28:101–104, 1974.

70. Miller JK, Laforest NT, Hedberg M, et al: Surveillance and control of Hubbard tank bacterial contaminants. *Phys Ther* 10:1482–1486, 1970.

71. Mansell RE, Borchardt KA: Disinfection hydrotherapy equipment. *Arch Phys Med Rehabil* 55:318–320, 1974.

72. *Disposal of Solid Wastes from Hospitals.* Atlanta, Centers for Disease Control, 1980.

73. Environmental Protection Agency: Hazardous waste management system. *Fed Reg* 45:33063–33285, 1980.

74. *Guidelines: Nosocomial Infections—Housekeeping Services and Waste Disposal.* Atlanta, Centers for Disease Control, 1982.

75. Fahlberg WJ: Floor disinfection in the United States. *Infect Control* 3:281, 1982.

76. Anderson RL, Mackel DC, Stoler BS, et al: Carpeting in hospitals: An epidemiological evaluation. *J Clin Micro* 15:408–415, 1982.

77. Scheffler GL: Patient and personnel safety, in Bond RG, Michaelsen GS, DeRoos RL: *Environmental Health and Safety in Health-Care Facilities,* 1st ed. New York, Macmillan, 1973.

78. *Health and Safety Guide for Hospitals,* publication no. 78-150. National Institute of Occupational Safety and Health, US Dept. of Health, Education, and Welfare, 1978.

79. *Life Safety Code.* Quincy, Mass., National Fire Protection Association, 101, 1981.

80. *General Industry Safety and Health Standards* (29 CFR 1910), rev. ed. US Dept. of Labor, Occupational Safety and Health Administration, 1981.

CHAPTER 16

INFECTION CONTROL MEASURES: TRANSMISSION—ISOLATION AND BEYOND

Walter J. Hierholzer, Jr.
R. Michael Massanari
Dorothy A. Rasley

Extended care facilities are faced today with the need to receive and care for many residents who in the past would have been viewed as unacceptable for admission because of infectious disease problems. Others enter with conditions severely compromising their ability to combat infection. The modern nursing facility must recognize the potential for problems in this combination and rise to the responsibility of dealing with it through appropriate precautions.

Current methods offer limited ability to modify the common defects in host defense mechanisms prevalent in the elderly; therefore, prevention of transmission of potentially infectious microorganisms to these compromised residents must be a priority feature of daily care.

This program should begin with a preplacement evaluation *before* the resident is accepted for admission to the extended care facility and must continue through the resident's first days in the institution as additional data are acquired. Once the individual's short- and long-term care plans are clarified and implemented, an institutionalized framework of periodic evaluation and protection must be applied as new infectious disease situations arise. This program will be made up of two parts: the formal evaluation and control features of a standard isolation program similar to components of the Centers for Disease Control's Guideline for Isolation Precautions in Hospitals (1), and the informal procedures of daily care that key and augment the formal program.

In support of these programs there should be a coordinated educational effort centered in the bedside control of transmission and an employee health program with strong elements of individual worker responsibility.

Above all, these recommendations must be simple, realistic, and practical, recognizing the unique problems of the geriatric or extended care resident and the modest resources available for care as compared to acute facilities.

EVALUATION ON ADMISSION TO THE EXTENDED CARE FACILITY

Admission to an extended care facility is often precipitated by changes in the physical or social well-being of the resident. Infections constitute an acute physical illness that may precipitate need for nursing care among older individuals. All new admissions to an extended care facility should be considered potential risks for introducing and transmitting infections within the facility. This is a particular problem when a patient is transferred to the institution from a hospital. When the hospital stay exceeds 30 days, as many as 75% of patients will have acquired a nosocomial infection. Not only do these patients present a risk of transmitting infections in extended care facilities, they may also introduce highly resistant nosocomial pathogens into the environment of the facility. To reduce the risks of transmission, several simple control measures are suggested. Preadmission screening for clinical or occult infections should be provided by the referring physician or by the acute care institution before admission to the extended care facility. The primary purpose of preadmission screening is to identify individuals who harbor communicable diseases and to identify factors that place the resident at high risk for nosocomial events. In addition, the screening procedure should identify residents who carry multiply resistant organisms that may be transmitted to other residents. Because information obtained from preadmission screens may be incomplete, protocols for evaluation at the time of admission should also be instituted. A sample admission form is shown in Chapter 12 (Fig. 12.4).

The admission evaluation should include the collection and recording of pertinent historical information, physical findings, and a modest laboratory screen in order to identify active infections. For infection control purposes, the subjective inquiry should focus on a history of active infection with particular emphasis on infections of the urinary tract, skin, respiratory tract, and gastrointestinal tract. Where such can be documented, inquiry regarding the etiologic agent is important. Information regarding ongoing therapy with antibiotics should also be ascertained and assessed. It is important to determine from where the resident is being admitted—that is, community or hospital. Inquiries should be made into underlying diseases, particularly those that may predispose to infection, such as level of activity, diabetes mellitus, or dysphagia due to cerebral vascular disease. Finally, a complete immunization history should be obtained in order to determine what additional immunizations may be necessary.

The admission physical examination should include a thorough review of all organ systems, with particular attention devoted to skin, lungs, and urinary tract.

Laboratory screening procedures can be kept to a minimum, particularly when information is available from previous hospitalizations or visits to the physician's office. When there is a previous history of urinary tract infection or when the resident is admitted with a Foley catheter, a standard urinalysis should be obtained and urine cultures and sensitivities requested. Stool cultures may be helpful if the resident presents with diarrhea. If the resident has open wounds or drainage sites, it is prudent to determine the predominant organisms and identify any multiply resistant organisms that may be a risk to other residents (see Chapter 11).

Chest x-rays should not be routinely ordered unless there is a history of respiratory disease. Any resident entering an extended care facility whose response to a purified protein derivative (PPD) test is uncertain or who has had a negative PPD more than one year prior to admission should be tested at the time of admission (see Chapter 5). Residents with recent PPD conversions or documented positive reactions and who have not had a chest x-ray within the previous year should have a radiological examination at the time of admission. Those with x-ray evidence of active tuberculosis or with chronic cough and sputum production should have sputum examined for evidence of active tuberculosis. Residents with a presumptive diagnosis of active tuberculosis should be isolated until the diagnosis is ruled out or until the resident has received appropriate antituberculosis therapy for 7 to 10 days. Finally, when indicated by the medical history, additional laboratory analysis should be requested, such as screening for hepatitis B antigenemia among patients admitted to or from extended care facilities for the retarded.

Transmission of infection from new admissions may have serious implications for other residents in the institution. For this reason, it is suggested that the new resident be segregated, that is, housed in a private room for a period of 72 hours following admission, if this is feasible for the nursing home. This will allow sufficient time to complete the initial evaluation protocol and to obtain any laboratory data that may be pertinent to the diagnosis and treatment of infections. During this time, it is also suggested that temperature be monitored on a daily basis, in the evening, as an additional means of identifying occult infections.

Admission screening has thus far focused on prevention of introduction of new infections into the institution from recent admissions. Steps should also be taken to prevent the spread of communicable diseases to the new resident following admission to the institution. The use of immunizations to protect patients against pneumococcal and influenza infections is discussed in Chapter 14. In brief, if the admission history indicates that the resident has not received recent immunizations for influenza and pneumococcal infections, these vaccinations should be administered at this time.

HANDWASHING

It is inevitable that some residents will acquire infections during their stay in extended care institutions. Whether the organisms responsible for the infection are acquired from the community, from the environment of the institution, or from the endogenous flora of the resident, it is important that steps be taken to control the spread of the infection. Employees of chronic care facilities should be cognizant of several simple and inexpensive measures that will reduce the risk of transmission of infection.

The single most important factor in preventing transmission of infections is handwashing. It is imperative that dietary, housekeeping, and nursing personnel recognize the need for good handwashing practices. This is a task that is frequently overlooked and needs repeated emphasis in policies and procedures.

To promote proper handwashing practices, administrators responsible for planning new construction should take into account the placement of sinks and bathrooms relative to work activities of staff. Ideally, there should be two sinks per resident room, one for use by staff and located near an exit and a second located in the bathroom. Staff will then rarely interrupt a resident using the bathroom in order to wash their hands after caring for other residents in the room. Placement of the faucet and size of the sink should be adequate to allow rinsing without recontamination.

The procedure for proper handwashing is outlined in Table 16.1. Instructions and practice in handwashing should be stressed during the orientation period for new staff. Furthermore, they should be reminded to wash their hands before and after resident contact, after using the bathroom, before eating or smoking, and before administering medications. Handwashing is also discussed in Chapter 15.

Table 16.1. Handwashing

Purpose
To prevent the spread of bacteria

Equipment
Hot and cold running water
Antiseptic soap solution
Paper towels

Procedure[a]
1. Adjust running water to comfortable force and temperature to prevent contamination of surrounding area by splashing water.
2. Wet hands and lather well with soap or other agent. Wash hands thoroughly using an interlacing motion and friction, paying particular attention to the medial areas of the fingers.
3. Dry hands, using paper towel.
4. Turn off water, using a paper towel, to protect hands from contaminated faucets.

Notes
A. Depending on the activity having been performed, it may be necessary also to wash the forearm and elbow before proceeding to the next activity.
B. If bar soap is used, the soap should remain in your hand throughout step 2.
C. Skin should be kept soft and intact. Hand lotion or creams may be used after handwashing only if the next activity does not involve direct patient contact, as lotions and creams are potential media for bacterial growth.
D. If, during the handwashing procedure, your hands become contaminated, the complete procedure must be repeated.
E. Handwashing is performed before and after all patient care, before meals and breaks, and after personal hygiene measures (blowing nose, handling hair, going to bathroom, etc.).

[a]See Figure 15.1.

CONTROL OF INFECTION BY ISOLATION

General Principles

Interrupting the transmission of pathogenic organisms by isolation and precautions is another effective, relatively inexpensive method for reducing infections in extended care facilities. The development and implementation of isolation policies for residents who acquire acute or chronic transmissible infections is strongly encouraged.

Authority for implementing isolation procedures should reside with nursing personnel as well as physicians. It is essential that nursing staff be granted the authority to make these decisions since they are most intimately acquainted with the resident and will probably be the first to identify an infection. Implementation of isolation procedures should be considered for any resident whose condition suggests a possible transmissible infection. The decision to isolate the resident should take into account all of the following factors: the site of the infection—for example, open draining wound versus urinary tract infections; the etiologic agent, if known; the usual modes of transmission (based upon a knowledge of the etiologic agent or site of the infection); availability and access to susceptible hosts; the coherence and mobility of the infected resident.

Category-Specific Isolation

Acute care institutions employ different levels of isolation based upon the nature of the organism and the source of the infection (1). This approach may be practical at larger or skilled nursing facilities. The various levels of isolation precautions are designated by cards placed on the door to the patient room:

1. *Strict isolation* requires a private room; the wearing of masks, gowns, and gloves by all persons entering the room; and discarding or disinfection of articles in the room. This form of isolation is indicated, for example, in diphtheria.

2. *Respiratory isolation* also requires a private room. Masks should be worn by those entering the room, but gowns and gloves are not needed. Respiratory isolation is recommended for meningococcal meningitis.

3. *Enteric precautions* require gowns and gloves to be worn by those having direct patient contact. A private room is not necessary. Articles contaminated with urine or feces should be discarded or disinfected. These measures are recommended for many types of infectious gastroenteritis and hepatitis A.

4. *Contact isolation* is suggested for wounds with purulent drainage not contained by dressings and for wounds containing group A streptococci or *S. aureus*. A private room is desirable, and gowns and gloves need to be worn by those having direct contact with the infected material. This category is appropriate for a major decubitus ulcer infection.

5. *Drainage/secretion precautions* are less stringent, involving double-bagging of soiled dressings and laundry but no private room. Gowns are indicated for touching infective material. This would be indicated for conjunctivitis or a minor infection of a decubitus ulcer.

6. *Blood/body fluid precautions*, as suggested for hepatitis B, also do not require a private room, but entail needle and syringe precautions and labeling of blood specimens.

7. *Tuberculosis isolation,* for patients with pulmonary tuberculosis, is similar to respiratory isolation. A private room with special ventilation is indicated.

All the above categories assume good handwashing on entering and leaving the room. Caps and booties are not necessary in any category of isolation precautions.

Disease-Specific Isolation

In order to simplify isolation procedures for extended care facilities, a single basic approach to isolation (disease-specific isolation) may be used. Minor alterations in the basic procedure may be instituted in accordance with the nature of the infecting organism and the site of the infection. This assumes that residents with communicable diseases requiring strict isolation will be transferred from a nursing home to an acute care facility. Using this approach, the infection precautions recommended for reducing the risk of transmitting infectious diseases in nursing homes are outlined in a *single* isolation card (see Fig. 16.1). In general, private rooms

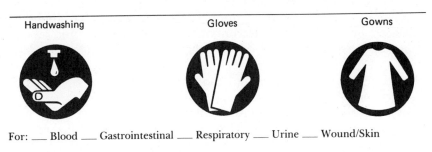

| Handwashing | Gloves | Gowns |

For: ___ Blood ___ Gastrointestinal ___ Respiratory ___ Urine ___ Wound/Skin

1. Private room—Not necessary*
2. Gowns—Only when soiling of uniform likely
3. Mask—Not necessary*
4. Hands—*Must* be washed on entering and following patient care
5. Gloves—Yes, for contact with infected area or drainage
6. Articles—Special precautions for contaminated instruments, dressings, and linen
7. Housekeeping—Routine cleaning
8. Specimens—Double-bagged, label container and outside bag "Contaminated"

*Unless otherwise indicated by guidelines in Table 16.2.

Figure 16.1. Summary of infection precautions for segregating a patient with presumed infection in a nursing care facility. This information can be prepared as a 5 × 8 card for placement outside the patient's room, above the bed, and on the patient's record in order to indicate need for special precautions.

are not necessary; however, several exceptions should be noted. Residents with respiratory infections that are spread by aerosolization should be confined to a private room. This includes residents with presumptive or active tuberculosis and residents with lower respiratory infections due to antibiotic-resistant organisms. Residents with disseminated herpes zoster infections—that is, involvement of more than one dermatome— should also be placed in a private room. Finally, residents with diarrhea or draining skin infections who are incoherent or unable to care for themselves should be placed in private rooms.

In general, gowns, masks, and gloves are not necessary unless the health care worker comes in direct contact with drainage or secretions from the infected site. For residents with infections that are transmitted primarily through blood, only gloves are necessary for nursing personnel who come in direct contact with blood or secretions. In addition, special precautions should be exercised in disposing of syringes and needles that may have been used in the care of the resident.

Processing of linen and the resident's clothing should include double-bagging of all material to be laundered before leaving the room, followed by standard laundering procedures with hot water and soap. Personal effects, including books, magazines, and monies, require no special attention unless visibly contaminated by infected secretions. Any laboratory specimens (e.g., sputum, feces, or discharge from the wound) should be enclosed in an impermeable container, double-bagged, and labeled "contaminated" before removal from the room and transport to the laboratory. For routine cleaning of the room, housekeeping personnel should be instructed regarding handwashing and any necessary attire before entering the room. Cleaning procedures should otherwise follow routine procedures. It is recommended that when cleaning rags are used in the room of an infected resident, they should either be discarded or removed and placed in the contaminated laundry for cleaning before leaving the room. Finally, all visitors entering the room should be instructed regarding necessary measures for preventing transmission of infection.

Terminal cleaning of isolation rooms is not usually different from terminal cleaning of any resident room. It involves emptying all receptacles, discarding disposable items, wet-vacuuming or mopping floors, and washing grossly soiled areas on walls. Equipment, furniture, and mattress covers should be washed with a germicidal detergent solution (see Chapter 15).

To assist in the execution of proper infection precautions, the reader is referred to Table 16.2. The table is organized according to the infectious agent or site of infection. Columns on the right indicate necessity

Table 16.2. Category-Specific Isolation Precautions

Agent/Site of Infection	Precautions or Isolation Indicated? (1 = no; 2 = yes)	Private Room Indicated? (1 = no; 2 = yes for patient who cannot use good hygiene; 3 = yes; 4 = yes with special ventilation)	Mask Indicated? (1 = no; 2 = yes for those who get close to patient; 3 = yes)	Gown Indicated? (1 = no; 2 = yes when soiling of clothes likely; 3 = yes)	Gloves Indicated? (1 = no; 2 = yes for contact with infected area or drainage; 3 = yes)	Comments (Including Duration of Precautions or Isolation)
Abscess, etiology unknown						
Draining	2	1	1	2	2	Maintain for duration of illness. Emphasize pus (drainage) precautions.
Not draining	1	—	—	—	—	—
Amebiasis						
Dysentery	2	2	1	2	2	Maintain for duration of illness. Emphasize stool precautions.
Bronchitis	2	1	1	1	1	Maintain respiratory secretion precautions for duration of illness.
Campylobacter gastroenteritis	2	2	1	2	2	Maintain for duration of illness. Emphasize stool precautions.
Candidiasis, all forms, including mucocutaneous (moniliasis, thrush)	1	—	—	—	—	—

(Continued)

Table 16.2. (Continued)

Agent/Site of Infection	Precautions or Isolation Indicated? (1 = no; 2 = yes)	Private Room Indicated? (1 = no; 2 = yes for patient who cannot use good hygiene; 3 = yes; 4 = yes with special ventilation)	Mask Indicated? (1 = no; 2 = yes for those who get close to patient; 3 = yes)	Gown Indicated? (1 = no; 2 = yes when soiling of clothes likely; 3 = yes)	Gloves Indicated? (1 = no; 2 = yes for contact with infected area or drainage; 3 = yes)	Comments (Including Duration of Precautions or Isolation)
Cellulitis						
Intact skin	2	—	—	—	—	—
Open, draining	2	2	2	2	2	Maintain for duration of illness. Emphasize pus (drainage) precautions.
Closed-cavity infection						
Draining	2	2	2	2	2	Maintain for duration of illness. Emphasize pus (drainage) precautions.
Not draining	2	—	—	—	—	—
Clostridium perfringens						
Food poisoning	2	—	—	—	—	
Gas gangrene	2	2	2	2	2	Maintain for duration of illness. Emphasize pus (drainage) precautions.
Other	2	2	2	2	2	Maintain for duration of illness. Emphasize pus (drainage) precautions.
Common cold	2	—	—	—	—	Maintain respiratory secretion precautions for duration of illness.

Disease					Precautions
Conjunctivitis, acute bacterial (sore eye, pink eye)	2	1	1	2	Maintain for duration of illness. Emphasize pus (drainage) precautions.
Conjunctivitis, viral (acute hemorrhagic and swimming pool conjunctivitis)	2	1	1	2	Maintain for duration of illness. Emphasize pus (drainage) precautions.
Coxsackie viral disease	2	2	2	2	Maintain for 7 days. Emphasize stool precautions.
Creutzfeldt–Jakob disease (see Jakob–Creutzfeldt disease)					
Cytomegalovirus, immunosuppressed patient	2	1	1	1	Maintain urine and respiratory secretion precautions for duration of hospitalization.
Decubiti (infected)	2	1	1	2	Maintain for duration of illness. Emphasize pus (drainage) precautions.
Diarrhea, acute—infective etiology suspected (see Gastroenteritis)	2	2	1	2	Maintain for duration of illness. Emphasize stool precautions.
Echovirus disease	2	2	1	2	Maintain for 7 days. Emphasize stool precautions.

(Continued)

Table 16.2. (Continued)

Agent/Site of Infection	Precautions or Isolation Indicated? (1 = no; 2 = yes)	Private Room Indicated? (1 = no; 2 = yes for patient who cannot use good hygiene; 3 = yes; 4 = yes with special ventilation)	Mask Indicated? (1 = no; 2 = yes for those who get close to patient; 3 = yes)	Gown Indicated? (1 = no; 2 = yes when soiling of clothes likely; 3 = yes)	Gloves Indicated? (1 = no; 2 = yes for contact with infected area or drainage; 3 = yes)	Comments (Including Duration of Precautions or Isolation)
Encephalitis or encephalomyelitis	2	2	1	2	2	Maintain for duration of illness or 7 days, whichever less. Likely causes include enteroviral and arthropodborne viral infections.
Enterobiasis (pinworm disease, oxyuriasis)	1	—	—	—	—	—
Enterocolitis						
Clostridium difficile	2	2	1	2	2	Maintain for duration of illness. Emphasize stool precautions.
Staphylococcal	2	2	1	2	2	Maintain for duration of illness. Emphasize stool precautions.
Enteroviral infection	2	2	1	2	2	Maintain for duration of illness or 7 days, whichever less. Emphasize stool precautions.

	1	2	3	4	5	Comments
Escherichia coli gastroenteritis (enteropathogenic, enterotoxic, or enteroinvasive)	2	2	1	2	2	Emphasize stool precautions.
Fever of unknown origin (FUO)	1	—	—	—	—	Patients usually need not be isolated; appropriate however, to isolate patient with signs and symptoms compatible with a disease that calls for isolation.
Food poisoning						
Botulism	1	—	—	—	—	—
Clostridium perfringens food poisoning	1	—	—	—	—	—
Salmonellosis	2	2	1	2	2	Maintain for duration of illness. Emphasize stool precautions.
Staphylococcal food poisoning	1	—	—	—	—	—
Furunculosis, staphylococcal	2	1	1	2	2	Maintain for duration of illness. Emphasize pus (drainage) precautions.
Gangrene—gas gangrene (due to any bacteria)	2	1	1	2	2	Maintain for duration of illness. Emphasize pus (drainage) precautions.

(Continued)

Table 16.2. (Continued)

Agent/Site of Infection	Precautions or Isolation Indicated? (1 = no; 2 = yes)	Private Room Indicated? (1 = no; 2 = yes for patient who cannot use good hygiene; 3 = yes; 4 = yes with special ventilation)	Mask Indicated? (1 = no; 2 = yes for those who get close to patient; 3 = yes)	Gown Indicated? (1 = no; 2 = yes when soiling of clothes likely; 3 = yes)	Gloves Indicated? (1 = no; 2 = yes for contact with infected area or drainage; 3 = yes)	Comments (Including Duration of Precautions or Isolation)
Gastroenteritis						
Unknown etiology	2	2	1	2	2	Maintain for duration of illness. Emphasize stool precautions.
Campylobacter spp.	2	2	1	2	2	Maintain for duration of illness. Emphasize stool precautions.
Clostridium difficile	2	2	1	2	2	Maintain for duration of illness. Emphasize stool precautions.
E. coli (enteropathogenic, enterotoxic, or enteroinvasive)	2	2	1	2	2	Maintain for duration of illness. Emphasize stool precautions.
Giardia	2	2	1	2	2	Maintain for duration of illness. Emphasize stool precautions.
Salmonella spp.	2	2	1	2	2	Maintain for duration of illness. Emphasize stool precautions.

Shigella spp.	2	2	1	2	Maintain until 3 consecutive feces cultures taken after ending antimicrobial therapy, negative for infecting strain. Emphasize stool precautions.
Vibrio parahaemolyticus	2	2	1	2	Maintain for duration of illness. Emphasize stool precautions.
Viral	2	2	1	2	Maintain for duration of illness. Emphasize stool precautions.
Yersinia enterocolitica	2	2	1	2	Maintain for duration of illness. Emphasize stool precautions.
Giardiasis	2	2	1	2	Maintain for duration of illness. Emphasize stool precautions.
Hepatitis, viral					
Type A (infectious epidemic hepatitis)	2	2	1	2	Maintain for 7 days after onset of jaundice.
Type B (serum hepatitis), including antigen carrier	2	1	1	1	Maintain blood precautions until patient is hepatitis B antigen–negative.
Non-A, non-B	2	1	1	1	Maintain blood precautions for duration of illness.

(Continued)

Table 16.2. (Continued)

Agent/Site of Infection	Precautions or Isolation Indicated? (1 = no; 2 = yes)	Private Room Indicated? (1 = no; 2 = yes for patient who cannot use good hygiene; 3 = yes; 4 = yes with special ventilation)	Mask Indicated? (1 = no; 2 = yes for those who get close to patient; 3 = yes)	Gown Indicated? (1 = no; 2 = yes when soiling of clothes likely; 3 = yes)	Gloves Indicated? (1 = no; 2 = yes for contact with infected area or drainage; 3 = yes)	Comments (Including Duration of Precautions or Isolation)
Unspecified type, consistent with viral etiology	2	2	1	2	2	Maintain blood precautions for duration of illness.
Herpangina	2	2	1	2	2	Maintain for duration of illness.
Herpesvirus hominis (herpes simplex)						
Encephalitis	1	—	—	—	—	—
Mucocutaneous, disseminated or primary, severe (skin, oral, and genital)	2	3	1	2	2	Maintain for duration of illness. Emphasize secretion precautions with lesions.
Mucocutaneous, recurrent (skin, oral, and genital)	2	1	1	1	2	Maintain for duration of illness. Emphasize secretion precaution with lesions.
Herpes zoster						
Localized in immunocompromised patient or disseminated	2	4	3	3	2	Maintain for duration of illness.

Disease						Comments
Localized in normal patient	2	3	1	1	2	Maintain for duration of illness. Personnel susceptible to herpes zoster (chickenpox) should wear mask.
Influenza	1	—	—	—	—	Respiratory secretions may be infectious.
Jakob–Creutzfeldt disease	2	1	1	1	1	Use caution when handling blood, brain tissue, or spinal fluid.
Keratoconjunctivitis, infectious	2	1	1	1	2	Maintain for duration of illness. Emphasize pus (drainage) precautions.
Legionnaires' disease	2	1	1	1	1	Maintain respiratory secretion precautions for duration of illness.
Meningitis						
Aseptic (nonbacterial, abacterial viral, or serous meningitis)	2	2	1	2	2	Maintain for duration of illness or 7 days, whichever less. Emphasize stool precautions.
Bacterial, etiology unknown	2	3	2	1	1	Maintain for 24 hours after start of effective therapy. Emphasize respiratory secretion precautions.
Neisseria meningitidis (meningococcal)	2	3	2	1	1	Maintain for 24 hours after start of effective therapy. Emphasize respiratory secretion precautions.

(Continued)

Table 16.2. (Continued)

Agent/Site of Infection	Precautions or Isolation Indicated? (1 = no; 2 = yes)	Private Room Indicated? (1 = no; 2 = yes for patient who cannot use good hygiene; 3 = yes; 4 = yes with special ventilation)	Mask Indicated? (1 = no; 2 = yes for those who get close to patient; 3 = yes)	Gown Indicated? (1 = no; 2 = yes when soiling of clothes likely; 3 = yes)	Gloves Indicated? (1 = no; 2 = yes for contact with infected area or drainage; 3 = yes)	Comments (Including Duration of Precautions or Isolation)
Pneumococcal	1	—	—	—	—	—
Tuberculous	2	1	1	1	1	Maintain for 24 hours after start of effective therapy. Emphasize respiratory secretion precautions.
Other diagnosed bacterial	1	—	—	—	—	—
Meningococcemia (meningococcal sepsis)	2	3	2	1	1	Maintain for 24 hours after start of effective therapy. Emphasize respiratory secretion precautions.
Multiply resistant organisms, infection or colonization						
GI	2	3	1	2	2	Maintain until off antibiotics and culture negative twice. Emphasize stool precautions.

					Comments
Respiratory	2	3	2	2	Maintain until off antibiotics and culture negative twice. Emphasize respiratory secretion precautions.
Skin	2	3	1	2	Maintain until off antibiotics and culture negative twice. Emphasize pus (drainage) precautions.
Urine	2	3	1	1	Maintain until off antibiotics and culture negative twice. Emphasize urine precautions, especially if patient has indwelling urinary catheter.
Mycobacteria, nontuberculous (atypical)					
Pulmonary	1	—	—	—	—
Wound	2	1	1	2	Maintain for duration of illness. Emphasize pus (drainage) precautions.
Mycoplasma pneumonia	2	1	1	1	Maintain for duration of illness. Emphasize respiratory secretion precautions.

(Continued)

Table 16.2. (Continued)

Agent/Site of Infection	Precautions or Isolation Indicated? (1 = no; 2 = yes)	Private Room Indicated? (1 = no; 2 = yes for patient who cannot use good hygiene; 3 = yes; 4 = yes with special ventilation)	Mask Indicated? (1 = no; 2 = yes for those who get close to patient; 3 = yes)	Gown Indicated? (1 = no; 2 = yes when soiling of clothes likely; 3 = yes)	Gloves Indicated? (1 = no; 2 = yes for contact with infected area or drainage; 3 = yes)	Comments (Including Duration of Precautions or Isolation)
Pediculosis	2	2	1	1	1	Maintain for duration of illness. Close contact with infected patients or their personal effects can result in transmission; effective treatment of patient rapidly reduces this hazard.
Pharyngitis, etiology unknown	2	1	1	1	1	Maintain oral secretion precautions for duration of illness.
Pinworm infection	1	—	—	—	—	—
Pleurodynia	2	2	1	2	2	Maintain for duration of illness. Emphasize stool precautions.
Pneumonia						
Etiology unknown	2	—	—	—	—	Maintain precautions necessary for the infection that is most likely. Use respiratory secretion precautions.

Bacterial—not listed elsewhere (included gram-negative bacterial)	2	1	1	1	1	Maintain for duration of illness. Emphasize respiratory secretion precautions.
Mycoplasma (primary atypical pneumonia)	2	1	1	1	1	Maintain for duration of illness. Emphasize respiratory secretion precautions.
Pneumococcal	1	—	—	—	—	Maintain respiratory secretion precautions until 24 hours after start of effective therapy.
Resistant bacteria	2	3	2	2	2	Maintain until off antibiotics and culture negative twice. Emphasize respiratory secretion precautions.
Staphylococcus aureus	2	3	2	2	2	Maintain for duration of illness. Emphasize respiratory secretion precautions.
Streptococcus, group A	2	3	2	2	2	Maintain until 24 hours after start of effective therapy. Emphasize respiratory secretion precautions.
Viral	2	1	1	1	1	Maintain sputum precautions for duration of illness.
Resistant bacterial (see Multiply resistant bacteria)						

(Continued)

Table 16.2. (Continued)

Agent/Site of Infection	Precautions or Isolation Indicated? (1 = no; 2 = yes)	Private Room Indicated? (1 = no; 2 = yes for patient who cannot use good hygiene; 3 = yes; 4 = yes with special ventilation)	Mask Indicated? (1 = no; 2 = yes for those who get close to patient; 3 = yes)	Gown Indicated? (1 = no; 2 = yes when soiling of clothes likely; 3 = yes)	Gloves Indicated? (1 = no; 2 = yes for contact with infected area or drainage; 3 = yes)	Comments (Including Duration of Precautions or Isolation)
Respiratory infectious disease, acute (if not covered elsewhere)	2	1	1	1	1	Maintain respiratory secretion precautions for duration of illness.
Ringworm (dermatophytosis, dermatomycosis, tinea)	1	—	—	—	—	—
Rotavirus infection	2	2	1	2	2	Maintain for duration of illness or 7 days, whichever less. Emphasize stool precautions.
Salmonellosis	2	2	1	2	2	Maintain for duration of illness. Emphasize stool precautions.
Scabies	2	2	1	2	2	Maintain for duration of illness. Gowns and gloves should be worn for close contact.

Disease					Comments
Shigellosis (including bacillary dysentery)	2	2	1	2	Maintain until 3 consecutive feces cultures, taken after ending antimicrobial therapy, negative for infecting strain. Emphasize stool precautions.
Staphylococcal disease (*S. aureus*)					
Enterocolitis	2	2	1	2	Maintain for duration of illness. Emphasize stool precautions.
Pneumonia or draining lung abscess	2	3	2	2	Maintain for duration of illness. Emphasize respiratory secretion precautions.
Skin, wound, or burn infection—limited or minor lesions	2	1	1	2	Maintain for duration of illness. Emphasize pus (drainage) precautions.
Skin, wound, or burn infection—major lesions	2	3	1	2	Maintain for duration of illness. Emphasize pus (drainage) precautions. Major lesions are those not covered by dressings or for which dressings do not adequately contain pus (drainage).

(Continued)

325

Table 16.2. (Continued)

Agent/Site of Infection	Precautions or Isolation Indicated? (1 = no; 2 = yes)	Private Room Indicated? (1 = no; 2 = yes for patient who cannot use good hygiene; 3 = yes; 4 = yes with special ventilation)	Mask Indicated? (1 = no; 2 = yes for those who get close to patient; 3 = yes)	Gown Indicated? (1 = no; 2 = yes when soiling of clothes likely; 3 = yes)	Gloves Indicated? (1 = no; 2 = yes for contact with infected area or drainage; 3 = yes)	Comments (Including Duration of Precautions or Isolation)
Streptococcal disease (group A streptococcus)						
Pharyngitis	2	1	1	1	1	Maintain for 24 hours after start of effective therapy. Emphasize respiratory secretion precautions.
Pneumonia	2	3	2	2	2	Maintain for 24 hours after start of effective therapy. Emphasize respiratory secretion precautions.
Skin, wound, or burn infection—limited or minor lesions	2	1	1	2	2	Maintain for 24 hours after start of effective therapy. Emphasize pus (drainage) precautions.
Skin, wound, or burn, infection—major lesions	2	3	1	2	2	Maintain for 24 hours after start of effective therapy. Emphasize pus (drainage) precautions. Major lesions are those not covered by dressings or for which dressings do not adequately contain pus (drainage).

Disease					Comments
Streptococcal disease (not group A or B), unless covered elsewhere	1	—	—	—	—
Syphilis					
Latent (tertiary) and seropositivity without lesions	1	—	—	—	—
Skin and mucous membrane, including congenital, primary, and secondary	2	1	1	3	Maintain until 24 hours after start of effective therapy. Blood from these patients may be infectious.
Tapeworm disease (*Hymenolepis nana*)	2	1	1	1	Maintain stool precautions for duration of illness.
Tetanus	1	—	—	—	—
Tinea (fungus infection)	1	—	—	—	—
Trichinosis	1	—	—	—	—
Trichomoniasis	1	—	—	—	—
Trichuriasis (whipworm disease)	1	—	—	—	—
Tuberculosis					
Extrapulmonary, draining lesion (including scrofula)	2	2	2	2	Maintain for duration of hospitalization. Emphasize pus (drainage) precautions.

(Continued)

Table 16.2. (Continued)

Agent/Site of Infection	Precautions or Isolation Indicated? (1 = no; 2 = yes)	Private Room Indicated? (1 = no; 2 = yes for patient who cannot use good hygiene; 3 = yes; 4 = yes with special ventilation)	Mask Indicated? (1 = no; 2 = yes for those who get close to patient; 3 = yes)	Gown Indicated? (1 = no; 2 = yes when soiling of clothes likely; 3 = yes)	Gloves Indicated? (1 = no; 2 = yes for contact with infected area or drainage; 3 = yes)	Comments (Including Duration of Precautions or Isolation)
Meningitis	1					—
Pulmonary (confirmed or suspected)	2	4	3	1	1	Maintain until patient improving and sputum negative for TB organisms. Mask necessary unless patient not coughing or always covers mouth during cough. Prompt use of effective antituberculous drugs is the most effective means to limit transmission.
Skin test positive with no evidence of pulmonary disease	1	—	—	—	—	—
Urinary tract infection (including pyelonephritis), with or without urinary catheter	1	—	—	—	—	See Multiply resistant bacteria if infection is with these bacteria.
Vibrio parahaemolyticus gastroenteritis	2	2	1	2	2	Maintain for duration of illness. Emphasize stool precautions.

Viral disease						
Pericarditis, myocarditis, or meningitis	2	2	1	1	2	Maintain for 7 days. Emphasize stool precautions.
Respiratory (if not covered elsewhere)	2	1	1	1	1	Maintain respiratory secretion precautions for 7 days.
Wound infection						
Limited or minor lesions	2	1	1	2	2	Maintain for duration of illness. Emphasize pus (drainage) precautions.
Major lesions	2	3	1	2	2	Maintain for duration of illness. Emphasize pus (drainage) precautions. Major lesions are those not covered by dressings or for which dressings do not adequately contain pus (drainage).
Yersinia enterocolitica gastroenteritis	2	2	1	2	2	Maintain for duration of illness. Emphasize stool precautions.

for private room, gowns, masks, and so on, depending upon the presumed infectious agent. Information on the necessary duration of isolation is available from Table 16.2 and other sources (1).

INSTRUCTION AND EVALUATION OF POLICIES AND PROCEDURES

Policies and procedures, in this instance procedures for isolation, are only effective if properly practiced by personnel who work within the institution (see Chapter 12). For this reason, education and dissemination of information regarding these techniques are necessary components of the infection control program. Persons requiring at least a minimal level of knowledge regarding prevention of spread of infectious disease in extended care institutions include any person who may come into contact with the infected resident. Education is essential for the following groups: health care personnel; personnel involved in support services, including housekeeping and dietary; visitors to the institution; and residents.

Familiarity with procedures and minimal acceptable levels of knowledge regarding infection control procedure will depend upon the frequency of exposure to the resident and upon the level of authority of the person for instituting and implementing these policies. Personnel involved in direct resident care should have the most comprehensive knowledge of infection control procedures. Support service personnel need not have a comprehensive understanding of these procedures; on the other hand, they should be sufficiently familiar with concepts so that when entering the room of an infected resident they will recognize the need for special precautions.

Education

Three methods are suggested for educating and informing employees regarding infection control procedures. First, at the time of orientation to their new position, each employee should receive both verbal and written instructions regarding procedures for controlling the spread of infection. These instructions should include a brief review of the risks of spread of infection within the institution, the objectives of isolation techniques for preventing spread of infection, and, finally, the specific steps necessary to prevent the spread of infection. A second method for educating employees should include timely in-service reviews of infection control procedures. For example, in the fall of the year and in anticipation of influenza epidemics, the institution may wish to conduct an in-service program regarding the spread of respiratory infections and measures for prevention, including both immunizations and isolation. A third technique, and perhaps the most important for informing and educating employees regarding infection control, is the use of identification and instruction cards posted on the door of the resident's room and on the medical record. This card (Fig. 16.1) identifies potential sources of infection, indicates the type of isolation being used, and lists the precautions that need to be taken when entering the room.

Visitors may transmit infection from person to person within the institution or may introduce community-acquired infections into the institution. For this reason, a modicum of information should be disseminated to visitors. It is suggested that education of visitors be carried out by the following two methods. First, visitors to rooms of infected individuals should be informed by nursing personnel of the nature of the infection, risk of spread of the infection, and the steps being taken to prevent spread of infection. Second, the card identification system outlined above should provide for the visitor an additional reminder of the risk of spreading infection and steps to be taken in order to prevent transmission.

Education of residents will also be important in reducing transmission of disease. This step in the education process is perhaps more important in extended care institutions than in acute care hospitals since residents are more likely to be ambulatory and moving from room to room. The nursing staff should be assigned the responsibility of disseminating information regarding the risks and steps to be taken in controlling transmission of infectious diseases within an extended care institution. Whereas education of the coherent, well-oriented individual should be sufficient, special steps will have to be taken for incoherent persons. For example, if the resident who is infected is also uncooperative, it is reasonable to restrict the activities of that individual to his or her room. This is particularly important for individuals with readily transmissible respiratory or gastrointestinal disease.

Quality Assurance

The final step in establishing a program to control transmission of infections is to assure that the recommended procedures are being practiced and that they are effective in achieving their objectives. Quality assurance can be measured by examining either the process or the outcome of the procedures. Neither of these measurements need entail significant expenditures of time or money on the part of the institution. To assure compliance with protocols for infection control, two steps should be taken. First, it should be the responsibility of health care personnel who are charged with authority for instituting or determining control measures to see that they are properly practiced. Nursing personnel should be quick to point out to coworkers, support personnel, visitors, or residents when they fail to comply with the institution's guidelines. An additional method for monitoring isolation techniques is to obtain data at the time of prevalence surveys or audits regarding the appropriate and inappropriate use of isolation techniques. If there is evidence from these surveys that isolation techniques are not being used when indicated or that inappropriate levels of isolation are being used for a given infection, additional in-service education should be provided to bring practices up to standard (see Chapter 13). Indications of the adequacy of outcome may be assessed simply by the presence or absence of epidemic and endemic infections within the institution. Furthermore, evidence that introduction of a resistant organism into the institution has spread from person to person over time suggests either that the infection control policies of the institution are inadequate or that adequate policies are not being practiced. Evidence of such problems should be sufficient cause for review of the institution's policies and for additional education regarding proper health care practices.

OCCUPATIONAL HEALTH: ROLE OF THE EMPLOYEE HEALTH PROGRAM IN PREVENTION OF INFECTION

The medical care worker in the extended care facility is both a continuing animate source of potentially transmissible infectious diseases for the person undergoing chronic care and rehabilitation and a transmitter of infectious microorganisms. Examples of transmission through chronic carriage (e.g., streptococcal, staphylococcal infections), chronic reactivated disease (e.g., tuberculosis, herpes simplex or herpes zoster), acute disease transmission (e.g., salmonellosis, shigellosis, influenza), and mechanical carriage through hand transmission are well documented in the medical literature. Specific diseases in employees are discussed further in Chapter 15.

Prevention of this transmission is best provided by a strong occupational health program supported by formal institutional medical and educational efforts. Such programs protect the patient and the worker from the potential effects of communicable and other occupational diseases and protect the institution from the costs and the liability of worker- and patient-related events.

The minimal occupational health program for an extended care facility should include a preemployment evaluation, an immunization program, a sick call information and evaluation program, and such periodic employee evaluations as are called for by the intensity of the care and services provided. This program need not be financially excessive, but must have important minimal information capabilities to be successful.

The preemployment evaluation should include an extensive self-administered medical history. This may be of the checklist type commonly used by the military and insurance organizations or a locally developed form based on experience in the individual setting. Questions should be especially focused on the areas of potentially transmissible infectious diseases of the skin, respiratory tract, and gastrointestinal tract but should not exclude questions on work history, absenteeism, drug abuse history, psychiatric history, or any disabilities related to vision, hearing, or the muscular–skeletal systems. An immunization history is also an important feature of this evaluation. This history should be carefully reviewed by a physician or a physician extender and any salient points clarified by interview and/or examination if necessary. Completion of the preemployment evaluation should be a condition for beginning employment. The cost of the examination may be borne either by the institution or by the individual worker.

Based on the immunization history, current immunization status for tetanus, diphtheria, and influenza A and B should be sought for each employee with resident contact. Tuberculin testing should be required or known from previous history.

Only such x-rays and laboratory tests deemed necessary from the medical history should be done. Routine x-rays, stool cultures, hematology, and other tests are not cost-effective unless supported by history and confirmatory examination.

Medical problems identified by the preemployment evaluation should be brought to the attention of the worker, and he or she should be encouraged to have them further evaluated through their personal physician. Preexisting conditions should be noted and their presence evaluated for their effect on employees' ability to safely work with residents or to perform on the available job without aggravating the preexisting problem.

The medical care worker should be encouraged to participate in an established personal preventive medicine program (weight control, screening exams, etc.), but the individual institution's ability to support such an effort unilaterally may be limited by funding constraints. Programs available to the employee in other local institutions or cooperative programs with other extended care facilities may solve this problem.

A limited and confidential medical file should be maintained on each employee. In addition to the preemployment evaluation information, this file should be updated with each acute disease event that appears to be significant for work in the extended care facility. Absences from work for medical reasons should be routinely documented by an entry into this record. Extended absences for illness should be further documented by information from the employee's private physician.

Any events that are related to potentially communicable diseases or that might impinge on the worker's ability to deliver medical care should have medical review to determine whether the worker continues to be able to safely provide patient care. Lower respiratory illness, diarrheal disease, and communicable skin conditions usually will preclude patient contact until the established period of communicability has passed and/or the condition has resolved. Recurrent undocumented illness may be grounds for medical or administrative review by the institution.

A periodic employee health evaluation should be used to update information on the employee. The periodicity of this evaluation should be judged by the risk nature of the worker environment (e.g., frequent in tuberculosis workers, infrequent in routine domiciliary care), the nature of the medical problems previously found in the worker, and the history of intervening illnesses. Such review may uncover unrecognized work hazards that require institutional procedural or functional changes.

The educational efforts necessary to encourage the employee to be responsible for personal health and to recognize and to assist in ethical determination of his or her ability to safely work with residents are probably the most important and least costly parts of a successful occupational health effort.

The extended facility, through its administration, must encourage this self-review by assisting in definitions of conditions requiring medical review, providing support for such review and not penalizing absences based on illnesses covered by these criteria. A successful effort should be judged by its success in protecting residents, employees, and the institution from risk.

REFERENCE

1. Centers for Disease Control: Guideline for Isolation Precautions in Hospitals. *Infect Control* July/Aug, 1983.

INDEX